Medical Assistant (CCMA) Certification Study Guide

EDITION 2.0

AUTHORS

Angie Kronlage, RT(R), MA

Dana L. Cardinal, CMAA

Margaret Garber, BA, RMA, CPC, CPPM

Mary Jane Janowski, RN, MA

Monica Cox, MHSA, CMA

Nancy Szwydek, RN, RHIA, RMA, CRAT, CMAC

Taiya Grannis, CCMA

REVIEWERS

Angie Kronlage, RT(R), MA

Elizabeth D. Gerber, MSN, MEd, RN

Kendra L. Williams, BS, CMA

Margaret Garber, BA, RMA, CPC, CPPM

Monica Cox, MHSA, CMA

Nancy Szwydek, RN, RHIA, RMA, CRAT, CMAC

Shateisha M. Phillips, CMA

Taiya Grannis, CCMA

INTELLECTUAL PROPERTY NOTICE

REPRINTED MARCH 2021

Director of content review: Kristen Lawler

Director of development: Derek Prater

Project management: Bertha Rucker-Ross

Coordination of content review: Angie Kronlage

Copy editing: Kelly Von Lunen, Bethany Phillips

Layout: Spring Lenox, Randi Hardy

Illustrations: Randi Hardy

Cover design: Kaitlyn Mackey

Interior book design: Spring Lenox

Online tutorial design: Charves Hervey

Online media: Morgan Smith, Ron Hanson, Nicole Lobdell, Brant Stacy

IMPORTANT NOTICE TO THE READER

The CCMA study guide provides the best insight on the type of content that will be included on the certification exam and can be an invaluable resource in your exam preparation. It is, however, a study guide. It should not be the only resource used in your studies, and it will not necessarily cover the specific construct of every question on the certification examination. Rather, it will provide the map to your success by presenting essential overviews of each topic included in the test plan.

INTRODUCTION

More than $3 trillion is spent on health care in the U.S. each year. Health care is a big business. Qualified medical assistants, like you, will continue to be in demand. Health care practitioners rely on skilled staff for the health of their business. Medical assistants qualify for employment in a variety of settings, including hospitals, clinics, and private provider offices. Accepting the challenge to become a part of this growing field requires dedication and a willingness to continually update your skills. Having a medical assistant certification will help you support a successful career in this field. This study guide will help you prepare for the National Healthcareer Association (NHA) Medical Assistant (CCMA) Certification examination. To sit for the CCMA examination, you must have a high school diploma or a GED and complete a training program. However, you may substitute 1 year of medical assistant experience in lieu of attending a formal training program. With this option, you must provide documentation that you worked as a medical assistant for at least 1 year. If you meet these criteria, you may register for the examination online at https://certportal.nhanow.com.

If your school is a registered NHA test site, you may be able to take a proctored exam via computer or in paper-pencil format. You also have the option to take the exam via computer at a PSI testing center. For more information about exam eligibility, see www.nhanow.com. The key instructional content, or body of each chapter, follows the CCMA test plan. Following the key instructional content, there is a chapter summary that recaps the main points within the chapter. At the end of this handbook, a glossary defines the key words highlighted throughout, and drill questions assess your knowledge of the chapter subjects.

NHA MEDICAL ASSISTANT (CCMA) CERTIFICATION DETAILED TEST PLAN

This test plan is based on the 2016 Job Analysis Study. The tasks under each content domain are examples that are representative of the content. Items reflective of these stated tasks may or may not appear on the examination. Additionally, items that are reflective of tasks other than those included in the outline below may appear on the examination, as long as they represent information that is considered part of the major content domain by experts in the medical assistant profession. Refer to the full test plan at www.nhanow.com.

Foundational Knowledge and Basic Science

Health care systems and settings
Knowledge Enablers

- Role and responsibilities of the medical assistant, other health care providers, and allied health personnel
- Scope of practice
- Titles and credentials
- Licensing and certification
- Health care delivery models (HMOs, PPOs, POS, PCMH, accountable care organizations [ACOs]/payment for performance, hospice, collaborative care model)
- General vs. specialties and services offered
- Ancillary services; alternative therapies
- Insurance fundamentals

Medical terminology
Knowledge Enablers

- Common abbreviations, acronyms, and symbols
- Conditions, procedures, and instruments
- Medical word building (prefixes, suffixes, plurals)
- Positional and directional terminology

Basic pharmacology

Knowledge Enablers

- Commonly prescribed medications and common approved abbreviations
- Drug classifications and schedules
- Side effects, adverse effects, indications, and contraindications
- Measurement (for metric and household systems), mathematical conversions, and dosage calculations
- Forms of medication (pill, capsule, ointment)
- Look-alike/sound-alike medications
- Routes of administration
- Pharmacokinetics (absorption, distribution, metabolism, excretion)
- Rights of drugs/medication administration
- *Physicians' Desk Reference* and online resources
- Principles of storage and disposal

Nutrition

Knowledge Enablers

- Dietary nutrients
- Dietary needs and patient education (general and related to diseases/conditions)
- Vitamins and supplements
- Eating disorders
- Food labels

Psychology

Knowledge Enablers

- Developmental stages
- End of life and stages of grief
- Psychology of the physically disabled, developmentally delayed, and people who have diseases
- Environmental and socioeconomic stressors
- Mental health screening
- Defense mechanisms

Anatomy and Physiology

Body structures and organ systems

Knowledge Enablers

- Anatomical structures, locations, and positions
- Structure and function of major body systems, including organs and their locations
- Interactions between organ systems, homeostasis

Pathophysiology and disease processes

Knowledge Enablers

- Signs, symptoms, and etiology of common diseases, conditions, and injuries
- Diagnostic measures and treatment modalities
- Incidence, prevalence, and risk factors
- Risk factors leading to high mortality and morbidity (complications, accompanying diseases)
- Epidemics and pandemics

Microbiology

Knowledge Enablers

- Cell structure (nucleus, cell wall, cell membrane, cytoplasm, ribosomes, mitochondria, lysosomes, nucleolus)
- Common pathogens and nonpathogens
- Organisms and micro-organisms
- Infectious agents, chain of infection, and conditions for growth

Clinical Patient Care

General patient care

Tasks

- Identify patient.
- Prepare examination/procedure room.
- Ensure patient safety within the clinical setting.
- Complete a comprehensive clinical intake process, including the purpose of the visit.

- Measure vital signs.
- Obtain anthropomorphic measurements.
- Identify/document/report abnormal signs and symptoms.
- Assist provider with general physical examination.
- Assist provider with specialty examinations.
- Prepare patient for procedures.
- Prepare and administer medications and/or injectables using nonparenteral and parenteral routes (oral, buccal, sublingual, intramuscular, intradermal, subcutaneous, topical, transdermal, inhalation), excluding IV.
- Perform staple and suture removal.
- Administer eye, ear, and topical medications.
- Perform ear and eye irrigation.
- Administer first aid and basic wound care.
- Identify and respond to emergency/priority situations.
- Perform CPR.
- Assist provider with patients presenting with minor and traumatic injury.
- Assist with surgical interventions (sebaceous cyst removal, toenail removal, colposcopy, cryosurgery).
- Review provider's discharge instructions/ plan of care with patients.
- Follow guidelines for sending orders for prescriptions and refills by telephone, fax, or email.
- Document relevant aspects of patient care in patient record.
- Operate basic functions of an EHR/EMR system.
- Enter orders into CPOE.

Knowledge Enablers

- Patient identifiers
- Elements of a patient medical/surgical/ family/social history
- Methods for obtaining vital signs (manual and electronic blood pressure; respirations; temperature; pulse; pulse oximetry)

- Normal and abnormal vital signs
- Methods for measuring height, weight, BMI; special considerations related to age, health, status, disability; growth chart
- Positioning and draping requirements for general and specialty examinations, procedures, and treatments
- Equipment, instruments, and supplies necessary to prepare the examination or procedure room
- Required equipment, supplies, and instruments related to general physical examinations
- Required equipment, supplies, and instruments related to specialty examinations
- Patient instructions specific to procedures, including pre- and postprocedure instructions
- Modifications to patient care depending on patient needs (assisting with ambulation and transfers for frail patients and patients who have disabilities; using easily understood terms for pediatric patients)
- Consent requirements (written and verbal)
- Immunization schedules and requirements
- Allergies (common drug and nondrug allergies [latex, bee stings]; type of reactions [mild, moderate, severe]; how to respond to allergic reactions or anaphylactic shock)
- Signs of infection
- Sterile techniques related to examinations, procedures, injections, and medication administration
- Dosage calculations related to oral medications and injectables
- Commonly used oral and parenteral medications (forms, packaging, routes of administration)
- Rights of medication administration
- Storage, labeling, and medication logs
- Techniques and injection site
- Supplies and equipment related to injections
- Storage of injectables

- Techniques and instruments for suture and staple removal; types and sizes of sutures
- Methods of administration, techniques, procedures, and supplies related to eye, ear, and topical medications
- Instruments, supplies, and techniques related to eye and ear irrigation
- Commonly occurring types of injuries (lacerations, abrasions, fractures, sprains)
- Treatment for commonly occurring types of injuries (bandaging, ice, elevation)
- Commonly occurring types of surgical interventions
- Signs and symptoms related to urgent and emergency situations (diabetic shock, heat stroke, allergic reactions, choking, syncope, seizure)
- Emergency action plans (crash cart, emergency injectables)
- Procedures to perform CPR, basic life support, and AED
- Computerized physician order entry (CPOE)
- Referral authorizations; insurance authorizations
- Legal requirements for content and transmission of prescriptions
- Prior authorizations for medication; electronic prescribing software
- Required components of medical records
- Medical necessity guidelines

Infection control

Tasks

- Adhere to regulations and guidelines related to infection control.
- Adhere to guidelines regarding hand hygiene.
- Perform disinfection/sanitization.
- Perform sterilization of medical equipment.
- Perform appropriate aseptic techniques for various clinical situations.
- Dispose of biohazardous materials as dictated by OSHA (sharps containers, red bags).

Knowledge Enablers

- Universal precautions
- Handwashing techniques
- Alcohol-based rubs/sanitizer
- Infectious agents, modes of transmission, precautions for blood-borne pathogens
- Personal protective equipment (PPE)
- Sterilization techniques (autoclave, instrument cleaner, germicidal disinfectants, disposables)
- Techniques for medical and surgical asepsis
- Order of cleaning and types of cleaning products
- Safety Data Sheets (SDSs)
- Cautions related to chemicals
- Disposal methods
- Exposure control plan
- Calibration of equipment
- Logs (maintenance, equipment servicing, temperature [refrigerator], quality control)

Testing and laboratory procedures

Tasks

- Collect nonblood specimens (urine, stool, cultures, sputum).
- Perform CLIA-waived testing (labs).
- Perform vision and hearing tests.
- Perform allergy testing.
- Perform spirometry/pulmonary function tests (electronic or manual).
- Recognize, document, and report normal and abnormal laboratory and test values.
- Match and label specimen to patient and completed requisition.
- Process, handle, and transport collected specimens.

Knowledge Enablers

- Point-of-care testing
- Information required on provider request or requisition form
- Specimen collection techniques and requirements

- CLIA-waived testing regulations
- COLA accreditation standards
- Controls/calibration/quality control
- Normal and abnormal laboratory test values
- Elements related to vision (color, acuity, distance, visual fields) and hearing tests (tone, speech and word recognition, tympanometry)
- Peak flow rates
- Common allergens
- Scratch test and intradermal allergy test
- Requirements for transportation, diagnosis, storage, and disposal of specimens (patient identifiers, site, test)
- Content of requisition (date, time, ICD-10)

Phlebotomy

Tasks

- Verify order details.
- Select appropriate supplies for tests ordered.
- Determine venipuncture site accessibility based on patient age and condition.
- Prepare site for venipuncture.
- Perform venipuncture.
- Perform capillary puncture.
- Perform postprocedure care.
- Handle blood samples as required for diagnostic purposes.
- Process blood specimens for laboratory.
- Match and label specimens to patient and completed requisition.
- Recognize and respond to abnormal test results.
- Prepare samples for transportation to a reference (outside) laboratory.
- Follow guidelines in distributing laboratory results to ordering providers after matching patient to provider.

Knowledge Enablers

- Patient identifiers (site, test) and content of requisition
- Requirements related to patient preparation for phlebotomy (fasting, nonfasting)
- Assessment of patient comfort/anxiety level with procedure
- Blood collection tubes required for chemistry, hematology, and microbiology testing
- Bloodborne pathogens
- Medical conditions or history and medications affecting collection of blood order of draw for venipuncture
- Anatomy, skin integrity, venous sufficiency, contraindications
- Phlebotomy site preparation (cleansing, wrapping, order of draw with microcollection tubes)
- Insertion and removal techniques
- Evacuated tube, syringe, and butterfly methods
- Types of tubes, tube positions, number of tube inversions, and fill level/ratios
- Additives and preservatives
- Bandaging procedures (allergies, skin types)
- Preanalytical considerations pertaining to specimen quality and consistency
- Special collections (timed specimens, drug levels, blood cultures, fasting)
- Centrifuge and aliquot
- Normal and abnormal test values, control values
- Equipment calibration
- Storage conditions related to sensitivity to light and temperature
- Requirements for transportation, diagnosis, storage, and disposal
- Processing and labeling requirements
- External databases (outside labs, reference sources)

EKG and cardiovascular testing

Tasks

- Prepare patients for procedure.
- Perform cardiac monitoring (EKG) tests.
- Ensure proper functioning of EKG equipment.
- Recognize abnormal or emergent EKG results (dysrhythmia, arrhythmia, artifact).
- Assist provider with noninvasive cardiovascular profiling (stress test, Holter monitoring, event monitoring).
- Transmit results or report to patient's EMR or paper chart, and provider.

Knowledge Enablers

- Procedures and instructions to minimize artifacts
- Artifacts, signal distortions, and electrical interference (fuzz, wandering baseline)
- Preparation, positioning, and draping of patient
- Supplies (paper, proper leads)
- Placement of limb and chest electrodes
- Techniques and methods for EKGs
- Signs of adverse reaction during testing (signs of distress, elevated blood pressure and respirations)
- Calibration of equipment
- Abnormal rhythms or dysrhythmias associated with cardiovascular testing
- Waveforms, intervals, segment

Patient Care Coordination and Education

Tasks

- Review patient record prior to visit to ensure health care is comprehensively addressed.
- Collaborate with providers and community-based organizations.
- Assist providers in coordinating care with community agencies for clinical and nonclinical services.

- Facilitate patient compliance (continuity of care, follow-up, medication compliance) to optimize health outcomes.
- Participate in transition of care for patients.
- Participate in team-based patient care (patient-centered medical home [PCMH], Accountable Care Organization [ACO]).

Knowledge Enablers

- Preventive medicine and wellness
- Education delivery methods and instructional techniques and learning styles
- Resources and procedures to coordinate care outpatient services
- Available resources for clinical services (home health care)
- Available community resources for nonclinical services (adult day care, transportation vouchers)
- Specialty resources for patient/family medical and mental needs
- Referral forms and processes
- Barriers to care (socioeconomic, cultural differences, language, education)
- Tracking and reporting technologies
- Roles and responsibilities of team members involved in patient-centered medical home

Administrative Assisting

Tasks

- Schedule and monitor patient appointments using electronic and paper-based systems.
- Verify insurance coverage/financial eligibility.
- Identify and check patients in/out.
- Verify diagnostic and procedural codes.
- Obtain and verify prior authorizations and precertifications.
- Prepare documentation and billing requests using current coding guidelines.
- Ensure that documentation complies with government and insurance requirements.

- Perform charge reconciliation (correct use of EHR software, entering charges, making adjustments, accounts receivable procedures).
- Bill patients, insurers, and third-party payers for services performed.
- Resolve billing issues with insurers and third-party payers (appeals, denials).
- Manage electronic and paper medical records.
- Facilitate/generate referrals to other providers and allied health professionals.
- Provide customer service and facilitate service recovery (follow-up patient calls, appointment confirmations, monitoring patient flow sheets, collecting on accounts, making up for poor customer service).
- Enter information into databases or spreadsheets (EHR, EMR, billing modules, scheduling systems).
- Participate in safety evaluations and report safety concerns.
- Maintain inventory of clinical and administrative supplies.

Knowledge Enablers

- Filing systems
- Scheduling software
- Recognition of urgency of appointment needs
- Requirements related to duration of visits (purpose of visit, physician preferences)
- Telephone etiquette
- Records management systems and software (manual filing systems [alphabetical, numeric], office storage for archived files, EMR/EHR software applications)
- Legal requirements related to maintenance, storage, and disposal of records
- Categories of the medical record (administrative, clinical, billing, procedural, notes, consents)
- Required documentation for patient review and signature
- Chart review

- E-referrals (how they are created, required information, how they are sent)
- Financial eligibility, sliding scales, and indigent programs
- Government regulations (meaningful use, MACRA)
- CMS billing requirements
- Third-party payer billing requirements
- Advance beneficiary notice (ABN)
- Specialty pharmacies (compounding and nuclear pharmacies; forms of medication available [liquid, elixir, balm, ointment])
- Insurance terminology (copay, coinsurance, deductible, tier levels, explanation of benefits)
- Aging reports, collections due, adjustments, and write-offs
- Online banking for deposits and electronic transfers
- Authorizations to approve payment processing
- Auditing methods, processes, and sign-offs
- Data entry and data fields
- Equipment inspection logs, required schedules, and compliance requirements, including inspection by medical equipment servicers

Communication and Customer Service

Tasks

- Modify verbal and nonverbal communication for diverse audiences (providers, coworkers, supervisors, patients, caregivers, external providers).
- Modify verbal and nonverbal communications with patients and caregivers based on special considerations (pediatric, geriatric, hearing loss, vision loss, mental handicap, disability).
- Clarify and relay communications between patients and providers.
- Communicate on the telephone with patients, caregivers, providers, and third-party payers.

- Prepare written/electronic communications/ business correspondence.
- Handle challenging/difficult customer service occurrences.
- Engage in crucial conversations with patients, caregivers, heath care surrogates, staff, and providers.
- Facilitate and promote teamwork and team engagement.

Knowledge Enablers

- Communication styles
- Patient characteristics affecting communication (cultural differences, language barriers, cognitive level, developmental stage, sensory and physical disabilities, age)
- Medical terminology and jargon, layman's terms
- Therapeutic communication
- Interviewing and questioning techniques (screening, probing, open- and closed-ended questions)
- Scope of permitted questions and boundaries for questions
- Active listening
- Communication cycle (clear, concise message relay)
- Coaching and feedback, positive reinforcement of effective behavior
- Professional presence (appearance, demeanor, tone)
- Patient satisfaction surveys
- When to escalate problem situations
- Techniques to deal with patients (irate clients, custody issues between parents, chain of command)
- Incident/event/unusual occurrence reports; documentation of event

- Cause-and-effect analysis (anxiety increases blood pressure or heart rate; risk management related to patient and employee safety)
- Email etiquette
- Business letter formats
- Telephone etiquette

Medical Law and Ethics

Tasks

- Comply with legal and regulatory requirements.
- Adhere to professional codes of ethics.
- Obtain, review, and comply with medical directives.
- Obtain and document health care proxies and agents.
- Provide, collect, and store medical order for life-sustaining treatment (MOLST) forms.
- Protect patient privacy and confidentiality, including medical records.
- Adhere to legal requirements regarding reportable violations or incidents.
- Identify personal or religious beliefs and values and provide unbiased care.

Knowledge Enablers

- Informed consent
- Advance directives (living will, DNR/DNI)
- Power of attorney
- Storage of medical records
- Conditions for sharing information/release of information
- Criminal and civil acts, and medical malpractice
- Mandatory reporting laws, triggers for reporting, and reporting agencies
- Hippocratic Oath

Table of Contents

CHAPTER 6
Body Structures and Organ Systems

CHAPTER 9
General Patient Care

CHAPTER 11
Testing and Laboratory Procedures — 195

CHAPTER 13

EKG and Cardiovascular Testing

CHAPTER 14
Patient Care Coordination and Education

CHAPTER 15
Administrative Assisting — 255

IN PRACTICE
Quizzes

National Healthcareer Association

CHAPTER 1

Health Care Systems and Settings

OVERVIEW

At first glance, the medical arena can seem overwhelming. New terminology, legal concerns, direct or indirect patient care, unique processes, and high expectations can contribute to initial apprehension for a new medical assistant. However, this new role can be better understood through a holistic approach, looking at the health care system from all sides. In addition to understanding the role and *scope of practice* for medical assistants, it is crucial to understand the importance of the entire health care team. Knowing the skills and responsibilities of the various allied health and specialty providers strengthens the effectiveness and cohesiveness of the health care team. Each team member needs to respect and assist others to provide the best possible care for the patient.

ROLES AND RESPONSIBILITIES

Medical assistants, along with other health care staff, function as members of a health care team that perform administrative and clinical procedures and responsibilities. Medical assistants often screen patients before the provider visit. The provider then assesses the patient and determines if further medical testing is necessary. Depending on the patient's current condition, the provider may send the patient for allied health services (phlebotomy, physical therapy). Whether services are provided in a hospital, *ambulatory* care center, home health agency, or hospice, medical personnel are ultimately responsible for the care and well-being of their patients.

Objectives

Upon completion of this chapter, you should be able to:

- Define the roles and responsibilities of the medical assistant, other health care providers, and allied health personnel.
- List professional traits or behaviors that are essential when working in health care.
- Define scope of practice and describe variables that affect what a medical assistant is able to perform.
- Define standard of care and describe how it applies to the medical assistant.
- List other titles or credentials medical assistants may obtain for career laddering opportunities.
- Compare and contrast licensure and certification.
- Describe types of health care delivery models available.
- Describe the roles of physician and nonphysician specialists in treating different types of patients.
- Describe types of ancillary services and alternative therapies that can assist patients in their journey to better health.
- Define common terms used in the insurance industry and describe various types of insurance plans available to patients.

---

scope of practice. Delegated clinical and administrative duties consistent with education, training, and experience
ambulatory. Able to walk

Roles and responsibilities of the medical assistant

The role of a medical assistant is primarily to work alongside a provider in an outpatient or ambulatory setting, such as a medical office. Depending on the size of the facility, the medical assistant might be cross-trained to perform administrative and clinical duties. Administrative duties include greeting patients, handling correspondence, and answering telephones. In addition, the medical assistant is often responsible for the clinical tasks of obtaining medical histories from patients, explaining treatments or procedures, drawing laboratory tests, and preparing and administering immunizations. A medical assistant can also achieve credentialing by passing a national certification exam.

Roles and responsibilities of health care providers

Medical doctors (MDs) are considered *allopathic* providers and are the most widely recognized type of doctor. They diagnose illnesses, provide treatments, perform procedures such as surgical interventions, and write prescriptions.

Osteopathic providers (DOs) complete requirements that are similar to those of MDs to graduate and practice medicine. In addition to using modern medicine and surgical procedures, DOs use *osteopathic* manipulative therapy (OMT) in treating their patients.

Nurse practitioners provide basic patient care services, including diagnosing and prescribing medications for common illnesses. Nurse practitioners require advanced academic training beyond the registered nurse (RN) degree and have an extensive amount of clinical experience. Generally, nurse practitioners focus on preventive care and disease prevention.

Physician assistants practice medicine under the direction and supervision of a licensed MD or DO. Additionally, physician assistants are able to make clinical decisions and be responsible for a variety of services.

Roles and responsibilities of allied health personnel

Medical laboratory technicians perform diagnostic testing on blood, bodily fluids, and other specimens under the supervision of a medical technologist.

Medical receptionists check patients in and out, answer phones, and perform filing, faxing, and other tasks.

Occupational therapists assist patients who have developed conditions that disable them developmentally, emotionally, mentally, or physically.

Pharmacy technicians assist pharmacists with duties that do not require the expertise or judgement of a licensed pharmacist.

Physical therapists assist patients in regaining their mobility and improving their strength and range of motion.

Radiology technicians use various types of imaging equipment to assist the provider in diagnosing and treating certain diseases.

---

allopathic. Homeopathic medicine; categorized by an effort to counteract the symptoms of a disease by administration of treatments that produce effects opposite to the symptoms

osteopathic. A type of medicine based on the concept that disturbances in the musculoskeletal system affect other bodily parts, causing many disorders that can be improved by various manipulative methods in combination with conventional medical, surgical, pharmacologic, and other therapeutic procedures

Professionalism

Professionalism consists of the skills, behavior, and appropriate judgment that represent the best qualities of a person in a specific profession. Medical assistants must exhibit a courteous, conscientious, and a businesslike manner in the workplace. Dependability, initiative, flexibility, confidentiality, and a good attitude are all necessary with a high level of professionalism.

Appropriate dress

The appropriate dress in a professional medical office includes good personal hygiene and appropriate work attire. Avoid perfumes and colognes due to possible patient sensitivities. Wear makeup conservatively, and keep nails clean (no acrylic) and at a reasonable length. Dress codes vary, but clothing should be comfortable and fit appropriately. Many facilities do not allow facial piercings, extreme hairstyles, or visible tattoos.

Personal phone use

Take personal phone calls and text messages during scheduled work breaks or lunch hours. Some offices issue a phone for professional use, but a medical assistant should never respond to a call or text while treating a patient. If a phone must be carried, put it on vibrate. Always step into a hall or break area if a call must be taken.

Punctuality

Punctuality and dependability are of key importance in maintaining professionalism in the health care environment. Arriving to work in a timely manner and performing all assigned duties each day are the basics of being a reliable employee. Good time-management skills are also needed in a fast-paced medical office. Learn to prioritize tasks and arrange schedules to perform all necessary duties efficiently and effectively.

Respect for boundaries

Setting appropriate boundaries in the workplace for coworkers and patients helps prevent awkward situations or misunderstandings. Most people's personal space ranges from 1½ to 4 feet. Respect this personal space and provide effective communication when interrupting it for a medical reason. Be aware of any nonverbal communication from the patient that might indicate she is feeling an invasion of personal space, and respond immediately.

Motivation

The power of motivation depends on the individual. Money, praise from others, self-fulfillment, and integrity are just a few of the different motivating forces that drive people to achieve their goals. There are two types of motivation. Intrinsic motivation originates within an individual and focuses on lifelong goals. Extrinsic motivation is physical in nature and driven by outside forces. Commonly, extrinsic motivation is short-lived and less fulfilling than intrinsic motivation. Remain motivated in the workplace to provide quality patient care and remain an important part of the health care team.

professionalism. The skills, behavior, and appropriate judgment that represent the best qualities of a person in a specific profession

Work ethic

Work ethic is a set of values based on the moral virtues of hard work and diligence. These values are based on an individual's diligence, virtues, morals, and desire to put forth a strong effort in their chosen profession. In the clinical or administrative work setting, always display initiative, be reliable, assist others, and be present and ready to work. When an employee consistently arrives late or is absent, their coworkers are shorthanded and must take on additional responsibilities that can hinder them from completing their own work. These types of behaviors are not welcome in the workplace and can be addressed with disciplinary action.

Integrity

Integrity is the quality of being honest and having strong moral principles. All members of the health care team must have a high level of integrity. Honesty, truthfulness, and equal treatment of all patients is a necessity for quality care in administrative and clinical settings.

Accountability

Accountability is being responsible for one's own actions. It also means being able to explain and answer questions relating to their actions. Medical assistants must be accountable for their actions regarding any clinical or administrative tasks at all times.

Flexibility

A medical assistant must be able to acclimate to a wide variety of situations. In the event of an emergency in the office, the staff must be flexible enough to adjust to schedule changes for all patients. Being flexible also means that staff members are willing to assist each other when workloads are uneven. A medical assistant should never say "That's not my job" to a task within their scope of practice.

Open-mindedness

Willingness to try new things and be considerate of others ideas is a welcome characteristic, personally and professionally. An open-minded individual listens to her opponent in a discussion rather than immediately shutting him out due to differences in opinion.

---

work ethic. A set of values based on the moral virtues of hard work and diligence

National Healthcareer Association

Scope of practice

Scope of practice describes the duties that can be delegated to medical assistants based on their education, training, and experience. The scope of practice for the medical assistant does not constitute the practice of medicine. Medical assistants should not perform duties that they have not been trained—or in some situations certified—to do. Prior to practice, review the duties and restrictions related to medical assisting, which vary by state. The medical assistant works under supervision of a provider and performs tasks allowed by state and provider approval.

Variables for the scope of practice

Variables that affect the scope of practice for medical assistants include the regulations and policies issues by state medical boards. A medical assistant with appropriate training may safely provide technical supportive services that are simple, routine medical tasks under the supervision of a licensed physician. In addition, the medical assistant may only provide technical supportive services that are clearly set forth by the medical office's organizational policies. These often include measuring height and weight, performing vital signs, and limited diagnostic and laboratory testing. Organizational policies must adhere to state and government guidelines to ensure they are in compliance with current applicable laws.

Standard of care

Standard of care is the degree of care or competence expected in a particular circumstance or role. Standard of care applies to all health care professionals who provide care to patients. Providers are extensively trained skilled professionals who are licensed to diagnose conditions and treat patients. Medical assistants cannot diagnose, treat, or instruct patients to take any course of action. Be careful to remain within the medical assistant scope of practice when carrying out duties at work.

standard of care. The degree of care or competence expected in a particular circumstance or role

TITLES AND CREDENTIALS

The Department of Labor projects that the medical assistant field will grow 23% from 2014 to 2024. This is much faster than the average occupation (7%). In the past, providers hired individuals without any training or education in the medical field for medical assistant roles. This often resulted in low wages and high turnover, and ultimately cost organizations money in the long run. Education and training that leads to advanced credentialing and certifications often have a positive effect for career advancement. Formal medical assisting programs often require an externship prior to graduation. This allows the medical assistant on-the-job training and hands-on experience to put skills and knowledge to work in actual clinical situations.

Additional credentials for medical assistants

There are several titles and credentials that a medical assistant can pursue for career-building opportunities.

Certified phlebotomy technician (CPT)

Certified EKG technician (CET)

Certified billing and coding specialist (CBCS)

Certified electronic health records specialist (CEHRS)

Certified health coach or patient navigator. A health coach or navigator often directs patients through the health care system. Navigators and patient coaches help organize patient care, connect patients to additional resources, and help patients understand the health care system. Many health coaches and patient navigators have a chronic disease focus area, such as cancer, heart disease, or diabetes.

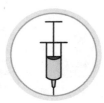 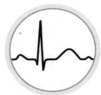 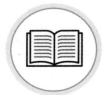 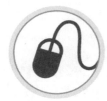 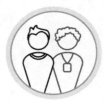

LICENSING AND CERTIFICATION

A medical school graduate must be licensed before beginning the practice of medicine. Being licensed by the state to practice medicine, diagnosing conditions, and providing treatment is essential for any medical doctor to maintain. It is important to understand the laws and regulations within each state to avoid violations of any kind.

Health care licensure

Licensure is regulated by state statutes through the medical practice acts. An MD, DO, or doctor of chiropractic degree is issued upon graduation from a medical or chiropractic institute. Licensure for physicians is mandatory and controlled by a state board of medical examiners. Licensure may be accomplished by examination, reciprocity, or endorsement. Every state requires a written examination for MDs to practice. Some states grant the license to practice medicine by reciprocity, which automatically recognizes that the requirements were already met from another state. Graduates of medical schools in the U.S. are licensed by endorsement of the national board certificate. Licensure by endorsement is granted on a case-by-case basis based on examinations. Graduates not licensed by endorsement must pass the state board exam.

As of 2016, no state requires medical assistants to be licensed. However, some states dictate that to complete specific services such as x-rays, individuals must have a license to perform that particular skill. For example, Florida does not require a medical assistant to have license to collect prescribed routine laboratory specimens. However, in the state of Washington, even nationally certified medical assistants must get licensing credentials through the Washington State Department of Health to perform phlebotomy or EKGs.

Certification

Certification is generally optional, but some states require official education and training for a medical assistant to administer medication or perform phlebotomy procedures. In addition, the government may require certification for the medical assistant to enter prescriptions into the **computerized physician order entry (CPOE)** program. Advantages of certification include increased initial job placement, higher wages, and career advancement opportunities. To keep credentials current, a medical assistant must perform continuing education units that give them credits toward courses that keep them up to date on procedures and developments in the medical field.

---

computerized physician order entry (CPOE). A process of electronic data entry of provider instructions for treatment

HEALTH CARE DELIVERY MODELS

Health care delivery (also known as the health care system) is the organization of individuals, establishments, and resources to deliver health care services and meet the health needs of specific populations. The payment model issues a single bundled payment to providers or health care facilities for all services rendered to treat a given condition or provide a given treatment. The Affordable Care Act promoted newer health care system and payment models by testing new methods of health care delivery and moving from a reimbursement structure (based on the amount of services rendered) to a method established on the value of care.

Types of health care delivery models

Accountable care organizations (ACOs): These groups of physicians, hospitals, and other health care providers come together voluntarily to provide coordinated high-quality care to their Medicare patients. When an ACO succeeds in delivering high-quality care and spending health care dollars wisely, it will share in the savings it achieves for the Medicare program.

Capitation (partial or full): In this payment model, patients are assigned a per-member, per-month payment based on their age, race, sex, lifestyle, medical history, and benefit design. Payment rates are tied to expected usage regardless of how often the patient visits. Like bundled payment models, providers have an incentive to help patients avoid high-cost procedures and tests to maximize their compensation. Under partial- or blended-capitation models, only specific types or categories of services are paid on a basis of capitation.

Global budget: This is a fixed total dollar amount paid annually for all care. However, participating providers can determine how money is spent. Global budgets limit the level and the rate of increase of health care cost. They typically include a quality component as well.

Health maintenance organization (HMO): This plan contracts with a medical center or group of providers to provide preventive and acute care for the insured person. HMOs generally require referrals to specialists, as well as precertification and preauthorization for hospital admissions, outpatient procedures, and treatments.

Patient-centered medical home (PCMH): In this care delivery model, a primary care provider (PCP) coordinates treatment to make sure patients receive the required care when and where they need it, and in a way they can understand.

Pay for performance: This reimbursement model compensates providers only if they meet certain measures for quality and efficiency. Generating quality benchmark measures connects provider reimbursement directly to the quality of care they provide.

Preferred provider organization (PPO): These plans have more flexibility than HMO plans. An insured person doesn't need a PCP, but can go directly to a specialist without referrals. Although patients can see providers in or out of their network, an in-network provider usually costs less.

General vs. specialty and services

A generalist provider is able to assess a wide range of symptoms, diagnoses, and conditions while using a variety of resources to build a treatment plan. A specialist provider assesses a more specific set of symptoms, diagnoses, and conditions.

Providers that practice general medicine

General practitioners (GPs) are medical doctors who treat acute and chronic illnesses and provide preventive care and health education to patients. A GP may take a holistic approach of general practice that takes into consideration the biological, psychological, and social aspects relevant to the care of each patient's illness.

Family practitioners offer care to the whole family, from newborns to older adults. They are familiar with a range of disorders and diseases. However, preventive care is their primary concern. This is one of the specialties most often chosen by physicians.

Internists provide comprehensive care of adults, often diagnosing and treating chronic, long-term conditions. They also offer treatment for common illnesses and preventive care. Internists must have a broad understanding of the body and its ailments to be able to diagnose conditions and provide treatment.

Providers that specialize

Allergists evaluate disorders and diseases of the immune system. This includes adverse reactions to medications and food, anaphylaxis, problems related to autoimmune disease, and asthma.

Anesthesiologists manage pain or use sedation during surgical procedures.

Cardiologists specialize in diagnosing and treating diseases or conditions of the heart and blood vessels.

Dermatologists specialize in conditions of the skin.

Endocrinologists specialize in hormonal and glandular conditions. They often work with patients who have diabetes mellitus.

Gastroenterologists specialize in managing diseases of the gastrointestinal tract: the stomach, intestines, esophagus, liver, pancreas, colon, and rectum.

Gynecologists specialize in the female reproductive system and fertility disorders.

Hematologists deal with blood and blood-producing organs. They often work with patients who have anemia, leukemia, and lymphoma.

Hepatologists specialize in the study of body parts such as the liver, biliary tree, gallbladder, and pancreas.

Neonatologists specialize in the care of newborns.

Nephrologists specialize in kidney care and treating diseases of the kidneys.

Obstetricians specialize in the care of women during and after pregnancy.

Oncologists specialize in the treatment and care of patients who have cancer.

Ophthalmologists specialize in eye conditions.

Orthopedists specialize in bones, joints, muscles, tendons, and ligaments.

Otolaryngologists specialize in the ear, nose, and throat.

Neurologists specialize in the nervous system.

Pathologists specialize in body tissues, blood, urine, and other body fluids to diagnose or treat medical conditions.

Pediatricians specialize in newborn, infant, child, and adolescent health care.

Psychiatrists specialize in mental disorders and conditions.

Radiologists specialize in the use of x-rays, ultrasound, nuclear medicine, computed tomography, and magnetic resonance imaging to detect abnormalities throughout the body.

Urologists specialize in disorders of the urinary tract.

Ancillary services and alternative therapies

Providing ancillary services in the provider's office adds convenience for patients and increases revenue for the organization. Ancillary services meet a specific medical need for a specific population. For example, an occupational therapist assists patients to acquire day-to-day physical tasks that they have never been able to do or recover those lost due to an illness or injury. An urgent care offers more locations and time flexibility to patients who might have cold-like symptoms.

Types of ancillary services

Urgent cares provide an alternative to the emergency department. They cost less, have a shorter wait time, and are often conveniently located. Most have flexible hours and offer walk-in appointments.

Laboratory services perform diagnostic testing on blood, body fluids, and other types of specimens to conclude a diagnosis for the provider.

Diagnostic imaging machines such as x-ray equipment, ultrasound machines, magnetic resonance imaging (MRI), and computerized tomography (CT) take images of body parts to further diagnose a condition.

Occupational therapy assists patients who have conditions that disable them developmentally, emotionally, mentally, or physically. Occupational therapy helps the patient compensate for loss of functions and rebuild to a functional level.

Physical therapy assists patients in regaining mobility and improving strength and range of motion, often impaired by an accident, injury, or as a result of a disease.

National Healthcareer Association

Alternative therapies

Acupuncture involves pricking the skin or tissues with needles to relieve pain and treat various physical, mental, and emotional conditions.

Chiropractic medicine diagnoses and treats mechanical disorders of the musculoskeletal system, particularly the spine.

Energy therapy is the calm method of clearing cellular memory through the human energy field promoting health, balance, and relaxation. It is centered on the idea of connection between the physical, emotional, mental states of life found in various holistic healing techniques.

Dietary supplements contain one or more dietary ingredients including vitamins, minerals, herbs, or other botanicals. A plant or part of a plant (flowers, leaves, bark, fruit, seeds, stems and roots, and amino acids) is used for its flavor, scent, or potential therapeutic properties.

INSURANCE FUNDAMENTALS

Medical insurance coverage is available to individuals and families through individual or group plans. Government plans or programs (Medicare, Medicaid, Tricare, Civilian Health and Medical Program of the Department of Veterans Affairs [CHAMPVA]) offer coverage to some people. Although health insurance is available, it is not always affordable to all people. In 2009, more than 46 million Americans did not have health care insurance. By 2014, a CDC survey showed that the number of uninsured Americans dropped to approximately 36 million. While the Affordable Care Act made improvements in this statistic, the number of Americans who lack health insurance is still high. Group, individual, and government-sponsored insurance; self-insured plans; and insurance terminology are discussed in *Chapter 15: Administrative Assisting.*

Insurance terminology

Advance beneficiary notice (ABN): A form provided to the patient when the provider believes Medicare will probably not pay for services received

Allowed amount: The maximum amount a third-party payer will pay for a particular procedure or service

Copayment: An amount of money that is paid at the time of medical service

Coinsurance: A policy provision frequently found in medical insurance whereby the policyholder and the insurance company share the cost of covered losses in a specified ratio, such as 80:20

Deductible: A specific amount of money a patient must pay out of pocket before the insurance carrier begins paying

Explanation of benefits: A statement from the insurance carrier detailing what was paid, denied, or reduced in payment; also contains information about amounts applied to the deductible, coinsurance, and allowed amounts

Participating provider (PAR): Providers who agree to write off the difference between the amount charged by the provider and the approved fee established by the insurer

Types of insurance plans

Federal and state government plans include Medicare, Tricare, CHAMPVA, Medicaid, *managed care* plans, and workers' compensation.

Medicare generally covers patients age 65 and older by Part A (hospitalization) or Part B (routine medical office visits) benefits.

Tricare authorizes dependents of military personnel to receive treatment from civilian providers at the expense of the federal government.

CHAMPVA covers surviving spouses and dependent children of veterans who died as a result of service-related disabilities.

Medicaid provides health insurance to the medically indigent population through a cost-sharing program between federal and state governments for those who meet specific eligibility criteria.

Managed care is an umbrella term for plans that provide health care in return for preset scheduled payments and coordinated care through a defined network of providers and hospitals.

Workers' compensation protects wage earners against the loss of wages and the cost of medical care resulting from an occupational accident or disease as long as the employee is not proven negligent.

Private insurance plans include Blue Cross Blue Shield, Aetna, and United Healthcare. Blue Cross Blue Shield is America's oldest and largest system of independent health insurers. Private insurance plans offer two basic managed care models: PPO and HMO. The preferred provider organization (PPO) allows more flexibility in the plan, such as not being required to choose a PCP. However, health maintenance organizations (HMOs) are comprehensive and most plans require their insured to choose a PCP.

CMS-1500 Form

Most health care payers use the CMS-1500 health insurance claim form for claims submitted by a provider or supplier. The medical assistant must have all the information needed to complete the form, including the patient's and guarantor's demographic and insurance information; diagnostic test, treatment, or procedure information; and billing information. The CMS-1500 form has 33 blocks or items, which are divided into three sections.

- *Section 1: Carrier Block* contains the address of the insurance carrier and is located at the top of the form.

- *Section 2: Patient/Insured Section* contains information about the patient or insured (if other than the patient); includes boxes 1 through 13.

- *Sections 3: Physician/Supplier Section* contains information about the physician or supplier: includes boxes 14 through 33.

managed care. An umbrella term for plans that provide health care in return for preset scheduled payments and coordinated care through a defined network of providers and hospitals

12

National Healthcareer Association

The Administrative Simplification Compliance Act (ASCA) requires that claims to Medicare be transmitted electronically. But if a provider uses a clearinghouse to submit claims, the draft sent to the clearinghouse may be completed on paper. For paper claims, the correct form to use is CMS-1500, which has been revised by the organization that maintains it, the National Uniform Claim Committee (NUCC). Any new version of the form must be approved by the White House Office of Management and Budget (OMB). OMB has approved the revised form, referred to as version 02/12, OMB control number 0938-1197.

It is very important to fill out the form correctly. The following section explains what information needs to go in each field.

Member information

Blocks 1 through 13 focus on basic information about the patient, the insured (if that person is different), and determining which plan is primary and which is secondary if the patient has two insurance plans (Block 11). This information must be entered exactly as specified.

1.1 CMS-1500 Form Blocks 1-8

SOURCE: NATIONAL UNIFORM CLAIM COMMITTEE

BLOCK 1   Check the box indicating what kind of insurance is applicable, such as Medicare.

BLOCK 1A   The patient's Medicare Health Insurance Claim Number (HICN). This number must be recorded whether Medicare is the primary or secondary payer.

BLOCK 2   The patient's first name, middle initial (if any), and last name, as shown on the patient's Medicare card.

BLOCK 3   The patient's eight-digit birth date recorded as MM|DD|CCYY and sex. For example, September 28, 1990, would be recorded 09|28|1990.

BLOCK 4   If there is insurance primary to Medicare, obtained through the patient's or spouse's place of work or through any other source, list the name of the insured here. If the patient and the insured are the same, write SAME. If Medicare is primary, leave this field blank.

BLOCK 5   The patient's mailing address and telephone number. Put the mailing address on the first line, the city and state on the second line, and the ZIP code and phone number on the third line.

BLOCK 6   Check the appropriate box for patient's relationship to the insured.

BLOCK 7   Enter the insured's address and phone number. If the insured is the same as the patient, write SAME. Complete this block only after blocks 4, 6, and 11 have been completed.

BLOCK 8   Leave blank.

1.2 CMS-1500 Form Blocks 9-13

9. OTHER INSURED'S NAME (Last Name, First Name, Middle Initial)	10. IS PATIENT'S CONDITION RELATED TO:	11. INSURED'S POLICY GROUP OR FECA NUMBER	
a. OTHER INSURED'S POLICY OR GROUP NUMBER	a. EMPLOYMENT? (Current or Previous) ☐ YES ☐ NO	a. INSURED'S DATE OF BIRTH MM DD YY SEX M ☐ F ☐	
b. RESERVED FOR NUCC USE	b. AUTO ACCIDENT? ☐ YES ☐ NO PLACE (State)	b. OTHER CLAIM ID (Designated by NUCC)	
c. RESERVED FOR NUCC USE	c. OTHER ACCIDENT? ☐ YES ☐ NO	c. INSURANCE PLAN NAME OR PROGRAM NAME	
d. INSURANCE PLAN NAME OR PROGRAM NAME	10d. CLAIM CODES (Designated by NUCC)	d. IS THERE ANOTHER HEALTH BENEFIT PLAN? ☐ YES ☐ NO *If yes*, complete items 9, 9a, and 9d.	
READ BACK OF FORM BEFORE COMPLETING & SIGNING THIS FORM. 12. PATIENT'S OR AUTHORIZED PERSON'S SIGNATURE I authorize the release of any medical or other information necessary to process this claim. I also request payment of government benefits either to myself or to the party who accepts assignment below. SIGNED _____ DATE _____		13. INSURED'S OR AUTHORIZED PERSON'S SIGNATURE I authorize payment of medical benefits to the undersigned physician or supplier for services described below. SIGNED _____	PATIENT AND INSURED INF

SOURCE: NATIONAL UNIFORM CLAIM COMMITTEE

BLOCK 9   Write the last name, first name, and middle initial (if there is one) of the Medigap enrollee if it is a different person from the one listed in Block 2. Otherwise, write SAME. If no Medigap benefits are assigned, leave blank.

BLOCK 9A   Enter the policy and/or group number of the Medigap insured preceded by MEDIGAP, MG, or MGAP.

BLOCK 9B   Leave blank.

BLOCK 9C   Leave blank.

BLOCK 9D   Write in the Coordination of Benefits Agreement Medigap-based identifier.

BLOCKS 10A-10C   Check "Yes" or "No" to indicate whether employment, auto liability, or other accident involvement applies to one or more of the services listed in block 24. A "yes" answer indicates there may be other insurance primary to Medicare.

BLOCK 11   This is an important field. This is the place to indicate that a good faith effort has been made to determine whether Medicare is the primary insurance. Information about insurance primary to Medicare should be listed in blocks 11a-11c.

Instances where Medicare is the secondary insurance include the following.

- Group health plan coverage
  - Working aged
  - Disability (large group health plan)
  - End-stage renal disease
- No-fault or other liability
- Work-related illness/injury
  - Workers' compensation
  - Black lung
  - Veterans benefits

BLOCK 11A   This is where the insured's birth date goes. Enter the sex as well if it is different from Block 3.

BLOCK 11B   For insurance primary to Medicare, enter employer's name, if applicable. If there is a change in the insured's insurance status (e.g., retired), enter either a 6-digit (MMDDYY) or 8-digit (MMDDCCYY) retirement date preceded by the word "RETIRED." For Tricare and CHAMPVA, enter the sponsor's branch of service, using abbreviations (e.g., United States Navy = USN). For commercial claims, check for payer-specific instructions.

BLOCK 11C   Enter the nine-digit payer ID number of the primary insurer. If there is no payer ID, then write in the primary payer's program or plan name. If the explanation of benefits (EOB) does not include the claim's processing address, then write it in.

BLOCK 11D   For Medicare, leave blank. For all other payers, enter an "x" in the correct box, if appropriate. If marked "YES," complete items 9, 9a, and 9d.

BLOCK 12   This is an important field. This is the place where the patient or an authorized person signs to authorize the release of medical information. The field must be dated and entered as a six- or eight-digit date. A signature on file or a computer-generated signature can also be used. The patient's signature authorizes release of information necessary to process the claim.

BLOCK 13   This signature authorizes payment of benefits to the provider or supplier. A signature on file is acceptable here.

Provider of service (POS) or supplier information

These fields (14 to 33) include information about the providers, services rendered, diagnoses made, procedures performed, and modifiers needed. Each field is described below.

1.3 CMS-1500 Form Blocks 14-18

14. DATE OF CURRENT ILLNESS, INJURY, or PREGNANCY (LMP) MM DD YY QUAL.	15. OTHER DATE QUAL.	MM DD YY	16. DATES PATIENT UNABLE TO WORK IN CURRENT OCCUPATION MM DD YY MM DD YY FROM TO
17. NAME OF REFERRING PROVIDER OR OTHER SOURCE	17a.		18. HOSPITALIZATION DATES RELATED TO CURRENT SERVICES MM DD YY MM DD YY
	17b. NPI		FROM TO

SOURCE: NATIONAL UNIFORM CLAIM COMMITTEE

BLOCK 14   For Medicare, for the current illness, injury, or pregnancy, enter either an 8-digit (MMDDCCYY) or 6-digit (MMDDYY) date. For chiropractic services, enter the date of the initiation of the course of treatment and enter the date of x-ray (if used to demonstrate subluxation) in item 19. Medicare does not use qualifiers.

For commercial claims: Enter the date of the first date of the present illness, injury, or pregnancy. For pregnancy, use the date of the last menstrual period (LMP) as the first date. Enter the applicable qualifier to identify which date is being reported (e.g., 431 Onset of Current Symptoms or Illness, 484 Last Menstrual Period).

BLOCK 15   For Medicare, leave blank (not required). For all other carriers, check for payer-specific instructions. When required, enter another date related to the patient's condition or treatment and the applicable qualifier to identify which date is being reported.

BLOCK 16   Dates patient is unable to work in his/her current occupation. This is required if the patient is eligible for disability or workers' compensation benefits. To fill out this field, enter the "From" and "To" dates as follows: MMDDYY (051512) or MMDDCCYY (05152012).

BLOCK 17   This is where the name of the referring or ordering provider goes. If Medicare requires that a supervising provider be listed, this is where to put that name. If a claim involves more than one referring, ordering, or supervising provider, a separate claim must be submitted for each one. Table 1.4 shows the qualifiers that should be used for each kind of provider.

1.4 Qualifiers for different kinds of providers

QUALIFIER	PROVIDER	DESCRIPTION
DN	Referring provider	The physician who requests the service for the patient.
DK	Ordering provider	A physician or, when appropriate, a nonphysician who orders nonphysician services for the patient. These services include diagnostic laboratory tests, clinical laboratory tests, pharmaceutical services, or durable medical equipment.
DQ	Supervising provider	The physician monitoring the patient's care.

BLOCK 17A Leave blank.

BLOCK 17B The NPI number goes here. As part of the enrollment process, all providers must apply for an NPI number. Authorized under the HIPAA Simplification Rule, the NPI is a unique identification number for all HIPAA-covered entities, including individuals, organizations, home health agencies, clinics, nursing homes, residential treatment homes, laboratories, ambulances, group practices, and health maintenance organizations (HMOs).

BLOCK 18 Dates entered in a six- or eight-digit format when a medical service rendered is a result of, or subsequent to, a related hospitalization.

1.5 CMS-1500 Form Blocks 19-23

SOURCE: NATIONAL UNIFORM CLAIM COMMITTEE

BLOCK 19 This block is used in numerous ways, based on the circumstances and payer type. Some common examples include:

- When modifier 99 (multiple modifiers) is used in block 24D, an explanation is given here in block 19 (e.g., 99 = 52 80 LT).

- When a claim needs to have a report or other documentation attached, enter "Additional Claim Information" in this block.

- Some payers require qualifiers in this block. Check with your private payer to see if this is required. NUCC provides a complete list on its website.

- Workers' compensation requires additional information in this block. Each state has an official website for workers' compensation, with claim form instructions. NUCC also lists the qualifiers used.

- Medicare also has specific instructions for various situations and specialty claims. Complete instructions can be found at www.cms.gov.

BLOCK 20 Mark "yes" to the question asked if lab tests were done by an entity other than the one doing the billing. If multiple tests are involved, each should be filed under a separate claim.

National Healthcareer Association

BLOCK 21   This is where the diagnosis codes go. Use ICD-10-CM codes to the greatest specificity possible.

BLOCK 22   Carrier-specific block; use for Medicaid claims.

BLOCK 23   The quality improvement organization (QIO) prior authorization number goes here for those procedures that require it. Enter the investigational device exemption (IDE) when an investigation device is used in an FDA-approved clinical trial.

Other information entered here includes the following.

- NPI of a home health agency or hospice when either is billed

- 10-digit Clinical Laboratory Improvement Act (CLIA) certification number for laboratory services billed by an entity performing CLIA-covered procedures

- ZIP code of a loaded ambulance's point of pick-up

IMPORTANT: Only one of these conditions can be listed per claim. If more than one apply, separate claims need to be submitted.

1.6 CMS-1500 Form Blocks 24A-J

SOURCE: NATIONAL UNIFORM CLAIM COMMITTEE

BLOCK 24A   Dates of service are listed here. Enter "From" and "To" dates in either a MMDDYY or MMDDCCYY format. When "From" and "To" dates are shown for a series of identical services, list them as a series of days in column G.

BLOCK 24B   This is where places of service codes go. These must be HIPAA-compliant. Codes are shown as two-digit numbers. For example, "01" should be used for a pharmacy; "02" is an unassigned number; "03" is for a school; and "04" is for a homeless shelter. For a complete list of codes, search www.cms.gov.

BLOCK 24C   Carrier-specific block; used by Medicaid. Enter an "x" when billing for emergency services, or the claim may be reduced or denied.

BLOCK 24D   Enter procedures, services, and supplies. For this field, use CPT or HCPCS codes. These will be described in *Chapter 15: Administrative Assisting.* This is also the place where *modifiers* go. Modifiers are additional information about types of services, such as surgical care or outpatient services. Modifiers are part of valid CPT or HCPCS codes.

BLOCK 24E   This field is for the diagnosis reference code, as shown in Block 21. This field matches the date of service to the procedures performed under the primary diagnosis code. Enter only one reference number per line. Do *not* enter the diagnosis code here.

BLOCK 24F   Enter the provider's billed charges for each service.

BLOCK 24G   Enter the number of days or units. This field is mostly used for multiple visits, units of supplies, anesthesia minutes, or oxygen volume. If only one service is performed, the number "1" must be entered.

BLOCK 24H Carrier-specific block. For Medicaid claims, refer to the Family Planning section of the Medicaid Providers Manual for detailed instructions.

BLOCK 24I Enter the ID qualifier 1C in the shaded portion.

BLOCK 24J Enter the provider's NPI in the unshaded portion.

1.7 CMS-1500 Form Blocks 25-33A

25. FEDERAL TAX I.D. NUMBER	SSN EIN	26. PATIENT'S ACCOUNT NO.	27. ACCEPT ASSIGNMENT? (For govt. claims, see back)	28. TOTAL CHARGE	29. AMOUNT PAID	30. Rsvd for NUCC Use
	☐ ☐		☐ YES ☐ NO	$	$	
31. SIGNATURE OF PHYSICIAN OR SUPPLIER INCLUDING DEGREES OR CREDENTIALS (I certify that the statements on the reverse apply to this bill and are made a part thereof.)		32. SERVICE FACILITY LOCATION INFORMATION		33. BILLING PROVIDER INFO & PH # ( )		
SIGNED DATE		a. NPI b.		a. NPI b.		

BLOCK 25 Enter the provider's or supplier's federal ID number or Social Security number and check the appropriate box.

BLOCK 26 Enter the patient's account number as assigned by the provider or supplier.

BLOCK 27 Check the appropriate box to indicate whether the provider or supplier accepts assignment of benefits. Be aware of which providers can only be paid on an assignment basis.

BLOCK 28 Enter total charges for all services.

BLOCK 29 For secondary claims only. Enter the total amount the patient's primary insurance paid.

BLOCK 30 Leave blank.

BLOCK 31 Enter the signature of the provider or the signature of an authorized representative.

BLOCK 32 Enter the name, address, and ZIP code of the facility where services were rendered.

BLOCK 32A Enter the NPI of the facility.

BLOCK 33 The provider's or supplier's billing name, address, ZIP code, and telephone number.

BLOCK 33A The NPI of the billing provider.

Other important considerations

Use an "x" for marking boxes. Special characters are not allowed on claim forms.

Medicare only accepts paper claims that use all capital letters.

Electronic submission of claims

Electronic claims can be submitted in several ways, such as direct billing or to a claims clearing house. Direct billing is the process by which an insurance carrier allows a provider to submit insurance claims directly to the carrier electronically. Clearinghouse submissions for claims allows a provider to submit all insurance claims using distinctive software. The clearinghouse then audits and sorts the claims and sends them in batches electronically to each of the insurance companies. Once the services have been rendered, the provider must submit the claims within timely filing limits. For example, Medicare/Medicaid claims must be filed to the appropriate carrier no later than 12 months after the date of service.

SUMMARY

Health care systems and settings include a variety of divisions in which health care providers, medical assistants, and allied health personnel work together as members of a health care team. All members of a health care system perform both clinical duties and administrative responsibilities. Medical assistants work under the supervision of health care professionals, such as MDs or DOs, to obtain a medical history and screen the patient. If the patient requires additional analysis, the provider may send the patient to see a specialist via the CPOE system. Whether the health care facility is a hospital, ambulatory care center, or other health care facility, the medical staff is accountable for the health and safety of patients, and the medical assistant is a crucial part of this process.

CHAPTER 2

Medical Terminology

OVERVIEW

Learning medical terminology might seem as daunting as learning another language. In a way, it is another language. When toddlers first start speaking actual words, they do not yet know what geography, philanthropy, or accountability mean. But with experience in listening and speaking, they learn to use and understand more words. They later begin to notice connections among words—their prefixes, roots, and suffixes. As their vocabulary continues to expand, children eventually master communication in their native language.

Medical assistants become fluent in medical terminology in much the same way, with one distinct advantage. They will first learn the basics in coursework and with learning activities such as this chapter. Here are the most common terms, abbreviations, acronyms, and symbols needed to begin to navigate communication in this new career. Learning how to dissect some terms into their prefixes, roots, and suffixes can also expand understanding of terminology much faster than learning each word individually, fast-tracking to mastery in medical terminology.

Objectives

Upon completion of this chapter, you should be able to:

- Recognize and use common medical abbreviations, acronyms, and symbols in written or electronic communication.
- Build and deconstruct medical terms, and define common word roots, prefixes, and suffixes in medical terms.
- Change medical terms from singular to plural.
- Provide medical suffixes for common conditions, procedures, and instruments.
- List and describe directional terms to use when referencing anatomical locations throughout the body.

COMMON ABBREVIATIONS, ACRONYMS, AND SYMBOLS

Medical assistants see and use many abbreviations (a term that will refer here to symbols as well) in everyday practice. The Joint Commission and the Institute for Safe Medication Practices have put some abbreviations on their "Do Not Use" and "Error-Prone Abbreviations" lists. Avoiding these abbreviations is essential because of their potential for misunderstanding and medical errors. The following table includes many abbreviations that should not be used. (For the full lists, go to the Joint Commission and the Institute for Safe Medication Practices websites.)

2.1 Error-prone abbreviation list

DO NOT USE	USE	DO NOT USE	USE
MS, MSO$_4$	morphine	q.o.d., QOD	every other day
MgSO$_4$	magnesium sulfate	Q6PM, etc.	6 p.m. daily or daily at 6 p.m.
abbreviated medication names (AZT, KCl, HCT, PTU, HCTZ)	full name of medication	TIW, tiw	3 times weekly
		mg., mL.	mg, mL (no period)
nitro	nitroglycerin	HS	half-strength, bedtime (hour of sleep)
decimal points without a leading zero (.5 mg)	smaller units (500 mcg) or a leading zero (0.5 mg)	BT, hs, HS, qhs, qn	bedtime or hour of sleep
		SC, SQ, sub q	subcutaneously
trailing zero (1.0 mg, 100.0 g)	no trailing zero (1 mg, 100 g)	IN	intranasal
		IJ	injection
u, U, IU	units	OJ	orange juice
µ, µg	mcg or microgram	> or <	greater than or less than
x3d	times 3 days	@	at
cc	mL	&, +	and
apothecary units	metric units	/	per
od, O.D., OD	daily or intended time of administration	AD, AS, AU	right ear, left ear, both ears
		OD, OS, OU	right eye, left eye, both eyes
q.d, qd, Q.D, QD, q1d, i/d	daily		

Common medical abbreviations and acronyms

It is acceptable to use the abbreviations in the following list. There are many others that are more facility-specific, but they are not necessarily universal. For example, one hospital might call its storage and processing area for medical products "central supply," while another might call it "materials management." So, "CS" has no meaning (or a different meaning) in Hospital B, and "MM" has no meaning (or a different meaning) in Hospital A. Likewise, Hospital A calls the surgery area the "operating room" (OR), while Hospital B calls it the "surgical suite" (SS). Yet another hospital uses "SS" to mean its department of social services.

Many acronyms go back to long-outdated usage. "Emergency room" became common parlance when there was literally one room—an emergency or accident room. Even though today's hospitals have enormous emergency departments, "ER" is still in prevalent use today. Other terminology changes over time. What was once the "recovery room" (RR) is now the "post-anesthesia care unit" (PACU). For this chapter, the focus will be on common abbreviations that reflect current clinical practice and are primarily universal. Providers use many of these when writing orders, often on prescription pads, for diagnostic tests and procedures.

Here is a list of many of those common abbreviations.

2.2 Acceptable abbreviations

ABBR.	MEANING	ABBR.	MEANING
abd	abdomen	BPM	beats per minute
ABGs	arterial blood gases	BRP	bathroom privileges
ac	before meals	BSA	body surface area
ACLS	advanced cardiac life support	BUN	blood urea nitrogen
ad lib	as desired	bx	*biopsy*
ADHD	attention deficit hyperactivity disorder	c̄	with
AKA	above-the-knee *amputation*	C	Celsius
AMA	against medical advice	C&S	culture and sensitivity
ASA	aspirin	ca	calcium, cancer
ASAP	as soon as possible	CABG	*coronary artery bypass graft*
BE	barium enema	CAD	*coronary artery disease*
BKA	below-the-knee amputation	CBC	complete blood (cell) count
BM	bowel movement	CC	chief complaint
BMI	body mass index	CDC	Centers for Disease Control and Prevention
BP	blood pressure		
BPH	benign prostatic hypertrophy	cm	centimeter

---

amputation. Surgical removal of all or part of a limb or extremity

biopsy. The removal and examination of tissue to diagnose a disease, such as cancer

coronary artery bypass graft. Surgery that eliminates a blockage in an artery going to the heart by replacing it with a section of a blood vessel from another area

coronary artery disease. A disorder that involves partial or complete blockage of the blood vessels that supply oxygen and nutrients to the heart

2.2 Acceptable abbreviations *continued*

ABBR.	MEANING
CNS	central nervous system
CP	chest pain
CPR	cardiopulmonary resuscitation
c/o	complains of
COPD	*chronic obstructive pulmonary disease*
csf	cerebrospinal fluid
CT	computed tomography
cv	cardiovascular
CVA	cerebrovascular accident (stroke)
CXR	chest x-ray
d	day
D&C	*dilation and curettage*
D/C, dc	discharge, discontinue
DM	diabetes mellitus
DNR	do not resuscitate
DOB	date of birth
DTap	diphtheria, tetanus, and acellular pertussis vaccine
dx	diagnosis
ECG, EKG	*electrocardiogram*
ED	emergency department
EEG	*electroencephalogram*
ENT	ear, nose, and throat
F	Fahrenheit
FBS, FBG	fasting blood sugar/glucose
f/u	follow up
FUO	fever of unknown origin
fx	fracture
GI	gastrointestinal

ABBR.	MEANING
GTT	glucose tolerance test
GU	*genitourinary*
GYN	*gynecology*, gynecologist
h, hr	hour
H_2O	water
Hct	*hematocrit*
HEENT	head, ears, eyes, nose, throat
HF	heart failure
Hgb	*hemoglobin*
HIV	human immunodeficiency virus
HPV	human papillomavirus
Htn, HTN	hypertension
hx	history
I&D	*incision* and drainage
I&O	intake and output
ICU	intensive care unit
IUD	intrauterine device
K	potassium
KUB	kidneys, ureters, bladder
L	liter
lb	pound
LLE	left lower extremity (left leg)
LLL	left lower lobe
LLQ	left lower quadrant
LMP	last menstrual period
LUE	left upper extremity (arm)
LUQ	left upper quadrant
mg/dL	milligrams per deciliter

chronic obstructive pulmonary disease. A persistent disorder that impairs breathing

dilation and curettage. Surgery involving the use of an instrument to open the cervix (entrance to the uterus) and then cutting away tissue inside the uterus for therapeutic purposes

electrocardiogram. A record of the heart's electrical impulses

electroencephalogram. A record of the brain's electrical activity

genitourinary. Referring to the urinary and reproductive organs

gynecology. The type of medical practice that deals with the female reproductive system

hematocrit. The percentage of a blood sample that is red blood cells

hemoglobin. The red, oxygen-carrying pigment of red blood cells

incision. A surgical wound that results from cutting into tissue

2.2 Acceptable abbreviations *continued*

ABBR.	MEANING	ABBR.	MEANING
MI	*myocardial infarction*	pt	patient
mL	milliliters	RA	*rheumatoid arthritis*
MM	mucous membrane	RBC	red blood cell
mm Hg	millimeters of mercury	RLE	right lower extremity (leg)
MRI	magnetic resonance imaging	RLL	right lower lobe
MS	multiple sclerosis	RLQ	right lower quadrant
N/V	nausea/vomiting	R/O	rule out
NB	newborn	ROM	range of motion
NG	*nasogastric*	RT	respiratory therapy or therapist
NKA	no known allergies	RUE	right upper extremity (right arm)
NPO	nothing by mouth (*nil per os*)	RUQ	right upper quadrant
NS	normal saline	Rx	prescription
NSAID	nonsteroidal anti-inflammatory drug	$\bar{s}$	without
O^2	oxygen	SOB	shortness of breath
OB	*obstetrics*	stat	immediately
OC	oral contraceptive	STI	sexually transmitted infection
OOB	out of bed	sx	symptoms
OP	outpatient	T&A	*tonsillectomy* and *adenoidectomy*
OT	occupational therapy or therapist	TB	*tuberculosis*
OTC	over-the-counter	TIA	*transient ischemic attack*
PA	posteroanterior, physician assistant	Tx	treatment
pc	after meals	UA	*urinalysis*
PE	physical examination	URI	upper respiratory infection
PID	*pelvic inflammatory disease*	UTI	urinary tract infection
PMS	premenstrual syndrome	VS	vital signs
PO	by mouth	WBC	white blood cell
PRN	as needed	WNL	within normal limits
PT	physical therapy or therapist	YO, y/o	years old

myocardial infarction. An interruption of blood flow to the heart, causing heart muscle damage; a heart attack

nasogastric. From the nose to the stomach

obstetrics. The type of medical practice that deals with women giving birth

pelvic inflammatory disease. A bacterial infection of the female reproductive organs

rheumatoid arthritis. An autoimmune disease that causes pain, swelling, and deformity especially in the hands and feet, due to inflammation in the joints

tonsillectomy. Surgical removal of the tonsils (small masses of lymphatic tissue)

adenoidectomy. The removal of small masses of lymphatic tissue near the opening into the pharynx

tuberculosis. A highly contagious infectious disease of the lungs that causes necrosis (death) of lung tissues

transient ischemic attack. A temporary interruption of blood flow to the brain

urinalysis. A diagnostic examination of urine; a physical, chemical and/or microscopic examination of urine

Common medical symbols

Some medical symbols have fallen out of use because of their tendency toward misinterpretation, especially in handwriting. Some of those are on the "Do Not Use" and "Error-Prone Abbreviations" lists. Examples are the symbols for "greater than" and "less than" (> and <), as well as those for "greater than or equal to" and "less than or equal to" (≥ and ≤). Those lists also advise against using @ and &, as people can mistake them for the numeral 2. Likewise, the plus sign should not be used, because it can look like the numeral 4. A good rule of thumb is when in doubt, spell it out. Here are a few symbols that medical assistants might still see in handwritten medical records. Keep in mind that these can also be risky: ↑ could look like the numeral 7, ↓ could look like the numeral 1, and ° could look like the numeral 0.

2.3 Symbols

SYMBOL	MEANING
#	pounds, number
↑	increase
↓	decrease
♂	male
♀	female
′	feet
″	inches
°	degrees

ENRICHMENT Abbreviation rules of thumb

Abbreviations, acronyms, and symbols are the shorthand of the medical field, and they can save some time. However, shorthand lends itself to miscommunication, so it is important to use extreme caution when considering these shortcuts.

Follow these three rules of thumb when using abbreviations, acronyms, and symbols.

- Become familiar with the "Do Not Use" and "Error-Prone Abbreviations" lists. Access them online and print them. Keep them handy as a reminder of what to avoid.
- Minimize your use of abbreviations, acronyms, and symbols. Don't set yourself up for misinterpretation of what you intend to communicate.
- Any time you have any doubts about what another staff member has communicated or documented within an abbreviation, go to that person and clarify the meaning. Remember, the safety of patients is always the primary concern.

MEDICAL WORD BUILDING FOR CONDITIONS, INSTRUMENTS, AND PROCEDURES

Roots, prefixes, suffixes, and plurals

As familiarity with medical terminology grows, it becomes easy to notice similarities among these terms. That is because many of them share common roots, prefixes, and suffixes. Putting together these components builds many medical terms. It's not foolproof; it doesn't work to just mix and match three components and find a word that is in universal use. For example, "hemi" means half, "narc" means sleep, and "ism" means condition. But if a patient chronically gets half the amount of sleep he should get, he doesn't have heminarcism. There is no such word. Also, with some combinations, the result requires interpretation, because the literal meaning might vary a little from the actual meaning. An example is antibiotic, a combination of the prefix "anti," meaning against, and the word root "bio," meaning life. Antibiotics are not incompatible with life. They kill a particular type of living organism, bacteria. Another thing to remember is that not all medical terms adhere to the prefix-root-suffix schema. However, looking at words that have any one of those word components in it can offer a clue to what the term means.

Common word roots by body system

Word roots are the core component of many words. Medical terms usually have one root but can have two or more. Sometimes, when a root attaches to a prefix or suffix, it needs an extra vowel to combine the components. For example, "hem" means blood and "rrhage" means excessive flow. The "o" between the two creates the medical term hemorrhage, meaning excessive blood flow. Not all word roots relate to a body system or a body part, but the following table lists some of the terms that do.

2.5 Word roots: Endocrine

WORD ROOT	MEANING
aden	gland
pancreat	pancreas
thyr	thyroid gland

2.6 Word roots: Hematologic

WORD ROOT	MEANING
hem, hemat	blood
phleb	vein
thromb	clot

2.4 Root words in use

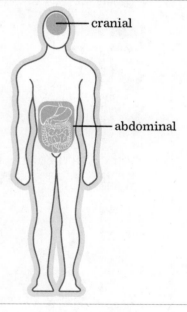

cranial

abdominal

2.7 Word roots: Musculoskeletal

WORD ROOT	MEANING	WORD ROOT	MEANING
arthr	joint	my	muscle
brachi	arm	oste	bone
cervic	neck	pod	foot
chondr	cartilage	sacr	sacrum (lower backbone)
cost	rib	spondyl	vertebra (backbone)
crani	skull	ten, tendin	tendon
dactyl	finger, toe	vertebr	vertebra
fibr	connective tissue		

2.8 Word roots: Gastrointestinal

WORD ROOT	MEANING	WORD ROOT	MEANING
abdomin	abdomen	hepat	liver
an	anus	icter	*jaundice*
appendic	appendix	ile	ileum (small intestine)
bil, chol	*bile*, gall	lapar	abdominal wall
col	colon (large intestine)	lingu	tongue
dent	teeth	pancreat	pancreas
enter	intestines	peps	digestion
esophag	esophagus	phag	eating, swallowing
gastr	stomach	proct	rectum
gingiv	gums	splen	spleen
gloss	tongue	stomat	mouth

2.9 Word roots: Genitourinary/reproductive

WORD ROOT	MEANING	WORD ROOT	MEANING
andr	men	oophor	ovary
colp	vagina	orchid	testicles
cyst	bladder	prostat	prostate gland
gravid	pregnant	pyel	pelvis of the kidney
gynec	woman	ren	renal (kidney)
hyster	uterus (womb)	salping	fallopian tube
mamm, mast	breast	ureter	ureters
metr	uterus	ur	urinary
nephr	kidney	vesic	bladder
ov	ovum (egg)		

2.10 Word roots: Respiratory

WORD ROOT	MEANING	WORD ROOT	MEANING
bronch	bronchial	pulmon	lung
laryng	larynx	rhin	nose
nas	nose	steth	chest
pleur	pleura	thorac	thorax (chest)
pneum, pneumon	lungs, air	trache	trachea (airway, windpipe)

bile. A yellow-green fluid the liver creates and the gall bladder stores that helps digest fats

jaundice. Yellowing of the skin, whites of the eyes, mucous membranes, and excretions as a result of liver disease

National Healthcareer Association

2.11 Word roots: Integumentary

WORD ROOT	MEANING
derm, dermat	skin
hidr	sweat
trich	hair
onych	nail
xer	dry

2.12 Word roots: Cardiovascular

WORD ROOT	MEANING
angi	blood vessel
arteri, arter	artery
cardi	heart
vas	vessel
ven	vein

2.13 Word roots: Neurological

WORD ROOT	MEANING	WORD ROOT	MEANING
blephar	eyelid	mening, meningi	membranes, meninges
cephal	head	myel	spinal cord, bone marrow
cerebr	cerebrum (part of the brain)	myring	eardrum, tympanic membrane
encephal	brain	neur	nerve
esthesi	sensation	ocul, ophthalm	eye
irid, ir	iris	ot	ear

Other common word roots

Here is a list of some of the word roots that apply in general clinical practice and/or across multiple body systems.

2.14 Root words in use

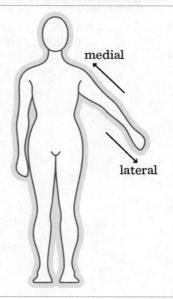

2.15 Other common word roots

WORD ROOT	MEANING	WORD ROOT	MEANING
adip	fat	lith	stone
bi	life	med, medi	middle
carcin	cancer	narc	numbness, stupor, sleep
cry	cold	necr	death
dors	back portion of body	onc	*tumor*
gluc, glyc	sugar	path	disease
herni	hernia	ped	child, foot
hist	tissue	psych	mind
hydr	water	py	pus
lact	milk	pyr	fever, heat
later	side	septic	infection
lip	fat	therm	heat

tumor. An abnormal mass of tissue that grows as a result of excessive cell division, either cancerous (malignant) or noncancerous (benign)

Combining forms

A combining form is a word root with a combining vowel. Often, the combining vowel makes the medical term easier to pronounce. In most cases, the combining vowel is an "o," but it is sometimes "i" or "e." A combining form should be used when the last word root in a medical term connects with a suffix that begins with a consonant. When the word root connects with a suffix that starts with a vowel, just the word root should be used. Refer to the examples below.

2.16 Word roots and combining forms

WORD ROOT	COMBINING VOWEL	COMBINING FORM	SUFFIX	MEDICAL TERM
col	o	col/o	-stomy	colostomy
cephal	o	cephal/o	-algia	cephalalgia
col	o	col/o	-ectomy	colectomy
cephal	o	cephal/o	-dynia	cephalodynia

Notice that when the suffix begins with a vowel, the word root is used. Examples include "cephalalgia" and "colectomy." However, when the suffix begins with a consonant, the combining form is used, as in "colostomy" and "cephalodynia." When connecting two word roots, always use the connecting vowel, even if the following word root begins with a vowel.

Common prefixes

Prefixes are word components that appear at the beginning of a word to change the meaning of the rest of the word. They generally mean the same thing in each word they modify. Some medical terms have no prefix. An example is splenectomy, a combination of the word root "splen," meaning spleen, and the suffix "ectomy," meaning removal. Here is a list of some of the common prefixes medical assistants will encounter.

2.17 Prefixes in use

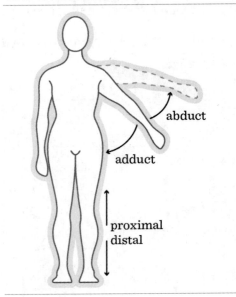

abduct

adduct

proximal
distal

2.18 Common prefixes

PREFIX	MEANING	PREFIX	MEANING
a-, an-	without	mega-	exceptionally large
ab-	away, from	meso-	middle
ad-	toward	meta-	over, beyond
ambi-	both	micro-	small
ante-	before	mono-	one
anti-	against	multi-	many
auto-	self	neo-	new
bi-	two, twice, double	nulli-	none
brady-	slow	peri-	around
circum-	around	poly-	many
contra-	against	post-	after, behind
de-	down	pre-, pro-	before, in front of
dys-	painful, abnormal, difficult, bad	presby-	older age
endo-	within, inside	primi-	first
epi-	above, on	pseudo-	false
eu-	normal, good	quadri-	four
ex, extra-, exo-	outside of	retro-	behind, in back of
hemi-	half	sten-	narrowed
hyper-	above, excessive, increased	sub-	under
hypo-	below, decreased, insufficient	super-, supra-	above, excess
infra-	beneath	sym-, syn-	together, with
inter-	between, among	tachy-	fast
intra-	within, during	trans-	across
levo-	to the left	tri-	three
macro-	large	ultra-	beyond, excess
mal-	bad	uni-	one

Common suffixes

Suffixes are word components that appear at the end of the word to change the meaning of the rest of the word. Some medical terms have no suffix, such as appendix. Some medical terms combine a prefix and a suffix with no word root. An example is hemiplegia, a combination of the prefix "hemi," meaning half, and the suffix "plegia," meaning *paralysis*. Here is a list of some of the common general suffixes medical assistants will encounter, as well as some that are more specific to clinical disorders and medical, surgical, and diagnostic procedures.

2.19 Suffixes in use

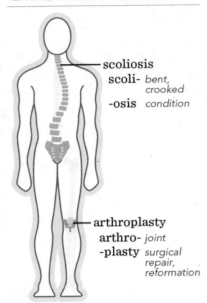

scoliosis
scoli- *bent, crooked*
-osis *condition*

arthroplasty
arthro- *joint*
-plasty *surgical repair, reformation*

2.20 Common suffixes: General

SUFFIX	MEANING	SUFFIX	MEANING
-age	related to	-logy, -logist	study of, one who studies
-cidal, -cide	pertaining to killing	-ole	little, small
-form	shape	-opia	vision
-fuge	driving away	-phylaxis	protection, prevention
-iatry, -iatrist	healing by a provider, healer		
-ical	pertaining to	-pnea	breathing
-ion	process	-therapy	treatment
		-uria	urine

2.21 Common suffixes: Surgery, procedures

SUFFIX	MEANING	SUFFIX	MEANING
-centesis	surgical puncture	-meter	device for measuring
-cise	cut, remove	-metry	process of measuring
-clasis	break down	-pexy	*fixation*, to put in place
-desis	stabilization, binding	-plasty	surgical repair, reformation
-ectomy	removal, excision	-scopy	visual examination
-gram	record	-spasm	involuntary twitch, contraction
-graph	instrument for recording	-stasis	stopping or controlling
-graphy	process of recording	-stomy	a new opening
-ion	process	-tomy	incision
-lepsy	seizure, convulsion	-tripsy	crushing
-lysis	destruction, separation		

paralysis. A loss of muscle movement due to nerve damage

fixation. The process of making bone immobile so it can heal

2.22 Common suffixes: Disorders, conditions

SUFFIX	MEANING	SUFFIX	MEANING
-algia	pain	-oma	tumor
-asthenia	weakness	-osis	condition, usually abnormal
-cele	swelling, *herniation*	-pathy	disorder, disease
-dynia	pain	-penia	deficiency, decrease
-ectasis	dilation expansion	-phagia	eating, swallowing
-emesis	vomiting	-phasia	speech
-emia	blood condition	-phobia	fear
-gen	producing	-plasia	formation of
-ia, -ism	condition	-plegia	paralysis
-iasis	presence of, formation of	-ptosis	drooping, falling
-itis	inflammation	-rrhage	bursting forth
-malacia	weakening of, softening of	-rrhea	flow, discharge
-mania	obsessive preoccupation	-rrhexis	rupture
-megaly	enlargement	-sclerosis	hardening condition
-oid	seeming like	-trophy	development
-ole	small		

herniation. The protrusion of a loop or portion of an organ or tissue through an abnormal opening

GAME Build the medical term

Choose one prefix, root, and suffix from the choices below to build the medical term for each of the following definitions. Remember that some medical terms require a connecting vowel between word parts.

1. The disorder that results from an excessive secretion of hormones from the gland that regulates metabolism. ____ _____ ___

2. The disorder that involves having stones in the gall bladder. ____ _____ ___

3. A medical provider who administers sedation for surgical procedures. ____ _____ ___

PREFIX		ROOT		SUFFIX	
an-	de-	thym	psych	-iasis	-ism
fore-	colo-	pyr	colp	-tomy	-logist
contra-	chole-	neur	lip	-therapist	-ia
pre-	hypo-	cerebr	thyroid	-ical	-iatrist
hyper-	anti-	cephal	esthesi	-desis	-age
cyst-	eu-	lith	enter	-osis	-sclerosis

Key: 1. hyperthyroidism; 2. cholelithiasis; 3. anesthesiologist

Rules for changing from singular to plural

Many medical terms are simply English words that follow standard rules for plural endings. Some just require adding an "s" to the end of the word. Examples are adhesions, lymphocytes, and *lacerations*. Others that end in "s" or "ch" require adding "es" to the end of the word. Examples are neuroses, viruses, and crutches. For nouns that end in "y" with a consonant in front of the "y," change the "y" to "i" and add "es." Examples are *colostomies*, ovaries, and arteries.

Many medical terms have their origins in other languages, often Latin, so they require a different approach. If they end in "a," just add an "e" to the end to make it plural. Examples are *conjunctivae*, vertebrae, and axillae. For words that end in "um," change the "um" to "a," like in bacteria, *diverticula*, and ova. If the words end in "is," change the "is" to "es." For example, *metastases*, diagnoses, and testes. When words end in "us," change the "us" to "i." Examples are fungi, *villi*, and alveoli. Words that end in "on" are made plural by changing the "on" to "a." For instance, *ganglia*, protozoa, and spermatozoa. Finally, for words that end in "ix" or "ex," change the "ix" or "ex" to "ices," as is the case with appendices, cortices, and *cicatrices*.

Keep in mind that there are exceptions to all these rules. Also, there are collective nouns that don't require singular and plural forms. Body fluids are good examples: blood, urine, saliva, and semen. Many conditions and disorders do not have a plural form: acne, pneumonia, and *hepatitis*.

---

laceration. A cut; a torn wound

colostomy. A surgical procedure in which an opening (stoma) is formed in the large intestine or colon through an incision in the anterior abdominal wall, which will allow stool to pass out of the body

conjunctiva. The delicate membrane that lines the eyelids and covers the external surface of the sclerae (the whites of the eyes)

diverticula. One of multiple pouches that can form in the walls of the large intestine

metastasis. The spread of disease, usually cancer, to body sites other than where the tumor originated

villus. One of many folds in the intestines

ganglion. A collection of nerve cell bodies in a place other than the central nervous system

cicatrix. A scar of a healed wound

hepatitis. Inflammation or infection of the liver

POSITIONAL AND DIRECTIONAL TERMS

Medical assistants also need a working knowledge of the medical terms that indicate directions and positions. For example, for various types of examinations and diagnostic procedures, they not only have to position patients correctly or optimally, but they also have to document how they positioned them and how the patients tolerated the positions that might be uncomfortable.

Here is a list of prefixes medical assistants can use to help understand directional terms, as well as a list of terms that are essential for positioning.

2.23 Directional prefixes

PREFIX	MEANING	PREFIX	MEANING
ab-	away from	intra-	inside
ad-	toward	ipsi-	same, equal
circum-	around	meso-	middle
contra-	against, in opposition to	meta-	after, beyond, over
de-	away from, down	para-	near, beside
ecto-, exo-	outside	peri-	surrounding, around
endo-	within	retro-	backward, behind
epi-	over, upon	sub-	under, near
extra-	outside	trans-	across, through
infra-	below, under		

2.24 Positional and directional terms

TERM	MEANING	TERM	MEANING
anterior	front	external	outside
bilateral	pertaining to both sides	flexion	bending a limb or body part at the joint
caudal	tail (coccygeal area)		
cephalic	head	Fowler's	raising the head of the bed up to 90 degrees
dextro	right		
distal	farther away from	inferior	below or directed downward
dorsal recumbent	lying on the back with knees up and feet flat on the table	internal	inside
		knee-chest, knee-elbow	drawing the knees up to the chest
eversion	turning outward or inside out	lateral	side, away from the middle
extension	bringing a limb to a straight position	lithotomy	on the back, flexing the legs on *abducted* thighs

abduct. Move away from the midline of the body

2.24 Positional and directional terms *continued*

TERM	MEANING	TERM	MEANING
medial	midline	recumbent	lying down
oblique	slanting, on an incline	rotation	turning around an axis
peripheral	outside the central area	Sims'	lateral with one knee and thigh up
posterior	back		
prone	lying on the abdomen	sinistro	left
proximal	toward the center or point of attachment	superior	above or directed upward
		supine	lying on the back
quadrant	dividing an area horizontally and vertically into four parts	Trendelenburg	lying with the head lower than the legs

Here are some of the common positions for patients undergoing physical examinations.

2.25 Positions for physical examinations

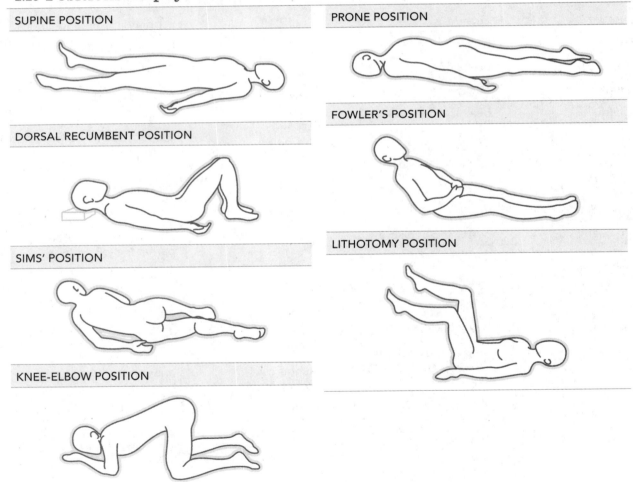

SUPINE POSITION

PRONE POSITION

DORSAL RECUMBENT POSITION

FOWLER'S POSITION

SIMS' POSITION

LITHOTOMY POSITION

KNEE-ELBOW POSITION

SUMMARY

Medical terminology is quite extensive and challenges medical assistants to develop fluency. This includes abbreviations, word components, and the terms themselves. With experience and a handy reference book, medical assistants will soon speak the language of medical professionals. Depending on the practice setting, the same core of terms will recur and become familiar quickly. With a little curiosity and a lot of initiative, mastery will soon follow.

CHAPTER 3
Basic Pharmacology

OVERVIEW

Pharmacology is the study of medications: how they act on the body (both good and bad), as well as their classifications and various properties. To assist patients with getting and understanding what they need to know about the medications they take, medical assistants need to know the basics of pharmacology as well as how to administer medications safely and effectively. This chapter introduces common medications and classifications, indications, contraindications, how to calculate dosages, administration routes, rights of medication administration, terminology and abbreviations in pharmacology in practice, and how to find out more about medications most often encountered in daily practice. Reading and interpreting medication prescriptions and metric conversions will also be covered.

COMMON MEDICATIONS AND ABBREVIATIONS

Thousands of medications are available for providers to prescribe, so it might seem overwhelming to learn about all of them. However, medical assistants tend to encounter the same commonly prescribed medications over and over. A working knowledge of those medications and the various common medication classifications will provide the knowledge and confidence needed to assist patients with medication therapy. For example, it is not necessary to know everything about every *antibiotic*, but a working knowledge of antibiotics in general is useful in encounters with patients who have bacterial infections.

Objectives

After completing this chapter, you should be able to:

- List 25 of the most commonly prescribed medications and their classifications.
- Recognize and use common pharmacological abbreviations in written or electronic communications.
- Describe medication classifications and their uses.
- Recognize and describe the five different medication schedules and the types of medications in each schedule.
- Describe common uses for medications, including therapeutic, diagnostic, curative, replacement, and prophylactic.
- Describe and differentiate between a side effect and an adverse effect.
- Define medication indication and contraindication.
- Convert within and between common systems of measurements (e.g., metric, household).
- Calculate adult and pediatric medication dosages.
- Describe different forms of medications.
- List a protocol for properly identifying medications that look alike and sound alike.
- List the routes of medication administration, their locations, and types of medications given by each route.
- Describe the four processes of pharmacokinetics.
- List the rights of medication administration.
- Properly use the *Physicians' Desk Reference* and online sources, and identify other resources available for referencing medications.

antibiotic. A medication that kills bacteria and thus treats bacterial infections

Commonly prescribed medications

Medication therapy changes often enough to make it essential to consult reference materials and websites often. New medications become available all the time, and medications go *off the market* often enough that it's helpful to make a habit of checking websites like drugs.com, rxlist.com, pdr.net, and fda.gov for the latest information. The U.S. Food and Drug Administration provides black box warnings that prominently state potential new and life-threatening risks of taking a specific medication. It is useful to subscribe to websites that send information about changes in medication therapy, such as medscape.com or webmd.com. Checking fda.gov can also provide the latest information about black box warnings.

The medications prescribed most often are a good place to start. Multiple websites list the top medications by sales, but this doesn't reflect common practice. That is because some *brand-name* medications do not have *generic forms* and are extremely expensive, so they might be on top, even if providers don't prescribe them as often as some other generic medications. These lists can still give a good idea of the most common medications. (Because there are multiple brand names for medications, these materials will only cover generic names. Medical assistants should be familiar with both.)

3.1 Commonly prescribed medications

GENERIC MEDICATION NAME: CLASSIFICATION	
albuterol: bronchodilator	esomeprazole: anti-ulcer agent, *proton-pump inhibitor*
amlodipine besylate: antihypertensive, *calcium channel blocker*	fenofibrate: antilipemic
amoxicillin: antibiotic	fluticasone/salmeterol: antiasthma, *glucocorticoid*, bronchodilator
aripiprazole: antipsychotic	furosemide: diuretic
atorvastatin: antilipemic, statin	gabapentin: anticonvulsant
azithromycin: antibiotic	hydrochlorothiazide: diuretic
celecoxib: anti-inflammatory	hydrocodone plus acetaminophen: opioid (narcotic) analgesic
cephalexin: antibiotic	
ciprofloxacin: antibiotic	insulin: hypoglycemic
clopidogrel: *antiplatelet* agent	levofloxacin: antibiotic
donepezil: anti-Alzheimer's	levothyroxine: thyroid hormone
duloxetine: antidepressant	lisinopril: antihypertensive, *ACE inhibitor*
enoxaparin: anticoagulant	losartan: antihypertensive
escitalopram: antidepressant	memantine: anti-Alzheimer's

off the market. No longer available for purchase or use

brand/trade name. Assigned by the medication's manufacturer, identifies the medication as the property of the company, begins with a capital letter

generic name. A noncommercial name for a medication, usually less complex than the medication's chemical name and often more complex than a brand or trade name

calcium channel blocker. A medication that prevents the entry of calcium ions into the cells of the body, which can lower blood pressure and treat cardiac pain and dysfunction

antiplatelet. A medication that helps delay blood clotting. This medication differs from an anticoagulant because it affects arterial as well as venous blood.

proton-pump inhibitor. A specific type of medication that reduces stomach acid

glucocorticoid. One of several hormones that have many functions, both naturally in the body and as a medication, including suppression of inflammation

ACE inhibitor. Angiotensin-converting enzyme inhibitor, a type of antihypertensive (blood pressure lowering) medication

3.1 Commonly prescribed medications *continued*

GENERIC MEDICATION NAME: CLASSIFICATION	
metformin: hypoglycemic	prednisone: glucocorticoid
methylphenidate: central nervous system stimulant	pregabalin: anticonvulsant
metoprolol succinate: antihypertensive, *beta blocker*	quetiapine: antipsychotic
	rosuvastatin: antilipemic, statin
metoprolol tartrate: antihypertensive, beta blocker	sildenafil: erectile dysfunction agent
montelukast: bronchodilator, *leukotriene inhibitor*	simvastatin: antilipemic, statin
olanzapine: antipsychotic	sulfamethoxazole/trimethoprim: antibiotic
omeprazole: anti-ulcer agent, proton-pump inhibitor	tramadol: analgesic
oxycodone: opioid (narcotic) analgesic	valsartan: antihypertensive
pioglitazone: hypoglycemic	warfarin: anticoagulant
pravastatin: antilipemic, statin	zolpidem: sedative-hypnotic (for sleep)

Commonly approved pharmacological abbreviations

Medical assistants see many pharmacological abbreviations daily. The Joint Commission and the Institute for Safe Medication Practices have identified some as "do not use" and "error-prone abbreviations." Avoiding these abbreviations is essential. For the full lists, see the Joint Commission and the Institute for Safe Medication Practices websites. The following abbreviations are acceptable.

3.2 Dosage forms

ABBREVIATION: MEANING				
amp: *ampule*	cr: cream	liq: liquid	sup: *suppository*	tab: tablet
cap: capsule	elix: elixir	lot: lotion	syr: *syrup*	ung: ointment

3.3 Strength and systems of measurement

ABBREVIATION: MEANING		
C: cup, Celsius	L: liter	oz: ounce
ds: double strength	lb: pound	qt: quart
g, gm: gram	mcg: microgram	tbsp: tablespoon
gr: grain	mEq: milliequivalent	tsp: teaspoon
gtt: drop	mg: milligram(s)	
kg: kilogram	mg/dL: milligrams per deciliter	

beta blocker. A medication that, by interfering with specific receptor sites in the heart, can help lower heart rate and blood pressure and treat many other cardiovascular disorders

leukotriene inhibitor. A specific type of medication that treats asthma by relaxing tight or constricted airways and inflammation in the airways

ampule. A small, sealed, single-use glass or plastic container containing sterile parenteral medications or solutions

suppository. A small, solid, cylinder-shaped medication for insertion into the rectum or vagina; solid at room temperature, dissolves at body temperature

syrup. A concentrated solution of sugar in water with a flavoring, sometimes with a medication in it

3.4 Route of administration

ABBREVIATION: MEANING		
ID: intradermally	IV: intravenously	r, rec: rectally
IM: intramuscularly	PO: by mouth, orally	subcut: subcutaneously
inj: inject, injection	PR: rectally	top: topically

3.5 Time or frequency of administration

ABBREVIATION: MEANING		
a: before	d: daily, day	q: every
ac: before meals	h, hr: hour	qam: every morning
ad lib: as desired	noct: night	q4h: every 4 hours
AM: morning	pc: after meals	qid: four times per day
bid: twice a day	PM: evening, nighttime	stat: immediately
c̄: with	PRN: whenever necessary	ut dict: as directed

3.6 Other abbreviations

ABBREVIATION: MEANING		
Agit: shake, stir	K: *potassium*	qs: sufficient amount
aq: water	MDI: *metered-dose inhaler*	rept: repeat
ASA: aspirin	med: medicine	rf: refill(s)
cmpd: *compound*	MO: mineral oil	rx: prescription, treatment
DAW: dispense as written	neb: *nebulizer*	s̄: without
dil: dilute	NKA: no known allergies	sig: write on the label
disp: dispense	NPO: nothing by mouth (*nil per os*)	susp: *suspension*
eq: equivalent	N/V: nausea/vomiting	sx: symptoms
ext: *extract*	nr: no refills	tinc: *tincture*
Fe: iron	OTC: *over-the-counter*	TO: telephone order
gen: generic	O$_2$: oxygen	tx: treatment
H$_2$O: water	per: by means of, through	VO: verbal order

compound. Combination of atoms of an element; pharmacologically, it refers to a mixture of medications or a medication with a specific base

extract. A concentrated combination of vegetable products and alcohol

potassium. A mineral that controls fluid volume, muscle and cardiac activity, and other bodily functions

metered-dose inhaler. A medication-delivery device that disperses the medication as an aerosol spray, mist, or powder into the airways via inhalation

nebulizer. A device for creating and delivering an aerosol spray for inhalation

over-the-counter. Available for purchase without a prescription

suspension. A liquid preparation consisting of solid particles dispersed throughout a liquid in which they are not soluble

tincture. A medicinal preparation in an alcohol base, sometimes for oral and sometimes for topical use

MEDICATION CLASSIFICATIONS AND SCHEDULES

A working knowledge of medication classifications and schedules is essential when assisting providers and helping patients understand what their medications should do. Learn the risks the federal government has identified with some medications and why it has limited their prescribing and dispensing patterns. The U.S. Drug Enforcement Administration (DEA) has designated some medications as controlled substances assigned to five schedules. These are primarily medications that have a potential for abuse and illicit use or do not have any approved medical use in the United States. The schedules change as new medications become available and the DEA determines that a medication already on the schedule has more or less potential for abuse. Prescribing rules also change. For some schedules, providers must issue handwritten prescriptions, but that might change as exclusively electronic prescribing (e-prescribing) becomes standard practice.

GAME Abbreviations

Match the abbreviation with its meaning.

ABBREVIATIONS	MEANINGS
1. ac	A. whenever necessary
2. gtt	B. immediately
3. NPO	C. after meals
4. stat	D. write on the label
5. PRN	E. drop
6. pc	F. every
7. q	G. twice a day
8. bid	H. nothing by mouth
9. qs	I. before meals
10. sig	J. sufficient amount

Key: 1. I; 2. E; 3. H; 4. B; 5. A; 6. C; 7. F; 8. G; 9. J; 10. D

Medication classifications and their uses

The classification of medications is complex. Primarily, a medication's therapeutic action dictates the classification, but sometimes it is done by chemical formulations, body systems they act on, or symptoms the medication relieves. Some medications fall into more than one category. Gabapentin and pregabalin are good examples. Both medications are anticonvulsants; they treat seizures. However, they are also analgesics, because they help relieve neuropathic (nerve) pain. Another example is hydrochlorothiazide, a diuretic—it helps eliminate excess fluid from the body. However, in doing so, it can help lower blood pressure; thus it is also an antihypertensive medication. Here are some of the most common classification of medications medical assistants are likely to encounter.

3.7 Medication classifications and their uses

MEDICATION CLASSIFICATION	ACTION	EXAMPLES
analgesics	relieve pain	acetaminophen, hydrocodone
antacids/anti-ulcer	neutralize stomach acid	esomeprazole, calcium carbonate
antibiotics	kill bacteria	amoxicillin, ciprofloxacin
anticholinergics	reduce *bronchospasm*	ipratropium, dicyclomine
anticoagulants	delay blood clotting	warfarin, enoxaparin, heparin
anticonvulsants	prevent or control seizures	clonazepam, phenytoin, gabapentin
antidepressants	relieve depression	doxepin, fluoxetine, duloxetine, selegiline
antidiarrheals	reduce diarrhea	bismuth subsalicylate, loperamide
antiemetics	reduce nausea, vomiting	metoclopramide, ondansetron

bronchospasm. Narrowing or constriction of the airways that interferes with breathing

3.7 Medication classifications and their uses *continued*

MEDICATION CLASSIFICATION	ACTION	EXAMPLES
antifungals	kill fungi	fluconazole, nystatin, miconazole
antihistamines	relieve allergies	diphenhydramine, cetirizine, loratadine
antihypertensives	lower blood pressure	metoprolol, lisinopril, valsartan, clonidine
anti-inflammatories	reduce inflammation	ibuprofen, celecoxib, naproxen
antilipemics	lower cholesterol	atorvastatin, fenofibrate
antimigraine agents	relieve migraine headaches	topiramate, sumatriptan
anti-osteoporosis agents	improve bone density	alendronate, ibandronate, calcitonin
antipsychotics	control psychotic symptoms	quetiapine, haloperidol, risperidone
antipyretics	reduce fever	acetaminophen, ibuprofen, aspirin
antispasmodics/ muscle relaxants	reduce or prevent muscle spasms	cyclobenzaprine, methocarbamol
antitussives/expectorants	control cough, promote elimination of mucus	dextromethorphan, codeine, guaifenesin
antivirals	kill viruses	acyclovir, interferon, oseltamivir
anxiolytics (antianxiety)	reduce anxiety	clonazepam, diazepam, lorazepam
bronchodilators	relax airway muscles	albuterol, isoproterenol, theophylline
central nervous system stimulants	reduce hyperactivity	methylphenidate, modafinil
contraceptives	prevent pregnancy	medroxyprogesterone acetate, ethinyl estradiol
decongestants	relieve nasal congestion	pseudoephedrine, mometasone
diuretics	eliminate excess fluid	furosemide, hydrochlorothiazide
hormone replacement	stabilize hormone deficiencies	levothyroxine, insulin, desmopressin, estrogen
laxatives, stool softeners	promote bowel movements	magnesium hydroxide, bisacodyl
oral hypoglycemics	reduce blood glucose	metformin, acarbose, glyburide
sedative-hypnotics	induce sleep/relaxation	zolpidem, temazepam, eszopiclone

Medication schedules

The federal Controlled Substances Act (CSA) created five schedules for controlled substances, according to their potential for abuse and addiction. Only controlled substances are scheduled.

Schedule I includes substances that have a high potential for abuse and no approved medical use in the United States. They are illegal, and providers may not prescribe them. These include heroin, mescaline, and lysergic acid diethylamide (LSD). Schedule I still includes cannabis (marijuana) even though it is legal in many states for medical use with a prescription.

GAME Medication classifications

Match the medication with the correct classification.

CLASSIFICATIONS	MEDICATIONS
1. diuretic	A. acetaminophen
2. antilipemic	B. lisinopril
3. analgesic	C. zolpidem
4. sedative-hypnotic	D. metformin
5. hypoglycemic	E. gabapentin
6. decongestant	F. diphenhydramine
7. antihypertensive	G. furosemide
8. antibiotic	H. pseudoephedrine
9. anticonvulsant	I. atorvastatin
10. antihistamine	J. ciprofloxacin

Key: 1. G; 2. I; 3. A; 4. C; 5. D; 6. H; 7. B; 8. J; 9. E; 10. F

Schedule II includes substances that have a high potential for abuse, are considered dangerous, and can lead to psychological and physical *dependence*. These include morphine, methadone, oxycodone, hydromorphone, hydrocodone, fentanyl, and methamphetamine. Providers must give patients a handwritten prescription with no refills (some states now allow schedule II to be prescribed via e-prescription). In health care facilities, staff members must keep these in a secure, locked cabinet or storage area separate from other medications.

Schedule III includes substances that have a moderate to low potential for physical and psychological dependence. These include ketamine, anabolic steroids, and testosterone. Prescriptions can be refilled up to five times within 6 months.

Schedule IV includes substances that have a low potential for abuse and dependence. These include diazepam, zolpidem, eszopiclone, alprazolam, chlordiazepoxide, and clonazepam. Providers must sign prescriptions for these substances, and patients may refill them five times in 6 months. Staff members may authorize refills over the phone.

Schedule V includes substances that contain limited quantities of some narcotics, usually for antidiarrheal, antitussive, and analgesic purposes. These include diphenoxylate with atropine, pregabalin, lacosamide, and opium/kaolin/pectin/belladonna. Providers must sign prescriptions for these substances, and patients may refill them five times in 6 months. Staff members may authorize refills over the phone.

For a current alphabetical list of all controlled substances and their CSA schedule number, go to the resources section of the Office of Diversion Control website.

dependence. Caused by repeated use of a medication and will result in withdrawal symptoms when the medication is discontinued

THERAPEUTIC EFFECTS, ADVERSE EFFECTS, INDICATIONS, AND CONTRAINDICATIONS

Medications have good and bad effects. The good effects—the ones providers prescribe them for—are known as the therapeutic effects. Side effects are undesirable unintended actions on the body, such as nausea or dry mouth, and can limit the usefulness of the medication. An adverse event is an unintended, harmful action of the medication, such as an *allergic reaction*, and prevents further use of the medications. Indications are the problems the provider prescribes a particular medication for. A contraindication is a symptom or condition that makes a particular treatment or medication inadvisable or even dangerous. In addition, precautions are problems that pose a lesser risk but require close observation and monitoring during medication therapy.

Common therapeutic effects, adverse effects, and allergic reactions

Therapeutic effects of medications tie very closely to their indications. An indication for an antihypertensive medication, for example, is high blood pressure. The provider might try to use conservative measures for lowering blood pressure, such as lifestyle changes (e.g., dietary salt reduction, moderate exercise, weight loss). If those measures do not work or the patient does not adhere to them, the provider might prescribe an antihypertensive medication, such as lisinopril.

The expected therapeutic effect of lisinopril is a sustained reduction in blood pressure. Unfortunately, lisinopril can cause many undesirable effects—some of them life-threatening. It is critical for medical assistants to review with a patient who is beginning medication therapy what side effects are the most common and which are serious enough to report to the provider immediately. With lisinopril, the patient might develop nausea, dizziness, or nasal congestion. These are common side effects and are likely to subside with time. However, if the patient develops swelling of the lips, face, and tongue, immediate medical care is imperative. These could potentially indicate a fatal reaction to the medication.

With lisinopril, facial swelling is a rare effect due to the accumulation of a substance in the body that mimics anaphylaxis (a serious allergic reaction). Most medications have the potential for causing an allergic reaction. Mild allergic reactions usually manifest as itchy rashes. Serious allergic reactions involve spasms of the airways, swelling of the face and throat, and serious decrease in blood pressure. The patient's allergy history can offer some clues to the possibility of an allergic reaction. For example, if a patient has had a previous serious allergic reaction to eggs, he could have a serious allergic reaction to the flu vaccine. Because allergic reactions can be life-threatening, it is important to advise all patients about seeking medical care immediately if they develop symptoms. An antihistamine, such as diphenhydramine, can help relieve a minor allergic reaction and is available over the counter. For a serious or anaphylactic reaction, the patient needs epinephrine and medical attention. Medication allergies should be discussed, reviewed, and updated at every visit. They should be confirmed any time a prescription is written and prior to medication administration.

allergic reaction. A hypersensitivity response to a medication, food, or other substance, ranging in intensity from mild itching to severe rash to anaphylaxis

Many people use side effects and adverse effects interchangeably, but there is a difference. Side effects develop predictably and nearly unavoidably, but aren't necessarily harmful. For example, a patient who takes diphenhydramine, an antihistamine, to relieve an itchy rash at bedtime sleeps better that night. Why? Because a side effect of diphenhydramine is *sedation* and sleepiness. So advise caution when taking this medication prior to driving or operating machinery.

For examples of medication indications, refer to the table of common medication classifications. Their actions apply to the common reasons for use, including pain, infection, muscle spasms, migraine headaches, anxiety, depression, or *insomnia*. Common potential adverse effects include gastrointestinal problems (e.g., nausea, vomiting, diarrhea, constipation). It helps some patients to take medications with food to minimize these effects. Furthermore, if stomach irritation is the problem, taking a formulation with an *enteric coating* can help minimize the negative effects on the stomach. Also common are central nervous system effects (e.g., dizziness, headache, sedation, insomnia). Many medications cause changes in heart rate, blood pressure, vision, and hearing.

Indications and contraindications for medication use

The most common contraindication is hypersensitivity (a previous allergic reaction) to that medication. Other frequent contraindications include damage to or malfunction of a body system. For example, cirrhosis of the liver is a contraindication for taking acarbose, and hepatitis is a contraindication for taking duloxetine. Many other medications are toxic to the liver and require extreme caution with patients who have liver disease. These include acetaminophen, phenytoin, fluconazole, bupropion, penicillin, erythromycin, rifampin, ritonavir, lisinopril, and losartan.

Another important consideration is how a medication interacts with food or other medications. It is easy to confuse contraindications with interactions. For example, medications that are in the classification of a specific type of antidepressant, monoamine oxidase inhibitors (MAOIs), interact dangerously with foods that contain *tyramine* (e.g., avocados, smoked meats, wine, most cheeses). MAOIs also interact adversely with other types of antidepressants, such as tricyclic antidepressants. Both of these interactions result in a hypertensive crisis. Examples of MAOIs are phenelzine, isocarboxazid, and tranylcypromine.

Grapefruit juice interacts with many medications, interfering with their metabolism, raising the levels of the medications, and producing *toxicity*. These medications include dextromethorphan, simvastatin, and sildenafil. Additionally, some herbal supplements interact with prescription medications. St. John's wort reduces the effectiveness of warfarin and oral contraceptives.

Even more common are the many medications that interact with other medications. For example, if patients take propranolol with albuterol, both medications lose their effectiveness. Aspirin and warfarin both have anticoagulant effects, so taking both puts patients at risk for hemorrhage (major bleeding). Many antibiotics—including ampicillin, sulfamethoxazole-trimethoprim, minocycline, and metronidazole—reduce the effectiveness of oral contraceptives.

sedation. A calm or sleepy state that results from taking a medication

insomnia. Difficulty falling asleep or staying asleep

enteric-coated. Containing an outer shell that prevents an oral tablet from dissolving until it reaches the intestines, often to prevent stomach irritation

tyramine. A substance in some foods and beverages, such as cheese and wine, that can have a life-threatening interaction with a specific type of antidepressant

toxicity. An adverse medication reaction resulting from excessive dosing

MEASUREMENTS, MATHEMATICAL CONVERSIONS, AND DOSAGE CALCULATIONS

Understanding systems of measurement and knowing how to calculate and verify medication dosages are essential skills for medical assistants. How often and what kinds of medications medical assistants will administer varies by practice setting, but these principles will help in discussions with patients about taking their medications at home. Patients might find measuring medications—especially liquid oral and injectable ones—challenging and might need some assistance.

Metric system

Most medication prescriptions and dosages will be in the metric system of weights and volume. However, there are still some medication formulations in the apothecary and household systems that require conversions. Also, some prescriptions require dosage calculations based on a patient's weight in kilograms, especially for pediatric doses. So, medical assistants need a working knowledge of conversions and calculations.

Units of the metric system

The metric system quantifies weight in kilograms (kg), grams (g), milligrams (mg), and micrograms (mcg). It measures volume in deciliters (dL), liters (L), and milliliters (mL). Length is in kilometers (km), meters (m), centimeters (cm), and millimeters (mm). There are other metric values, but these are the ones most likely to be seen and used in practice.

Prescriptions do not usually include length measurements, but there are exceptions. For example, the amount of nitroglycerin ointment to squeeze onto the application paper is a length measurement. It might be a half inch, but that the patient or provider might the metric equivalent of 1.25 cm. Metric lengths are common in other clinical applications (e.g., measurements of wounds, distances to use in procedures).

The equivalency tables show the relationship various metric measurements have to each other.

3.8 Units of the metric system

UNIT	RELATIONSHIP TO BASE UNIT	DECIMAL VALUE/WHOLE NUMBER
micro-	÷ 1,000,000	0.000001
milli-	÷ 1,000	0.0001
centi-	÷ 100	0.01
base unit	1	1
kilo-	× 1,000	1,000

So for example, 1 gram = 1,000 mg and 1 mg = 1,000 mcg.

Apothecary measurements

It is very rare that medical assistants will encounter apothecary system measurements. They include weight measurements of grains and volume measurements in minims and drams. This system also includes household measurements of ounces, pints, and quarts. It is helpful to know that 15 grains = 1,000 mg, 1 minim = 1 drop, and 1 dram = 60 minims.

Household measurements

Household measurements of medications are still common, especially for liquid oral medications taken at home. Many liquid medications come with measuring cups that have household and metric equivalents marked. Still, patients could misplace the cups and ask about using a teaspoon or tablespoon to measure the dosage. The table shows the most common equivalents for liquids and weight in this system.

3.9 Household measurements

HOUSEHOLD VALUE	APOTHECARY VALUE	METRIC EQUIVALENT
15 drops (gtt)	15 to 16 minims	1 mL
1 teaspoon (tsp)	1 dram	5 mL
1 tablespoon (tbsp)	4 drams	15 mL
1 fluid ounce (oz), 2 tbsp	8 drams, 1 oz	30 mL
1 cup	8 oz	240 mL
1 pint	1 pint	480 mL (about 500 mL)
1 quart	1 quart	960 mL (about 1 L)
1 gallon	1 gallon	3,830 mL (about 1 gallon)
2.2 pounds (lb)	2.2 lb	1 kilogram (kg)

Mathematical conversions

There are several methods for converting one measurement to another within or between measurement systems. Within systems, simple arithmetic is usually sufficient. For example, if a provider prescribes 0.088 mg levothyroxine and the medication comes in mcg, the conversion is simple. There is a three–decimal–point difference between mg and mcg. Because the conversion is from a larger value (mg) to a smaller value, the decimal point moves three places to the right.

$0.088 \times 1,000 = 88$ mcg

The proportion method works well for other conversions between systems. This involves thinking of the conversion like this: if 2.2 lb equals 1 kg, then the number of pounds to convert 66 lb equals how many (X) kg? Another way to accomplish this calculation is to divide the weight in pounds by 2.2 (because 1 kg = 2.2 lb).

If a patient weighs 66 lb, how many (X) kilograms is this?

1 kg = 2.2 lb, therefore $\dfrac{66\ lb}{2.2\ lb} = \dfrac{66}{2.2} = 30$ kg

Or:

$\dfrac{2.2\ lb}{1\ kg} = \dfrac{66\ lb}{X\ kg}$

Cross-multiply and you should get the following.

$1 \times 66 = 2.2X$

$66 = 2.2X$

Then divide both sides of the equation by 2.2, and the result is 30 kg.

Here is another example.

The dosage of a medication is 15 mL, but the patient wants to measure it in teaspoons. If 5 mL equals 1 tsp, then 15 mL equals how many (X) tsp?

$\dfrac{5\ mL}{1\ tsp} = \dfrac{15\ mL}{X\ tsp}$

Cross-multiply and you should get the following.

$1 \times 15 = 5X$

$15 = 5X$

Then divide both sides of the equation by 5, and the result is 3 tsp.

Adult dosage calculations

With all dosage calculations, medical assistants should always take their time and recheck their calculations. If there is any doubt at all, ask the provider or another medical assistant to check calculations. The patient's well-being depends on accuracy in all calculations.

For calculating adult dosages, the proportion method works well. For example, a provider prescribes diphenhydramine 50 mg for a patient who is having a mild allergic reaction. Available are 25 mg capsules. Here is how to determine how many capsules to give the patient.

If 25 mg equals 1 capsule (cap), then 50 mg equals how many (*X*) capsules?

$$\frac{25\,mg}{1\,cap} = \frac{50\,mg}{X\,cap}$$

Cross-multiply and you should get the following.

$$1 \times 50 = 25X$$

$$50 = 25X$$

Then divide both sides of the equation by 25, and the result is 2 capsules.

Another common method for dosage calculation is the formula method, or "desired over have." This involves thinking of the calculation as what to give divided by what you have times the quantity you have. So, for that same prescription for diphenhydramine, the equation looks like this.

$$\frac{desired}{have} \times quantity = X$$

$$\frac{50\,mg}{25\,mg} \times 1\,cap = X$$

$$50 \div 25 \times 1 = 2\ capsules$$

Pediatric dosage calculations

The most accurate method to determine medication dosage calculations for children is to use weight calculations.

A provider prescribes diphenhydramine 5 mg/kg/day divided in four doses per day for a child who weighs 88 lb. Available is diphenhydramine oral liquid 12.5 mg in 5 mL. How much should the child receive per dose?

First, convert the child's weight to kg.

$$\frac{2.2 \text{ lb}}{1 \text{ kg}} = \frac{88 \text{ lb}}{X \text{ kg}}$$

Cross-multiply and you should get the following.

$1 \times 88 = 2.2X$

$88 = 2.2X$

Divide both sides of the equation by 2.2, and the conversion is 40 kg.

Multiply 5 mg by 40 kg to determine the daily dose.

5 mg × 40 kg = 200 mg/day

Divide the daily dose into four doses.

200 mg ÷ 4 = 50 mg/dose

Then use either method to determine the amount of liquid medication to give the child.

If 12.5 mg equals 5 mL, then 50 mg equals how many (X) mL?

$$\frac{12.5 \text{ mg}}{5 \text{ mL}} = \frac{50 \text{ mg}}{X \text{ mL}}$$

Cross-multiply and you should get the following.

$5 \times 50 = 12.5X$

$250 = 12.5X$

Divide both sides of the equation by 12.5, and the result is 20 mL.

Body surface area (BSA) is widely considered the most accurate way to calculate dose based on weight for children up to age 12. The provider might calculate BSA using a nomogram and then use a formula to determine the pediatric dosage. Several formulas can be used to figure the dose. The following is an example.

$$\frac{BSA \text{ of child in } m^2}{1.7 \text{ m}^2} \times adult \text{ } dose = child's \text{ } dose$$

Example using BSA of 0.7 and an adult dose of 50 mg

$$\frac{0.7 \text{ m}^2}{1.7 \text{ m}^2} \times 50 \text{ mg} = 20.5 \text{ mg is the child's dose (follow rounding rules of facility)}$$

FORMS OF MEDICATION

Medications are available in a variety of formulations. Here are some types that medical assistants might encounter.

3.10 Forms of medication and their routes

MEDICATION FORM: ROUTE(S)		
aerosols: inhalation	**injectable liquids:** IV, IM, subcut, ID	**solid extracts, fluid extracts:** oral
caplets: oral	*liniments:* topical	**solutions:** oral, topical, vaginal, urethral, rectal (enemas)
capsules: oral	**lotions:** topical	**sprays:** topical, nasal, inhalation, sublingual
creams: topical, vaginal, rectal	**lozenges:** oral	
drops: otic, ophthalmic, nasal	**mist:** inhalation, nasal	**steam:** inhalation
dry powder for inhalation: inhalation	**ointments:** topical, ophthalmic, otic, vaginal, rectal	**suppositories:** vaginal, rectal
elixirs: oral		**suspensions:** oral
emulsions: oral	**patches:** topical (transdermal)	**syrups:** oral
foams: vaginal	**powders:** topical	**tablets:** oral, buccal, sublingual, vaginal
gels: oral, topical, rectal	**powders for reconstitution:** IV, IM, subcut, ID	**tinctures:** oral, topical

LOOK-ALIKE/SOUND-ALIKE MEDICATIONS

Be very careful when handling and administering medications that have names or labels that look or sound alike. It is mandatory to check the medication label against the prescription to avoid making potentially serious medication errors. Make every effort to store these medications away from each other, or add a labeling system to point out the extra caution staff should use when administering these medications. Often it is a medication's brand name that might be similar to another medication's generic name, such as *clonidine* and the brand name of clonazepam, *Klonopin*. Other pairs that can cause confusion are *hydroxyzine* and *hydralazine*, or *hydrocodone* and *hydromorphone*. For an extensive list of look-alike, sound-alike medications, see the tools section of the Institute for Safe Medication Practices website.

Here are some additional strategies to help avoid errors in handling these medications.

- Do not use abbreviations for medication names.

- Use "tall man" (mixed case) letters to emphasize parts of medication names that could cause confusion (e.g., *cefoTEtan* and *cefOXitin).*

- Change the appearance of look-alike medication names to alert staff to their differences.

- Create labels with indications or purposes for use, such as adding a "diuretic" label to hydrochlorothiazide packaging.

- Store look-alike or sound-alike medications in separate areas in medication cabinets or rooms.

- Alter computer selection screens to avoid having look-alike medication names appear consecutively.

elixir. A fragrant, sweet, often alcoholic liquid that has a medication in it

emulsion. A mixture of water and oil that improves the taste of something distasteful, such as fish oil

liniment. A liquid or semiliquid preparation containing oil, alcohol, or water for application to the skin, often as a counterirritant

ROUTES OF ADMINISTRATION

Medical assistants use and discuss many different routes for using medications with patients. Providers must include the route of administration on every prescription to avoid undesirable effects that can occur with giving a medication by the wrong route.

The most common routes fall into two general categories: enteral (through the gastrointestinal tract) and parenteral (outside the gastrointestinal tract). Literally, parenteral would include routes like topical and vaginal. However, in common usage, parenteral refers to injections—intramuscular, intradermal, subcutaneous, and intravenous. Medical assistants do not give medications by routes that require nurses or providers: intravenous, epidural, intrathecal, and others.

3.11 Routes of administration: Parenteral

ROUTE	LOCATION(S)	MEDICATION FORMULATIONS	CCMA PERMITTED TO ADMINISTER
epidural	epidural space (spine)	injectable liquid	No
intra-arterial	arteries (to break up clots)	injectable liquid	No
intra-articular	within a joint space	injectable liquid	No
intradermal	skin of the upper chest, forearms, upper back	injectable liquid	Yes
intramuscular (IM)	deltoid, vastus lateralis, ventrogluteal muscles	injectable liquid	Yes
intraosseous	bone marrow	injectable liquid	No
intraperitoneal	peritoneal cavity (abdomen)	injectable liquid	No
intrapleural	pleural space (lungs)	injectable liquid	No
intrathecal	subarachnoid space (brain)	injectable liquid	No
intravenous (IV)	major veins, most often in the arms and hands, or via central venous access devices	injectable liquid	No
subcutaneous*	under the skin of the abdomen, anterior thighs, upper outer arm, upper back (under the shoulder)	injectable liquid	Yes

This includes implantable devices, such as those that deliver insulin to treat diabetes mellitus.

3.12 Routes of administration: Enteral

ROUTE	LOCATION(S)	MEDICATION FORMULATIONS	CCMA PERMITTED TO ADMINISTER
buccal*	against the cheek	tablets	Yes
oral	mouth, stomach (nasogastric, gastrostomy tubes), intestines (nasoenteric tube)	tablets, capsules, caplets, lozenges, syrups, suspensions, emulsions, elixirs, solutions	Yes
sublingual*	under the tongue	tablets	Yes

Some sources consider buccal and sublingual routes to be oral administration; others consider them mucous membrane administration, along with nasal, inhalation, ophthalmic, rectal, and vaginal routes.

mucous membrane. The moist inner lining of various tubular structures, including the mouth, esophagus, stomach, and intestines

3.13 Routes of administration: Other

ROUTE	LOCATION(S)	MEDICATION FORMULATIONS	CCMA PERMITTED TO ADMINISTER
nasal	nose	sprays, mist, drops	Yes
ophthalmic	eyes	drops, ointment	Yes
otic	ears	drops, ointment	Yes
rectal	anus/rectum	solutions, suppositories, creams, ointments, gel	Yes*
respiratory/inhaled	airways	sprays, aerosols, mists, steam, dry powder for inhalation	Yes
topical/transdermal	on the skin	gels, tinctures, solutions, ointments, lotions, creams, liniments, powders, patches, sprays	Yes
vaginal	vaginal/vulva	tablets, suppositories, creams, foams, solutions	Yes*
urethral	urethra	solutions	Yes*

According to office policy.

GAME Routes of medication administration

Match the route with its location.

ROUTES		LOCATIONS	
1. buccal	6. subcutaneous	A. on the skin	F. spine
2. topical	7. sublingual	B. under the tongue	G. ear
3. otic	8. epidural	C. into the skin	H. airways
4. ophthalmic	9. intradermal	D. cheek	I. under the skin
5. nasal	10. inhaled	E. eye	J. nose

Key: 1. D; 2. A; 3. G; 4. E.; 5. J; 6. I.; 7. B; 8. F; 9. C; 10. H

PHARMACOKINETICS

Pharmacokinetics is the study of how medications move through the body. Understanding the four actions pharmacokinetics involves—absorption, distribution, metabolism, and excretion—helps with understanding a medication's onset of activity, the peak time of its effects, and how long its effects will last.

Absorption

Through the process of absorption, the body converts the medication into a form the body can use and moves it into the bloodstream. For example, oral tablets or capsules move through the stomach or intestines to be absorbed. Oral liquids are absorbed the same way, but have faster absorption because the fluids in the stomach do not have to break them down into an absorbable form.

3.14 Absorption

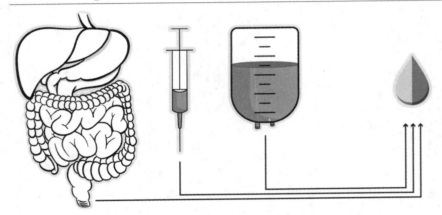

The medication goes from the site of entry into the body through the gastrointestinal tract, subcutaneous tissue, veins, other sites, and into the bloodstream.

The process of absorption also varies with the route. With IV administration, the medication goes directly to the bloodstream, so the onset of action is much quicker. IM medication has to go through muscle tissue, topical and intradermal go through the skin, and inhaled medications go through the airways. At least some of every medication, even those for application on a skin rash or as eye drops, winds up in the bloodstream.

The speed of absorption depends on other factors as well, such as how easily the medication dissolves in fat. Medications that are highly fat-soluble pass more readily through cell membranes into the blood. Medications injected into muscle tissue are absorbed more quickly by the body due to blood circulation throughout skeletal muscle. Another factor is the surface area available for absorption. The stomach has a smaller inner surface area than the intestines, so intestinal absorption is faster. Food slows the absorption of many medications and can inactivate some medications. Medications that are negatively affected by the gastrointestinal system require parenteral administration, such as by injection.

National Healthcareer Association

Distribution

Distribution is the transportation of the medication throughout the body. The bloodstream carries the medication to the body's tissues and organs. There are some barriers to medication distribution. The blood–brain barrier protects the brain from dangerous chemicals but can also make it difficult to get some therapeutic substances into brain tissues. On the other hand, some medications cross the placental barrier very easily, which is why many medications are risky for pregnant women to take.

Metabolism

Metabolism changes active forms of the medication into harmless metabolites ready for excretion through urine or feces. The liver is the primary organ of metabolism, but the kidneys also metabolize some medications.

Many factors affect the ability to break down the chemicals in medications. These include the patient's age, how many medications she takes, the health of various organs and tissues, and even genetic makeup. Infants and older adults have the least efficient metabolism, so medication dosages must be modified to compensate for this variation.

3.15 Distribution

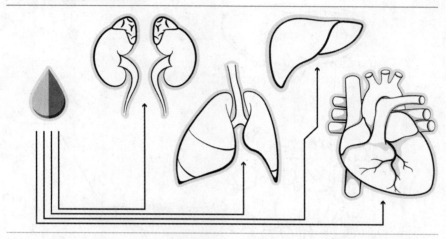

The medication goes from the bloodstream to the various sites of action: organs and tissues in the body.

3.16 Metabolism

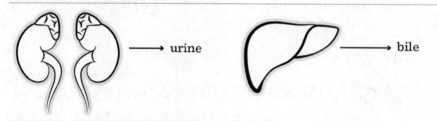

The liver and kidneys break down the medication to prepare it for excretion.

Excretion

Excretion is the removal of a medication's metabolites from the body. The kidneys accomplish most of this through urine, but feces, saliva, bile, sweat glands, breast milk, and even exhaled air also eliminate some medications. A medication's half-life is how long it takes for the processes of metabolism and excretion to eliminate half a dose of a medication. Some medications have very short half-lives, such as a few minutes, while others take days to leave the body. Knowledge of half-lives helps determine dosing intervals. If a patient does not receive the next dose before the half-life time, the therapeutic level of the medication will be too low (below the *therapeutic range*) to be effective.

3.17 Excretion

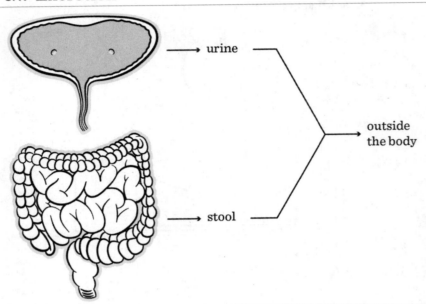

The bladder and large intestines eliminate the metabolites of the medication through urine and feces.

RIGHTS OF MEDICATION ADMINISTRATION

The rights of medication administration are a collection of safety checks that everyone who administers medications to patients must perform to avoid medication errors. It began as "the five rights"—the right patient, medication, dose, time, and route. But depending on the source, there are now up to twice that many. Most sources agree that the original five, plus the right technique and the right documentation, are the absolute essentials every time a person administers a medication to a patient.

The right patient

Medical assistants should use two patient identifiers to verify that they are about to administer a medication to the right patient. Then verify that data with the information on the medical record or medication administration record. The most common verification methods are asking patients to state their full name and date of birth. Other acceptable identifiers pertain only to that patient, such as a mobile phone number or a photo identification card.

---

therapeutic range. The amount of a medication the body must have available to produce the desirable effects for which the provider prescribed it

The right medication

Check the label three times to verify the medication, strength, and dose—often referred to as the "three befores." The first time to check the medication label is when taking the medication container from the storage cabinet or drawer. The second is when taking the medication from its container to prepare to administer it. The third check is when putting the container back in storage or discarding it. This triple check is essential every time a person gives a medication to a patient. While checking the label, it is also important to check the medication's expiration date to make sure it is a future date. Otherwise, the medication might be ineffective or even dangerous due to factors such as bacterial contamination. Never administer expired medication.

The right dose

Compare the dosage on the prescription in the patient's medical record with the dosage on the medication's label. If the dosage form available does not match what the provider prescribed, medical assistants must perform the mathematical calculations for administering the right dosage or find a medication container with a dosage form that matches the prescription. They must also double-check any calculations that seem questionable or they are uncertain about, and have another medical assistant or the provider check them as well.

The right route

Medical assistants must compare the route on the prescription in the medical record with the administration route they are planning to use. It is essential to determine that the route is appropriate for the patient and that the medication formulation is right for that route. The correct route of administration can be confirmed with the medication's product insert, the *Physicians' Desk Reference*, or another reliable medication reference. The route of administration, as dictated by the medication's manufacturer, must be adhered to.

The right time

In most office and clinic settings, medical assistants give medications right after the provider writes the prescription. Nevertheless, it is essential to confirm whether the medication has any timing specifications, such as the patient having an empty stomach or waiting several hours after taking another medication (such as an antacid) that might interact with the new medication. Make sure to prepare the patient for any immediate effects of the medication. For example, eye drops that dilate the pupils for an eye examination cause blurry vision and photophobia (sensitivity to light) after administration. The patient might not be able to drive until the effects wear off. If the patient does not have an escort or cannot wait in the facility long enough for the medication's effects to wear off, this is the wrong time to administer this medication.

The right assessment

Before administering any medication, ask the patient about any allergies that might make it unsafe for receiving the medication. New allergies can develop, so it is essential to ask and not just rely on previous data in the medical record. Also ask about any unusual reactions the patient has had to medications, as well as any problems that might affect the pharmacokinetics of the medication. Some medications require a vital-sign check or a review of laboratory results before administration. Review past experiences with medications, such as fainting after receiving an injection, and document in the medical record if the patient has any complications following medication administration.

The right to refuse

Patients have the right to refuse any prescribed medication or treatment. Never attempt to coerce or even persuade patients to take a medication they have refused. If this happens, document the refusal and notify the provider.

The right technique

Medical assistants must know the correct techniques for administering every medication they give by every route.

The right documentation

Always document administering a medication after the patient receives it, not before. If the medical assistant does not administer a medication as prescribed, the documentation must include this and why the patient did not receive it. Proper documentation includes date, time, quantity, medication, strength, lot number, manufacturer, expiration date, and patient outcome.

The right reason

Inform patients about why the provider has prescribed the medication for them. If the patient is unclear about the purpose of the medication or is unable/unwilling to give consent, the provider should be notified prior to administration.

The right to know

Inform patients about the medication they are receiving, as well as any precautions or adverse effects to watch for and to report to the provider. If patients will continue to take the medication at home, they must understand the timing, dosage, and any special requirements (e.g., the time of day to take it, whether to take it with food). Review at-home directions verbally and give the patient a copy in writing. Document understanding of at-home directions in the patient's chart. Provide vaccine information sheets to patients (or parents/guardians) receiving any vaccine.

The right evaluation

Evaluate for effects and intervene as appropriate, especially for medications that require observing for a reaction before allowing the patient to leave the facility. At subsequent encounters, document any adverse effects the patient reports developing after starting a new medication, as well as how effective the medication has been.

PHYSICIANS' DESK REFERENCE AND ONLINE RESOURCES

It is not possible for any one health care professional to know everything about every medication. Because of this, it is essential for medical assistants to have access to reliable, medically approved references they can refer to easily to find information regarding medications they give. In addition to books and online resources, there are phone apps that have extensive information about thousands of medications. Medical assistants can also find extensive information in the package inserts that come with medications.

Physicians' Desk Reference

A new edition of the *Physicians' Desk Reference* becomes available each year. Publishers send free copies to providers' offices, and it is available for purchase. It contains current, detailed information about thousands of medications. The *Physicians' Desk Reference* also has a product identification guide with color photographs of many medications. This is useful when a patient brings medications to the office in secondary medication containers instead of pharmacy-issued packaging.

Online medication references

Online sources are easy to access when medical assistants have a question about a medication or just need more information to share with patients. Examples are drugs.com, rxlist.com, pdr.net, webmd.com, nlm.nih.gov, mayoclinic.org, medicinenet.com, fda.gov, and manufacturers' websites. Use only approved online resources to research medication information, especially when relating that information to patients. Consult providers regarding their preferred sites.

SUMMARY

A working knowledge of how medications act on the body helps medical assistants administer medications safely and effectively. This also helps patients with safely self-administering their medications. Knowing the indications, contraindications, therapeutic and adverse effects, and how to calculate dosages provides a sound basis for learning how to administer medications by various routes and how to follow up with patients about the effectiveness and adverse effects of the medications. Medical assistants also need to know how to access all the information they need to answers patients' questions proficiently and to continue to build their own knowledge base of the basics of pharmacology.

CHAPTER 4
Nutrition

OVERVIEW

Although the slogan "You are what you eat" dates back to the 1820s, it became part of American pop culture during the 1960s. It is still relevant today, as experts have learned so much about the connections between nutrition and health.

Many patients have medical issues and disorders that changes in nutrition could improve. Dietary modifications can reduce the risk of *hypertension* and other heart diseases, stroke, some types of cancer (such as colon cancer), and *type 2 diabetes mellitus*. It can also assist with recovery from surgeries, injuries, and infections. Many other diseases and disorders require specific dietary modifications to improve the patient's quality of life and reduce the risks of complications.

Support patients in understanding and following principles of good nutrition, and reinforce efforts to manage disorders that nutrition and specific guidelines can help prevent or control. An important aspect of this support is making sure patients understand how to read food labels and the importance of making this a regular practice.

Objectives

Upon completion of this chapter, you should be able to:

- Define nutrient, and list common nutrients and their functions.
- List major food groups and their health benefits.
- List major vitamins, their functions, and food sources.
- List major minerals, their functions, and food sources.
- Describe dietary modifications necessary for specific patient populations.
- Educate patients about good nutrition and how to read a food label.
- Describe different types of eating disorders and contributors that lead to these disorders.

Another area of growing concern is the prevalence of eating disorders. Anorexia and bulimia are well known, but the most common eating disorder in the U.S. is overeating, or binge eating disorder, currently affecting millions of adults. This problem is challenging to uncover, because many people who have it just think they "like to eat" or "overdo it sometimes." Medical assistants can help spot the warning signs so the provider can intervene.

hypertension. A common cardiovascular disorder, often with no symptoms, with which the blood exerts an abnormal amount of force on the inside walls of the arteries persistently so blood pressure readings increase

type 2 diabetes mellitus. A disorder involving too little insulin (the hormone that regulates blood sugar) secretion and/or a resistance to the effects of insulin, resulting in the need for therapy that includes diet, exercise, oral medications, and possibly injectable medication

DIETARY NUTRIENTS

Nutrients are essential food substances—the *organic* and *inorganic* materials the body needs for energy and for cellular activities like growth, repair, disease resistance, fluid balance, and *thermoregulation*. Some nutrients are essential, meaning the body cannot produce them. For example, some protein components have to come from foods. Nonessential nutrients are those the body can make. Examples are vitamin D and *cholesterol*, which do not have to come from the diet.

The body has to break down all the nutrients in the diet into substances it can use. This process begins with *digestion*. Nutrients that contain *calories* are proteins, carbohydrates, and fats (lipids). Other nutrients might be in foods that contain calories, but water, vitamins, minerals, and fiber themselves do not contain calories. A balance of these nutrients in the diet is essential for everyone, but especially for children, pregnant patients, and older adults.

The body needs energy for every function it performs—even during sleep, because its organs and systems are still functioning. Energy comes from the three nutrient groups that contain calories: proteins, carbohydrates, and fats. How much energy (or how many calories) a person needs depends on multiple factors, including *basal metabolism*, activity level, age, sex, and various disorders.

Most young adults need 1,800 to 2,200 calories per day. Those who exceed that caloric intake regularly can gain weight and might become *obese*. Those who do not meet their caloric requirements routinely can lose weight and possibly become malnourished. A quick way to get an estimate of where a patient falls on the continuum between underweight and obese is to calculate body mass index (BMI). Many such calculators are available online or in mobile apps. The formula is divide the patient's weight (in kilograms) by height (in meters) squared.

4.1 BMI categories

BMI	WEIGHT CATEGORY
Less than 18.5	Underweight
18.5 to 24.9	Healthy weight
25.0 to 29.9	Overweight
30.0 or greater	Obese

$$BMI = \frac{Mass}{Height^2} = \frac{kg}{m^2}$$

Q: A medical assistant determines a patient's BMI to be 26.3. Is this patient underweight, of healthy weight, overweight, or obese?

A: A BMI between 25.0 and 29.9 indicates that the person is overweight.

organic. Obtained from living things; not made with artificial chemicals

inorganic. Made from or containing material that does not come from living things

thermoregulation. The control or maintenance of body temperature

cholesterol. An essential substance in the body that can increase adversely with ongoing fat intake and block blood flow through blood vessels, causing impairment in heart, blood vessel, and brain function

digestion. The process by which the gastrointestinal system breaks down foods to increasingly smaller components to prepare nutrients for absorption

calorie. A unit that provides a measurement for energy; the amount of heat it takes to raise the temperature of 1 kg of water 1 degree Celsius; also called a kilocalorie

basal metabolism. The amount of energy necessary for maintaining life-sustaining activities for a specific period of time

obese. Having a body mass index of 30 or greater

Encourage patients to follow a diet that is low in fat, high in fiber from plant sources and whole grains, stays within caloric limits, provides a healthy balance of nutrients, and avoids highly processed foods. Healthful diets can go off track occasionally. It is common to consume sugary beverages instead of water with and between meals. Restaurant dining typically results in servings that exceed caloric recommendations (portion distortion). It is a challenge to help patients who frequently indulge in these habits to undo them and get back on track nutritionally, but their lives, health, and well-being depend on it.

Major nutrients and their functions

Water

The human body is 50% to 80% water. People can survive longer without food than they can without water—that is how essential it is. Although almost every food and beverage contains water, it is recommended that people still drink 2 to 3 L (64 to 96 oz) each day for optimal health.

Water has many functions, including transporting nutrients and oxygen throughout the body, helping remove wastes, regulating body temperature though perspiration, and providing the basic component of blood and other bodily fluids. The body loses water throughout the day in urine, stool, sweat, and water vapor in breath—a total of 1,750 to 3,000 mL each day. Ideally, the body needs to balance intake and output, replenishing fluids the body eliminates with drinking water.

With the exception of oils, almost all foods contain water. Fruits and vegetables contain the most water, but people should not just rely on the fluid that food and flavored beverages contain. Thirst is a good indication that the body needs more water, and pale-colored urine (nearly clear) is a good indication of adequate hydration. It is especially important to consume adequate water during extreme exercise, in hot environments, and during illness.

Drinking too little water can result in dehydration, which can adversely affect body temperature, heart rate, and mental and physical functioning. Without correction, dehydration can cause fatigue, weakness, dizziness, loss of balance, delirium, and exhaustion. Dehydration can also result from vomiting and *diarrhea*.

Drinking too much fluid will not adversely affect healthy people; the body will eliminate it in urine. Excessive intake in infants, athletes, and people who have some medical conditions can cause *hyponatremia* if sodium losses are not replaced.

Bottled water is popular and convenient, but public water supplies are adequate for providing the water the body needs. Added vitamins, minerals, herbs, flavorings, sugar, caffeine, and coloring are unnecessary. Caffeine can act as a diuretic, eliminating water the body might need.

4.2 Portion distortion

french fries portion 1990s
210 calories
2.4 ounces

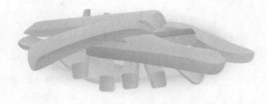

french fries portion today
610 calories
6.9 ounces

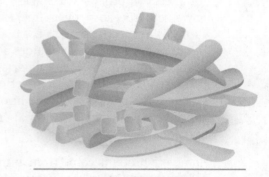

calorie increase: 190%

diarrhea. Frequent passage of loose, watery bowel movements

hyponatremia. A low level of sodium in the blood

Proteins

Proteins are large, complex molecules the body makes from amino acids, which are the natural compounds that plants and animal foods contain. There are three types of amino acids.

- Essential amino acids are ones the body cannot produce.

- Nonessential amino acids are ones the body can make from essential amino acids or as proteins break down.

- Conditional amino acids are not usually essential but might become essential when the body is undergoing stress or illness.

Nonessential does not mean unnecessary; the body needs all 20 amino acids for optimal functioning. The body uses amino acids to repair and build tissues. The body can also use protein for energy, if other sources (carbohydrates, fats) are not readily available. Using protein for energy is wasteful, because, over time, the body will lose lean tissues and muscle strength will diminish. Proteins also contribute to the body's structure, fluid balance, and creation of transport molecules. Because the body does not store amino acids, it is important to consume protein every day. Each gram of protein provides 4 calories. Too little protein causes weight loss, malnutrition, fatigue, and increased susceptibility to infection. Too much protein will wind up as body fat or be converted to glucose. The body requires additional protein when recovering from burns, major infections, major trauma, and surgery. Additional protein is also important during pregnancy, breastfeeding, infancy, and adolescence.

Complete proteins come from animal sources and contain all nine essential amino acids. Soy is the only plant food that is a source of complete protein. Incomplete proteins come from plant sources and do not contain all the essential amino acids. Certain combinations of incomplete protein foods can create complementary proteins, which means together they provide the essential amino acids. The following are some examples of such combinations.

- Black beans and rice
- Pea soup with toast
- Peanut butter sandwich
- Wheat and soybeans
- Corn and beans

The U.S. Department of Agriculture's (USDA's) MyPlate recommends 5 to 6 oz of protein daily for healthy adults. (Check www.choosemyplate.gov periodically, because its recommendations can change.)

Ounce equivalents for proteins are 1 oz meat, poultry, or fish; ¼ cup cooked beans; 1 egg; 1 tbsp peanut butter; or ½ oz nuts or seeds. The recommended serving size for animal proteins is 2½ to 3 oz. In general, protein sources should be lean or low-fat and prepared without skin or excessive amounts of fat and sodium. Many processed meats (ham, sausages, frankfurters, deli meats) have excessive amounts of sodium, fat, additives, and preservatives. This is one of the reasons it is important to read food labels.

Sources of animal protein include meat, seafood, poultry, milk, yogurt, eggs, and cheese. Sources of plant protein include legumes (beans, lentils, black-eyed peas), grains (cereals, pasta, bread), nuts, seeds, and some vegetables (broccoli, potatoes, leafy greens, green peas). MyPlate recommendations include selecting seafood rich in omega-3 fatty acids (salmon, trout, sardines, anchovies, herring, oysters, mackerel). Choose unsalted nuts and seeds to minimize sodium intake. Consume a variety of protein foods.

It is a common belief that athletes who want to build muscle mass require an increase in protein intake. Although protein is essential for this process, relatively small amounts (6 g essential amino acids before or after exercise) are generally enough. More is not necessarily better, and the source should be from the diet, not protein supplements. From a nutritional standpoint, the most important requirement for building muscle mass is calories, not specifically protein.

Carbohydrates

Carbohydrates are organic compounds that combine carbon, oxygen, and hydrogen into sugar molecules and come primarily from plant sources. Carbohydrates comprise the majority of the calories in most diets. Depending on their structure, they are either simple sugars (honey, candy, cane sugar) or complex carbohydrates (fruits, vegetables, cereal, pasta, rice, beans, whole-grain products). Simple sugars have one or two sugar molecules, while complex carbohydrates are long chains of hundreds to thousands of sugar molecules. Complex carbohydrates include starch, which is the glucose plants do not need immediately for energy. It is stored in seeds, roots, and stems. Sources of starch include potatoes, wheat, rice, corn, barley, oats, and some other vegetables. Fiber is another complex carbohydrate.

The body uses carbohydrates primarily for energy for its cells and all their functions. Glucose is the simple sugar the body requires for energy needs, and the body burns it more completely and efficiently than it does protein or fat. Therefore, it has the important function of sparing protein so that it is available for functions such as replenishing blood cells and healing wounds.

Through digestion, the body converts all other digestible carbohydrates into glucose. When the supply of glucose exceeds the demand, the body stores glucose in the liver as glycogen, a ready source of energy when the body needs it. The body can use glucose to create nonessential amino acids from available essential amino acids. It can also use glucose to make some other compounds in the body; but after that, excess glucose becomes body fat. Each gram of carbohydrate provides 4 calories. Too little carbohydrate in the diet results in protein loss, weight loss, and fatigue. Too much can lead to weight gain and tooth decay.

MyPlate quantifies requirements for fruits, vegetables, and grains separately. Protein foods also contain carbohydrates. Dairy is a separate category, because dairy products typically contain protein, fat, and carbohydrates. MyPlate discourages sweet desserts and snacks, soft drinks, candy, and other products that have added sugars, because they are high in calories but low in nutritional value. The added sugar provides "empty calories." These should be treats to consume in small portions only.

Other tips MyPlate offers for limiting the consumption of added sugars include the following.

- Drinking water, unsweetened tea or coffee, or other calorie-free beverages instead of sodas or other sweetened beverages

- Choosing beverages that will help fulfill daily requirements in the dairy and fruit group, such as low-fat or fat-free milk and 100% fruit juice

- Choosing fruit as a naturally sweet dessert or snack instead of foods with added sugars

- Choosing packaged foods that have low or no added sugars (plain yogurt, unsweetened applesauce, frozen fruit without added sugar or syrup)

Q: In addition to weight gain, too much carbohydrate in the diet can lead to what complication?

A: Sugary treats can cause dental caries, or tooth decay.

Fats

Fats, or lipids, are a highly concentrated source of energy the body can use as a backup for available glucose. Like carbohydrates, they are made of carbon, hydrogen, and oxygen, but the arrangement is different. Fat molecules contain fatty acids. Chemically, the distinctions between fatty acids and the types of fats they form are complex. For dietary purposes, the important difference is the degree of saturation.

- Unsaturated fatty acids are less dense and heavy. They are basically oils, and have less potential for raising cholesterol levels (thus causing heart disease) than saturated fats do. Unsaturated fats can be monounsaturated (olive, canola, and peanut oil) or polyunsaturated (corn, sunflower, and safflower oil).

- Trans fat is a fatty acid used to preserve processed food products. It is a byproduct of solidifying polyunsaturated oils (a process called hydrogenation) and raises LDL ("bad") cholesterol levels.

- Saturated fats are solid at room temperature. Primarily from meat products as well as palm and coconut oil, this type of fat also raises LDL. There is no cholesterol in other plant foods.

Fat is an important nutrient that is essential for the absorption of fat-soluble vitamins. Fats provide structure for cell membranes, promote growth in children, maintain healthy skin, assist with protein functions, and help form various hormone-like substances that have important roles like preventing blood clots and controlling blood pressure. Stored fat has a protective function of insulating and protecting organs. Each gram of fat provides 9 calories. Too little fat in the diet can cause vitamin deficiencies, fatigue, and dry skin. Too much fat can cause heart disease and obesity.

MyPlate recommends minimizing intake of saturated and trans fats. Foods that are high in saturated fats include whole-milk dairy products, egg yolks, butter, cream, ice cream, mayonnaise, whole-milk cheeses, meat (especially red meat), oil-packed fish, shortening, lard, and coconut and palm oils. Read food labels and look for products that specify "no trans fat." A label that reads "zero trans fat" could have up to 0.5 g (numbers less than 0.5 round to zero), so it is best to avoid those products. Even small amounts of trans fats can add up.

Q: How many calories does each gram of fat provide?

A: 1 g of fat = 9 calories. By comparison, 1 g of protein or carbohydrate = 4 calories.

Fiber

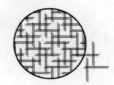

Fiber is a complex carbohydrate that humans cannot digest. There are many chemical names for various types of fiber, such as cellulose and pectin, but a common name for fiber is roughage. It has important functions.

- Slowing the time food takes to pass through the stomach, thus providing a feeling of fullness that discourages overeating

- Adding bulk to the stool to promote normal *defecation*

- Absorbing some wastes for easier elimination in the stool

- Lowering cholesterol levels

- Slowing glucose absorption

A diet rich in fiber helps prevent *constipation*, *gallstones*, *hemorrhoids*, *irritable bowel syndrome*, and *diverticulosis*. It also helps with managing diabetes mellitus and reducing the risk for colon cancer.

Although fiber itself does not provide calories, the reactions it causes in the intestines can produce some fatty acids. So fiber provides an estimated 1.5 to 2.5 calories per gram. Too little fiber increases cancer risk and blood glucose levels after eating, and also causes constipation. Too much fiber can interfere with mineral absorption and cause gastrointestinal problems (bloating, diarrhea).

Sources of fiber include whole grains, beans, nuts, fruits, and vegetables. A tip from MyPlate is that a product that provides at least 3 g of fiber per serving is a good source of fiber. A product that contains 5 or more grams of fiber per serving is an excellent source of fiber. It is also important to note that fiber needs water to perform its essential functions in the body. Adequate intakes of fiber and water go hand in hand.

Vitamins

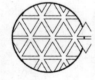

Vitamins are organic substances the body needs for various cellular functions. Each vitamin has a specific role. With the exception of vitamins D, A, and B_3, the body cannot make them or cannot make enough of them, so they have to be part of dietary intake to promote health and avoid deficiencies. Vitamins do not provide energy, but they are necessary for the body to metabolize energy.

Some manufacturers add vitamins to products to make them more nutritious. Examples are fortified cereals, juices, and milk. Some vitamins (C, E) can help some foods last longer. Vitamin E can help keep vegetable oils from becoming rancid. In large doses, some vitamins have medicinal purposes. For example, large doses of niacin can help lower cholesterol, and vitamin C can help with bone and wound healing.

The major classification of vitamins is according to their solubility. This means that their absorption, transportation, storage, and excretion depend on the availability of the substance in which they dissolve.

- Fat–soluble vitamins: A, D, E, K

- Water–soluble vitamins: B_1, B_2, B_3, B_6, folate, B_{12}, pantothenic acid, biotin, C

defecation. Excretion (elimination) of solid waste from the body

constipation. Condition of having hardened stool that is difficult to eliminate and causes discomfort and excessive straining

gallstones. The formation of stones in the gall bladder, which is the pear-shaped organ behind the liver that stores and concentrates bile (a substance that helps digest fats)

hemorrhoid. A mass of dilated veins in swollen tissue at the anus or within the rectum

irritable bowel syndrome. A recurrent bowel dysfunction that causes abdominal pain, diarrhea, bloating, and flatulence (expulsion of gas from the rectum)

diverticulosis. Disorder that involves multiple small pouches forming in the walls of the large intestine

4.3 Vitamins

VITAMIN	MAJOR FUNCTIONS	FOOD SOURCES
A (retinol)	night vision cell growth and maintenance health of skin and mucous membranes	milk fat, meat, butter, leafy vegetables, egg yolks, fish oil, yellow and orange fruits
B$_1$ (thiamine)	carbohydrate metabolism heart, nerve, and muscle function	whole grains, meat, legumes, nuts, seeds, yeast, rice
B$_2$ (riboflavin)	fat and protein metabolism	organ meat; dairy products; fortified grains; green, leafy vegetables; eggs
B$_3$ (niacin)	carbohydrate and fat metabolism	fish, meat, poultry, fortified grains
B$_6$ (pyridoxine)	enzyme assistance in amino acid synthesis	fish, meat, poultry, grains, nuts, beans, legumes, avocados, bananas, prunes
B$_{12}$ (cobalamins)	protein and fat metabolism nerve-cell maintenance cell development	meats, seafood, dairy products, eggs, molasses, yeast
biotin	carbohydrate, protein, and fat metabolism	liver, cereals, grains, yeast, legumes
C (ascorbic acid)	immunity iron absorption structure of bones, muscle, and blood vessels	berries, citrus fruits, green peppers, mangoes, broccoli, potatoes, cauliflower, tomatoes
D (calciferol)	calcium absorption bone and tooth structure support of heart and nerve function	sunlight, fortified milk, eggs, fish, butter, liver
E	protection of cells from destruction formation of blood cells	fortified cereal; nuts; vegetable oils; green, leafy vegetables
folate	maintenance of red blood cells genetic material development	liver; green, leafy vegetables; beans; asparagus; legumes; some fruits
K	normal blood clotting bone growth	green, leafy vegetables; dairy and grain products; meat; eggs; fruits
pantothenic acid	release of energy from carbohydrates and fats	meat, grains, legumes, fruits, vegetables

Minerals

Minerals are inorganic substances the body needs in small quantities for building and maintaining body structures. They are essential for life because they contribute to many crucial life functions, like those of the musculoskeletal, neurological, and *hematological system*s. They provide the rigidity and strength of the bones and contribute to muscle contraction and relaxation. They also help regulate the body's acid–base balance and are essential for normal blood clotting and tissue repair. They are cofactors for *enzymes*, which means they assist those substances in performing their *metabolic* functions.

The major classification of vitamins is according to how much the body needs each day.

- Major minerals should be consumed in amounts of 100 mg or more to promote health and avoid deficiencies. These include calcium, sodium, potassium, phosphorus, and magnesium.

- Trace minerals are needed in 20 mg or less each day. These include iron, iodine, zinc, copper, fluoride, selenium, chromium, manganese, and molybdenum.

Here is a table of major minerals, their functions, and common dietary sources. Iron is not a major mineral but is in this list because of its importance for the production of red blood cells. Iron deficiency anemia can cause problems, especially for infants and children.

4.4 Minerals

MINERALS	MAJOR FUNCTIONS	FOOD SOURCES
calcium	bone and tooth development nerve and muscle function normal blood clotting	dairy products; green, leafy vegetables; broccoli; kale; almonds; fortified cereal
magnesium	carbohydrate and protein metabolism muscle contraction and structure	legumes; nuts; bananas; whole grains; green, leafy vegetables
phosphorus	formation and maintenance of bones and teeth energy production	meat fish, dairy products, eggs, legumes, whole grains, carbonated beverages
potassium	muscle contraction fluid balance nerve, muscle, and heart function	bananas, raisins, oranges, vegetables, meat, dairy products, legumes, molasses, peanut butter, potatoes
sodium	fluid balance glucose transport acid-base balance muscle and nerve function	salt
iron	formation of hemoglobin in red blood cells for oxygen transport contributor to enzymes and protein	meat (especially organ meats), fortified cereals; green, leafy vegetables; molasses; legumes; dried fruit

hematological system. The structures and functions relating to the blood

enzyme. A chemical substance in animals and plants that causes or facilitates natural processes such as digestion

metabolic. Referring to metabolism, the set of processes by which the body uses nutrients it absorbs for energy and to form and maintain the body's structures and functions

Q: What major mineral is responsible for fluid balance, glucose transport, acid-base balance, and muscle and nerve function?

A: Sodium. Although patients who have cardiovascular disease should limit their salt intake, some sodium is essential for these major functions.

DIETARY NEEDS AND PATIENT EDUCATION

The amount of nutritional information available can feel overwhelming. What is important is to understand and become familiar with the information patients will need to hear often to assist them in maintaining optimal health and managing various diseases and disorders. Medical nutrition is a huge field, and patients should not expect medical assistants to be experts in all this field entails. Referrals to dietitians and nutritionists are an appropriate way to help patients who need nutritional overhauls to improve their health. The keys to optimal nutrition are balance, variety, and moderation.

Major food groups

Fruits

Fruits include berries, melons, stone fruits, and fruit juices. MyPlate lists the following benefits of eating fruits and vegetables every day.

- Reduces the risk for heart disease, including heart attack and stroke.

- Protects against some types of cancer.

- Reduces the risks of heart disease, obesity, and type 2 diabetes mellitus.

- Lowers blood pressure, helps reduce bone loss, and reduces the risk of developing kidney stones.

- Lowers calorie intake.

4.5 Recommended daily fruit consumption

AGE	FEMALE	MALE
2 to 3 years old	1 cup	
4 to 8 years old	1 to 1 ½ cups	
9 to 13 years old	1 ½ cups	
14 to 18 years old	1 ½ cups	2 cups
19 to 30 years old	2 cups	
31 to 50 years old	1 ½ cups	2 cups
51 years and older	1 ½ cups	2 cups

Any fresh, canned, frozen, or dried fruit or 100% fruit juice counts as part of MyPlate's fruit group. In general, 1 cup of fruit or 100% fruit juice, or ½ cup of dried fruit makes up 1 cup from the fruit group.

Q: In the MyPlate fruit group, how much dried fruit counts as 1 cup?

A: ½ cup. One cup of fruit or 100% fruit juice counts as 1 cup, but half of that amount of dried fruit counts as 1 cup.

Vegetables

The benefits of eating vegetables are similar to those for fruits. Any raw, cooked, fresh, frozen, canned, or dried/dehydrated vegetable or 100% vegetable juice is in the vegetable group. In general, 1 cup of raw or cooked vegetables or vegetable juice, or 2 cups of raw, leafy greens equals 1 cup from the vegetable group.

4.6 Recommended daily vegetable consumption

AGE	FEMALE	MALE
2 to 3 years old	1 cup	
4 to 8 years old	1 ½ cups	
9 to 13 years old	2 cups	2½ cups
14 to 18 years old	2½ cups	3 cups
19 to 30 years old	2½ cups	3 cups
31 to 50 years old	2½ cups	3 cups
51 years and older	2 cups	2½ cups

Q: How many cups of vegetables should a 45-year-old female patient consume each day?

A: Female patients aged 14 to 50 should consume 2½ cups of vegetables each day.

Grains

Grains include bread and other baked goods. MyPlate lists the following benefits of eating grains every day.

- Whole grains can reduce the risk of heart disease.

- Foods containing fiber, such as whole grains, can minimize or eliminate constipation.

- Whole grains can help with weight management.

- Grain products fortified with folate, consumed before and during pregnancy, help prevent neural tube defects during fetal development.

Any food made from wheat, rice, oats, cornmeal, barley, or another cereal grain is considered a grain product. In general, 1 slice bread; 1 cup ready-to-eat cereal; or ½ cup cooked rice, pasta, or cereal is a 1 oz equivalent from the grains group.

4.7 Minimum and recommended daily grains consumption

AGE	MINIMUM		RECOMMENDED	
	FEMALE	MALE	FEMALE	MALE
2 to 3 years old	1 ½ oz equivalents		3 oz equivalents	
4 to 8 years old	2 ½ oz equivalents		5 oz equivalents	
9 to 13 years old	3 oz equivalents		5 oz equivalents	6 oz equivalents
14 to 18 years old	3 oz equivalents	4 oz equivalents	6 oz equivalents	8 oz equivalents
19 to 30 years old	3 oz equivalents	4 oz equivalents	6 oz equivalents	8 oz equivalents
31 to 50 years old	3 oz equivalents	3 ½ oz equivalents	6 oz equivalents	7 oz equivalents
51 years and older	3 oz equivalents		5 oz equivalents	6 oz equivalents

Proteins

Protein foods include nuts, seeds, seafood, meat, poultry, beans, peas, eggs, and soy products. MyPlate lists the following benefits of eating protein foods every day.

- Meat, poultry, fish, dry beans and peas, eggs, nuts, and seeds provide protein, energy, B vitamins (niacin, thiamin, riboflavin, and B_6), vitamin E, iron, zinc, and magnesium.

- Proteins function as building blocks for bones, muscles, cartilage, skin, blood, enzymes, hormones, and vitamins.

- Many protein foods provide iron, which helps carry oxygen in the blood.

- Seafood provides omega-3 fatty acids, which can help reduce the risk for heart disease.

How much protein should patients consume each day? MyPlate suggests the following.

4.8 Recommended daily protein consumption

AGE	FEMALE	MALE
2 to 3 years old	2 oz equivalents	
4 to 8 years old	4 oz equivalents	
9 to 13 years old	5 oz equivalents	
14 to 18 years old	5 oz equivalents	6 ½ oz equivalents
19 to 30 years old	5 ½ oz equivalents	6 ½ oz equivalents
31 to 50 years old	5 oz equivalents	6 oz equivalents
51 years and older	5 oz equivalents	5 ½ oz equivalents

Q: How many ounce equivalents of protein should a 70-year-old female patient consume each day?

A: Female patients age 51 and older should consume 5 oz equivalents of protein foods each day.

Dairy

Dairy includes milk, cream, yogurt, cheese, sherbet, lassi, smoothies, and milkshakes. MyPlate lists the following benefits of consuming dairy products every day.

- Improves bone health and reduce the risk of osteoporosis.

- Especially important for bone health for children and adolescents because they are building bone mass.

- Reduces the risk of developing cardiovascular disease (including hypertension) and type 2 diabetes mellitus.

All fluid milk products and many foods made from milk are part of this food group. In general, 1 cup milk, yogurt, or soy milk; 1½ oz natural cheese; or 2 oz processed cheese equals 1 cup from the dairy group.

4.9 Recommended daily dairy consumption

AGE	
2 to 3 years old	2 cups
4 to 8 years old	2½ cups
9 years and older	3 cups

Oils

Oils include canola, corn, cottonseed, olive, safflower, soybean, walnut, sesame, and sunflower oil. Although not exactly a food group, MyPlate lists the following benefits of consuming oils every day.

- Oils provide essential nutrients, including essential fatty acids.

- Oils are necessary for the absorption of fat–soluble vitamins.

Oils are fats that are liquid at room temperature, like the vegetable oils used in cooking. Because they are liquids, they are measurable in teaspoons.

MyPlate notes that some people consume enough oil in the foods they eat, such as nuts and fish. Thus, they would not need to add oil to fulfill daily requirements. For example, 2 tbsp of peanut butter contain about 4 tsp of oil, while half of a medium–size avocado contains about 3 tsp of oil. MyPlate recommends oils only, not solid fats.

4.10 Recommended daily oil consumption

AGE	FEMALE	MALE
2 to 3 years old	3 tsp	
4 to 8 years old	4 tsp	
9 to 13 years old	5 tsp	
14 to 18 years old	5 tsp	6 tsp
19 to 30 years old	6 tsp	7 tsp
31 to 50 years old	5 tsp	6 tsp
51 years and older	5 tsp	6 tsp

**Q: A 25-year-old male patient should limit oil
to how many teaspoons per day?**

A: Male patients aged 19 to 30 should not consume more than 7 tsp of oil each day.

Educating patients about nutrition

When educating about nutrition, consider each patient's likes and dislikes, cultural traditions for food, and any health limitations or needs. Also consider each patient's age, readiness and ability to learn and change, lifestyle, and psychological and socioeconomic factors. It is helpful to set realistic goals, let the patient participate actively in the learning process, and reinforce learning and adherence to dietary modifications.

4.11 MyPlate

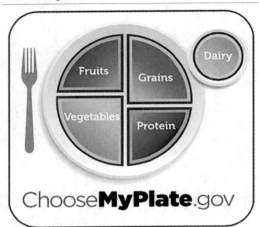

MyPlate (www.choosemyplate.gov) offers informational pages, publications, and online tools for supporting patients in improving their nutritional status. MyPlate also offers materials that can enhance patient education, such as printable handouts and a primer for creating nutrition education materials.

Reading food labels

To succeed in following strict guidelines for nutritional modifications (low sodium, adequate potassium), patients need to understand and use food labels. Reading food labels routinely can be a real eye-opener. Many people have no idea how much they are consuming each day compared to what they need.

4.12 Food labels

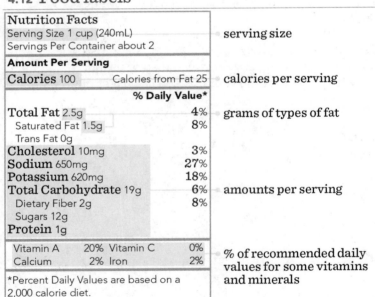

The USDA requires food products to contain labels that give details about their contents. These nutrition facts must include specific elements.

- Serving size

- Calories per serving

- Grams of different types of fat

- Amounts of sodium, potassium, cholesterol, total carbohydrates, sugar, and protein

- Percentage of recommended daily values for some vitamins and minerals

Other information is voluntary, and requirements change from time to time.

When showing patients how to read food labels, emphasize that they should check the serving size and number of servings in the package. It is easy to mistake the list of calories and nutrients as the amount in the entire container, when it might only be a small percentage of the container. Consider a bottle of a sports drink. After strenuous activity, thirst might dictate drinking the whole container, with the person thinking the amounts of sugar and sodium are reasonable. On closer inspection, those amounts are for one serving, and the bottle contains three servings.

Serving sizes often vary by manufacturer. One can of tomato soup, for example, might appear to have fewer calories and less fat than another. However, the first can might consider the portion size to be 4 oz while the other is 8 oz. These variations can be deceptive, so it is crucial to prepare patients to compare labels critically when choosing a food product. Low-fat products can contain more carbohydrates than a regular-fat product. It is also important to check ingredient lists. The ingredients begin with the one the product contains the most of and then others in descending order. It can be surprising to see sugar or corn syrup as a major component of foods many people think of as healthy, like cereal or fiber bars.

Some of the nutritional claims the federal government regulates are as follows.

4.13 Regulated nutritional claims

CLAIM	MEANING
light	reduced in fat by at least 50%; reduced in calories by at least one third; or reduced in sodium by at least 50%
fresh	never frozen, processed, or preserved
lean	less than 10.5 g fat and less than 3.5 saturated fat/serving
calorie-free	less than 5 calories/serving
fat-free	less than 0.5 g fat/serving
sugar-free	less than 0.5 g sugar/serving
sodium-free	less than 5 mg sodium/serving

Emphasize the components that are especially important for each individual patient's situation. Patients who are at risk for or have heart disease should be especially careful about sodium and cholesterol. On the other hand, patients who are at risk for bone loss will want to check calcium amounts and opt for choices to increase their dietary calcium intake.

It is also important to consider the % Daily Value column. One serving of ice cream, for example, can contain more than 25% of the daily allowance for total fat and half the daily limit for saturated fat—and that's for weight maintenance.

CHALLENGE Comparing nutrition labels

Carolyn loves vegetable soup but needs to reduce carbohydrates from her diet, especially sugar. Which of the following canned soups is the better option for Carolyn?

Nutrition Facts		Nutrition Facts	
Serving Size 1 can (240mL)		Serving Size 1 can (240mL)	
Servings Per Container 1		Servings Per Container 1	
Amount Per Serving		**Amount Per Serving**	
Calories 100	Calories from Fat 25	**Calories** 100	Calories from Fat 25
	% Daily Value*		**% Daily Value***
Total Fat 1g	4%	**Total Fat** 0g	0%
Saturated Fat 1g	4%	Saturated Fat 0g	0%
Trans Fat 0g		Trans Fat 0g	
Cholesterol 0mg	0%	**Cholesterol** 0mg	0%
Sodium 491mg	27%	**Sodium** 250mg	13%
Total Carbohydrate 15g	6%	**Total Carbohydrate** 35g	12%
Dietary Fiber 2g	8%	Dietary Fiber 2g	8%
Sugars 5g		Sugars 10g	
Protein 1g		**Protein** 1g	
Vitamin A 20% Vitamin C 0%		Vitamin A 20% Vitamin C 0%	
Calcium 2% Iron 2%		Calcium 2% Iron 2%	
*Percent Daily Values are based on a 2,000 calorie diet.		*Percent Daily Values are based on a 2,000 calorie diet.	

The first soup is the better choice because it has fewer carbohydrates and less sugar, even though it has more sodium. Avoiding prepackaged foods such as canned soups would be the best way to avoid added sodium and sugar. But for the times people do choose to eat prepackaged foods, it's important to know how to read the labels.

1. What are some things that are listed on a nutritional label?

2. Will every food product come with a nutritional label?

3. What changes would Carolyn need to make if she chose the second option for the vegetable soup?

Key: 1. Serving size, sugar, carbohydrates, ingredients, and calories. 2. Yes. If you are in a restaurant, you will have to request the nutritional information. 3. She would be able to have a whole portion due to the contents. A half-portion would have to be her serving size.

Dietary modifications for specific patient populations

Providers request dietary consultations with nutrition professionals for patients who have various disorders that require dietary modifications. The guidelines for diabetes mellitus, for example, are extensive and beyond the scope of this chapter. Thus, the following table lists common disorders and brief notes about major dietary guidelines.

4.14 Common dietary modifications

CARDIOVASCULAR DISEASE	CANCER	GASTROESOPHAGEAL REFLUX DISEASE (GERD)
balanced diet	high protein	low fat
low sodium	vitamin supplementation	not spicy
low fat	low-temperature foods	no coffee, mints, or chocolate
high fiber	favorite foods	**lactose sensitivity**
little or no alcohol	small meals frequently	no dairy products
DIABETES MELLITUS	**MALABSORPTION SYNDROMES**	**chronic constipation**
balanced diet	low fiber	high fiber
low sodium	supplements	
sweets in moderation	low fat	
calorie limitations	small meals frequently	

It is also important to understand the dietary modifications for patients who are postoperative and those who have mechanical impediments to regular diets, such as difficulty swallowing.

- Clear liquid: fluids that are transparent or translucent (broth, gelatin, plain tea, apple juice)

- Full liquid: clear fluids plus all juices, milk, ice cream, custard, cooked eggs

- Pureed: any blenderized food that does not contain particles or strands that could trigger choking (blenderized fruits, vegetables, meats)

- Soft: cooked or canned foods (cooked fish that flakes easily, canned fruits); no chewy, stringy, or tough foods

- Mechanical soft: chopped or blended foods that do not require a knife to cut (cooked, chopped cauliflower, soft meatloaf)

gastroesophageal reflux disease. A disorder that involves chronic or recurrent return of stomach contents into the esophagus, causing a burning sensation under the breastbone, as well as sometimes nausea and coughing

Eating disorders

Medical assistants are likely to encounter patients who have eating disorders, which are food patterns that can impair health and well-being. The most common are binge-eating disorder, anorexia nervosa, and bulimia nervosa.

Anorexia nervosa is most common in white females in their teens or early 20s, but it is becoming more common in childhood, middle age, and in males. Characteristically, patients are high achievers who exert severe control over eating. Often, there is a family history of anorexia and of alcohol use disorder. Some patients have histories of childhood trauma, depression, major life changes, and high stress levels.

Warning signs and symptoms of anorexia nervosa include the following.

- Self-starvation
- Perfectionism
- Extreme sensitivity to criticism
- Excessive fear of weight gain
- Weight loss of at least 15%
- Amenorrhea (no menstrual periods)

- Denial of feelings of hunger
- Excessive exercising
- Ritualistic eating behavior
- Extreme control of behavior
- Unrealistic image of the self as obese

Medical assistants who observe or suspect any of these manifestations should alert the provider immediately, as this disorder can be life-threatening. Treatment involves hospitalization with ***parenteral nutrition*** or ***nasogastric feedings***, plus ***psychotherapy***. Educating the patient and family about nutrition is also essential.

Bulimia nervosa involves eating large amounts of food (bingeing) and then purging by self-induced vomiting, laxatives, or diuretics. It is a controlling behavior, usually aimed at gaining control of weight. Sometimes it is caused by gaining some weight and dieting unsuccessfully to lose the weight. People who have bulimia can feel guilty when they eat too much or eat high-calorie foods, and then attempt to alleviate the guilt by eliminating the food they ate. Often, people who have this disorder define their value as being thin and might previously have been thin. For a variety of reasons, they cannot control their eating habits. Those who seek treatment are most often in their 20s.

Warning signs and symptoms of bulimia nervosa include the following.

- Buying and consuming large amounts of food
- Purging after eating excessive amounts of food
- When dining with others, using the bathroom immediately after eating
- Using laxatives and diuretics
- Keeping weight constant while overeating fattening foods
- Mood swings
- Depression and guilt after bingeing and purging

parenteral nutrition. Nutrients delivered intravenously (into a vein)

nasogastric feedings. Delivery of formula through a tube that goes from the nose to the stomach

psychotherapy. The treatment of mental or emotional disorders primarily with verbal, therapeutic communication

Medical assistants who observe or suspect any of these manifestations should alert the provider immediately. Although this disorder itself is not life-threatening, it can cause lesions in the esophagus, erosion of tooth enamel, and *electrolyte* and hormone imbalances. Treatment involves psychotherapy, medication for anxiety and depression, dental work, nutrition counseling, and support groups.

Binge-eating disorder is similar to bulimia nervosa, without the purging behavior. With this disorder, people chronically overeat. The major manifestation is weight gain and obesity. Obesity increases the risk for heart disease, as well as hypertension, type 2 diabetes mellitus, stroke, some forms of cancer, joint disorders, GERD, and *sleep apnea.* People who are obese often have heartburn, bloating, abdominal pain, diarrhea, and other gastrointestinal problems. With binge-eating disorder, patients do not restrict their diet between bingeing episodes, often eat quickly until they are uncomfortably full, eat when not hungry, and eat alone due to feelings of shame and guilt about overeating. Food becomes an addiction or a coping mechanism, and it predisposes patients to alcohol and substance use disorders.

Medical assistants who suspect this disorder should alert the provider immediately. Treatment involves focusing on eating healthful food, self-acceptance, awareness of hunger and fullness, and engaging progressively in enjoyable physical activity. For some, keeping a food diary helps provides a realistic picture of how much food they are consuming. Discussion with a counselor of feelings and emotions they associate with eating can also help. Psychotherapy is effective for reducing the frequency and severity of binge episodes.

SUMMARY

People are not just what they eat, but also how much they eat, why they eat, how often they eat, what meanings and emotions they attach to eating, and many other factors. Balanced nutrition plays a vital role in helping patients meet their greatest potential for health and wellness and also for managing many diseases and disorders.

Every dietary nutrient has an important function—proteins, carbohydrates, fats, vitamins, minerals, and water. With a good understanding of the necessary amounts of these nutrients, medical assistants can help patients correct deficiencies, manage weight, and gain better control of acute and chronic health problems. They can also use USDA resources and recommend them to patients.

electrolyte. A chemical substance that develops an electrical charge and can conduct an electrical current when placed in water, such as sodium and potassium

sleep apnea. A disorder in which muscles near the airways relax during sleep and cause a temporary cessation of breathing

CHAPTER 5

Psychology

OVERVIEW

There are many basic psychology principles and guidelines medical assistants can follow to enhance their relationships with patients and coworkers. It begins with learning about the patterns people follow throughout their life span, from developmental stages to end-of-life considerations and responses. With this basic understanding, medical assistants can help patients who have special needs and those who are struggling to deal with some common sources of stress.

PSYCHOLOGY

Psychology is the study of the mind and behavior. A *psychologist* is a health care professional who conducts evaluations of behavior and practices individual, group, and family therapy. A *psychiatrist* is a physician who assesses behavior, conducts and prescribes interventions, provides ongoing therapy, and can prescribe medications. A medical assistant may work directly with a mental health professional, but all medical assistants can benefit from having a basic working knowledge of psychological theories, principles, and how to apply them in everyday practice. When working with patients, it is important to understand their physical challenges as well as their developmental, emotional, socioeconomic, and psychological challenges. Understanding the interplay of all these factors that effect a patient's personality and behavior can help medical assistants adjust the style and content of their communication to best meet that patient's needs.

Objectives

Upon completion of this chapter, you should be able to:

- List and describe Erik Erikson's stages of psychosocial development.

- List and explain Benjamin Maslow's Hierarchy of Needs.

- List and explain the stages of grief (the Kübler-Ross model).

- Describe psychological and social aspects affecting patients who have physical disabilities, patients who have developmental delays, and patients who have a chronic or terminal disease.

- Discuss environmental and socioeconomic stressors that can lead to depression and other psychological impairments.

- Describe what a mental-health screening includes and the medical assistant's role in facilitating the screening.

- List common defense mechanisms that shield the mind from unpleasant thoughts or painful memories.

---

psychology. The study of behavior and of the functions and processes of the mind

psychologist. A person who specializes in the study of the structure and function of the brain and related mental processes.

psychiatrist. A physician with additional medical training and experience in diagnosis, prevention, and treatment of mental disorders

DEVELOPMENTAL STAGES

Developmental theories abound, usually taking into consideration some of the most basic ideas about human growth and development. *Growth* generally refers to physical growth from infancy to adulthood and then the *physiological* changes that take place as people age. *Development*, however, encompasses physiological, emotional, mental, social, interactive, spiritual, and physical or maturational changes. These theories take into account the activities of the conscious mind—the thoughts, beliefs, and emotions people are aware of—and the *unconscious* mind—the emotions that lie beneath the surface and beyond awareness but profoundly affect the conscious mind.

Erikson's stages of psychosocial development

One of the most generally accepted developmental theories is the work of Erik Erikson. His eight stages of development offer a guideline for identifying the *psychosocial* challenges patients face at different periods in their lives and the tasks they must master before successfully transitioning to the next stage of development. Erikson believed that society and culture affect how the personality of an individual develops and that successful completion of each stage supports the healthy development of the person's *ego*.

Trust vs. mistrust

This is the psychosocial crisis for infants (birth to 18 months). Trust is the successful outcome of this stage; mistrust is the unsuccessful outcome. The developmental tasks for infants are to form an attachment with and develop trust in their primary caregiver—usually the mother—and then generalize those bonds to others. They also begin to trust their own body as they learn gross and then fine motor skills. Achieving the tasks of this stage results in self-confidence and optimism that caregivers will meet the infant's basic needs. Nonachievement leads to suspiciousness and struggles with interpersonal relationships.

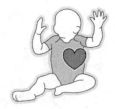

Autonomy vs. shame and doubt

This is the psychosocial crisis for toddlers (2 to 3 years). *Autonomy* is the successful outcome of this stage; shame and doubt are the unsuccessful outcome. During this stage, toddlers begin to develop a sense of independence, autonomy, and self-control. They also acquire language skills. Parents should be firm but tolerant with toddlers. Achieving the tasks of this stage results in self-control and voluntary delaying of gratification. Nonachievement leads to anger with self, a lack of self-confidence, and no sense of pride in the ability to perform tasks.

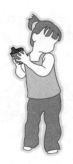

physiological. Referring to the body and its functions

psychosocial. Referring to the relationship between and interplay of mental health and interpersonal relations

ego. A part of the mind that senses and adapts to reality

autonomy. The right to make one's own personal decisions, even when those decisions might not be in that person's own best interest

Initiative vs. guilt

This is the psychosocial crisis for preschoolers (3 to 6 years). *Initiative* is the successful outcome of this stage; *guilt* is the unsuccessful outcome. During this stage, children look for new experiences but will hesitate when adults reprimand them or restrict them from trying new things. Preschoolers have an active imagination and are curious about everything around them. Eventually they will start feeling guilt for some of their actions, which is part of the natural development of moral judgment. Achieving the tasks of this stage results in assertiveness, dependability, creativity, and personal achievement. Nonachievement leads to feelings of inadequacy, defeat, guilt, and the belief that they deserve punishment.

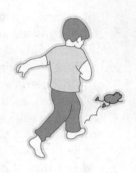

Industry vs. inferiority

This is the psychosocial crisis for school-age children (7 to 12 years). *Industry* is the successful outcome of this stage; *inferiority* is the unsuccessful outcome. During this stage, children need to receive recognition for accomplishments to provide reinforcement and build self-confidence. If the achievements are met with a negative response, inferiority can be established. Children require acknowledgment of their successes. Achieving the tasks of this stage results in feelings of competence, self-satisfaction, and trustworthiness in addition to increased participation in activities and taking on more responsibilities at school, home, and the community. Nonachievement leads to feelings of inadequacy and the inability to compromise or cooperate with others.

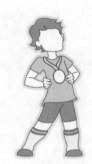

Identity vs. role confusion

This is the psychosocial crisis for adolescents (12 to 20 years). Identity is the successful outcome of this stage; role confusion is the unsuccessful outcome. During this stage, adolescents try to figure out where they fit in and what direction their life should take. If role confusion sets in, adolescents become followers, which can lead to poor decision-making. Achieving the tasks of this stage results in emotional stability, ability to form committed relationships, and sound decision-making. Nonachievement leads to a lack of personal goals and values, rebelliousness, *self-consciousness,* and a lack of self-confidence.

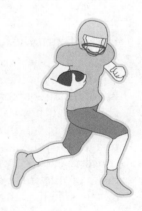

initiative. The ability and tendency to start an action

guilt. A remorseful awareness of having done something wrong

industry. Competence in performing tasks

inferiority. A personal feeling or sense of being inadequate

self-consciousness. A feeling of anxiety or constant awareness of others' perception of oneself

Intimacy vs. isolation

This is the psychosocial crisis for young adults (20 to 35 years). Intimacy is the successful outcome of this stage; isolation is the unsuccessful outcome. During this stage, young adults begin to think about partnership, marriage, family, and career. Lack of fulfillment in this key area of life can lead to isolation and withdrawal. Achieving the tasks of this stage results in the ability for mutual self-respect and love, intimacy, and commitment to others and to a career. Nonachievement leads to social isolation and withdrawal; multiple job changes or lack of productivity and fulfillment in one job; and an inability to form long-term, intimate relationships.

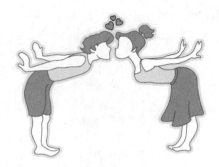

Generativity vs. stagnation

This is the psychosocial crisis for middle adults (35 to 65 years). *Generativity* is the successful outcome of this stage; *stagnation* is the unsuccessful outcome. During this stage, adults continue raising children and some become grandparents. They want to help mold future generations, so they often involve themselves in teaching, coaching, writing, and social activism. Achieving the tasks of this stage results in professional and personal achievements and active participation in serving the community and society. Nonachievement occurs when development ceases which leads to self-preoccupation without the capacity to give and share with others.

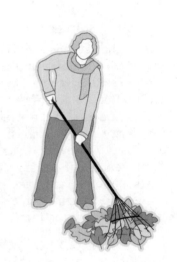

Ego integrity vs. despair

This is the psychosocial crisis for older adults (65 years and older). Ego *integrity* is the successful outcome of this stage; despair is the unsuccessful outcome. During this stage, most adults retire; their children, if they have any, no longer live at home. Many will volunteer to retain a feeling of usefulness. Their bodies succumb to age-related changes, and health problems become a major concern, especially as friends and loved ones die. Achieving the tasks of this stage results in wisdom, self-acceptance, and a sense of self-worth as life draws to a close. Nonachievement leads to dissatisfaction with one's life, feelings of worthlessness, helplessness to change, depression, anger, and the inability to accept that death will occur.

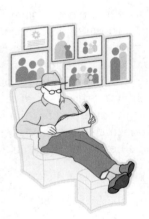

generativity. The concern for establishing and guiding the next generation that stems from a sense of optimism about humanity

stagnation. The result of stopping progression or forward movement

integrity. The state of being whole, honest, or fair

Maslow's Hierarchy of Needs

Another theory used frequently in health care is Maslow's Hierarchy of Needs. This theory is based upon the idea that all individuals have needs ranging from basic to complex. This is usually represented as a triangle or pyramid, with each step becoming smaller going up. This represents the fact that not all individuals will achieve the higher and more complex needs.

Maslow's Hierarchy of Needs begins with the needs that sustain life: the physiological. Needs such as food, air, water, homeostasis, reproduction, rest, and physical activity are at this level. All individuals who have an illness or health issue are at this step. Once all these needs are met, the individual can move to the next level: safety. Achievement of this level means the individual feels emotionally and physically safe in their environment. There is a level of protection in their surroundings, and they have adequate housing and a safe work environment. Once this is accomplished, the next step is love and belonging. Meaningful relationships and connections with others is the paramount accomplishment with this step. When met, the individual moves up to the next level of self-esteem. Recognition of accomplishments from others gives the individual a sense of confidence and independence resulting in self-esteem. Illness can affect this by changing the individual's appearance (limb loss, disfigurement) or by role changes (inability to perform activities of daily living, changes required for employment). The final step is that of self-actualization. At this step, the individual has attained personal growth and reached their full potential as a human being. They have developed wisdom and wish to share their knowledge with others.

5.1 Maslow's hierarchy of needs

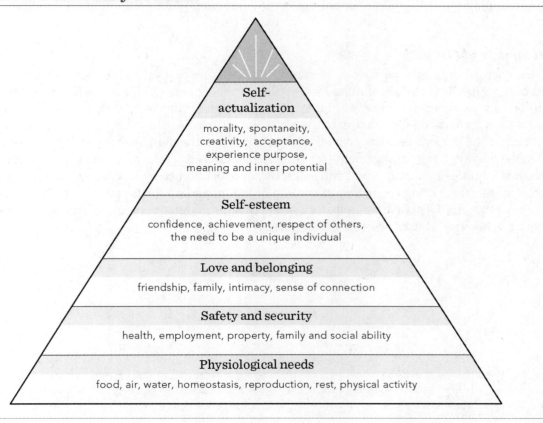

END OF LIFE AND STAGES OF GRIEF

As people age and their physiologic abilities and reserves dwindle, they tend to seek more health care services. With the exception of pediatric settings, many of the patients who medical assistants will encounter in their daily practice will be in their last few decades of life.

After age 60, many people start to think about their own mortality. They realize that so much of their life is behind them, and they begin to wonder how many "good years" they have left. For many, their adult children live long distances away and have families and careers of their own. It gradually becomes more difficult for older adults to continue to work, maintain their home, and—depending on what health conditions they have—participate in activities they enjoy (gardening, tennis) as well as activities of daily living. They worry that minor issues, like forgetting to buy an item they need at the grocery store or misplacing their keys, means they are developing *dementia*. Those whose capacity for independent living has diminished can become victims of elder abuse, which can involve neglect or physical abuse, often perpetrated by caregivers or family members who are overwhelmed with the burden of caring for the aging individual.

Many older adults deal with constant grief, as older friends, neighbors, and family members die. They may also grieve for themselves—for their younger, healthier days and for the abilities they are losing or have lost. They hear many clichés, such as "Just take one day at a time," "Don't worry about what hasn't happened yet," and "You're only as old as you feel." But the reality is that these platitudes offer little comfort to older adults grappling with the grim realities of aging.

All patients need support when they encounter the health care system, but medical assistants must realize that older adults are a unique population because they face so many challenges toward the end of life. The physical challenges are real, and the feelings of grief can be overwhelming. This leads to a major health concern for older adults: depression.

End-of-life struggles

Many older patients have chronic or even terminal illnesses that influence them to prepare for the end of their life. It is not uncommon for a provider to tell a patient who has a life-threatening illness, such as advanced cancer or kidney disease, that it is time to "get their affairs in order." This means that patients should make arrangements for end-of-life care, funeral, burial, and cremation services. If the person has a dependent, such as a partner, the dying person will want to make financial or caregiving arrangements for the dependent. The person also needs to have *advance directives* in place, as well as a will and a *durable power of attorney for health care* document available. These preparations bring the reality of the end of life into sharp focus, and generally put the patient and loved ones into a state of anticipatory grief. This means that they are feeling the emotions and reactions that grief causes before the loss actually occurs.

---

dementia. A progressive mental disorder characterized by decline of mental functioning and impairment of memory, judgement, and impulse control

advance directives. A document that communicates a patient's specific wishes for end-of-life care should the patient become unable to do so

durable power of attorney for health care. A document in which patients designate someone to make health care decisions for them if they are unable to do so themselves

Stages/cycle of grief (Kübler-Ross)

Just like with developmental stages, several theorists have defined the various stages of grief. The most well-known theory is the five stages of grief Elisabeth Kübler-Ross defined as a result of her extensive experience in working with dying patients. Awareness of these stages can help medical assistants understand what grieving patients are experiencing, whether the loss is the death of a loved one, a loss of a body part or function, a financial loss, the loss of a home, or any number of other losses that have a strong and lasting effect on the person.

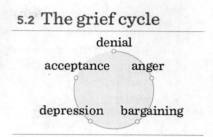

5.2 The grief cycle

denial

acceptance   anger

depression   bargaining

It is important to understand that not everyone grieves in the same way. While one person might navigate through the stages of grief one by one and in sequence, others can be in more than one stage simultaneously. Some might even skip one of the stages. The duration of the process is also highly variable. There is no "right way" to grieve. The stages of grief that Kübler-Ross defined are as follows.

Denial

During this stage, the grieving person cannot or will not believe that the loss is happening or has happened. He might deny the existence of the illness and refuse to discuss therapeutic interventions. Thought processes reflect the idea of "No, not me." The medical assistant should try to support the patient without reinforcing the denial. It might help to give the patient written information about the disease and treatment options.

Anger

During this stage, the grieving person might aim feelings of hostility at others, including health care staff (because they cannot fix or cure the disease). Thought processes reflect the idea of "Why me?" The medical assistant should not take the patient's anger personally but should instead help him understand that becoming angry is an expected response to grief.

Bargaining

During this stage, the grieving person attempts to avoid the loss by making some kind of deal, such as wanting to live long enough to attend a particular family occasion. The patient might also be searching for alternative solutions. He is still hoping for his previous life, or life itself, or at least a postponement of death. Thought processes reflect the idea of "Yes, me, but..." The medical assistant should listen with attention and encourage the patient to continue expressing his feelings.

Depression

During this stage, the reality of the situation takes hold, and the grieving person feels sad, lonely, and helpless. For example, he might have feelings of regret and self-blame for not taking better care of himself. He might talk openly about it or might withdraw and say nothing about it. Thought processes reflect the idea of "Yes, it's me." The medical assistant should sit with the patient and not put any pressure on him to share his feelings but instead convey support and understanding. Referrals to a support group or for counseling can be helpful.

Acceptance

During this stage, the grieving person comes to terms with the loss and starts making plans for moving on with life despite the loss or impending loss. He is willing to try to "make the best of it" and formulate new goals and enjoy new relationships. If death is imminent, he will start making funeral and burial arrangements and might reach out to friends and family who have not been a part of his recent years of life. There might still be some depression, but there might also be humor and friendly interaction. Thought processes reflect the idea of "Yes, me, and I'm ready." The medical assistant should offer encouragement, support, and additional education to the patient and his family and friends during this time.

CHALLENGE Stages of grief

A patient says, "I lost my husband to cancer last week. I know he was sick, but we kept praying hard for a cure. I don't know why God couldn't spare him. We always did such good work for the church. We deserve better than this."

What stage of grief is the patient in at this time?

Answer: Anger. During this stage of grief, "Why me?" is the prevalent attitude. The patient feels that, because she and her husband have served their church diligently, God should not have taken him from her.

PHYSICAL DISABLITY, DEVELOPMENTAL DELAY, AND DISEASE

A major focus of psychology is communication. This occurs with patients who have a wide variety of problems and communication barriers. A general understanding of the principles of *therapeutic communication* is helpful when working with all patients. For example, medical assistants can encourage patients to express their feelings by reflecting patients' statements back to them in a way that promotes further communication. It is also helpful to make observations and offer recognition of positive changes. These techniques promote positive communication. Patients can also have specific types of problems that require special consideration and techniques. The medical assistant helps build and nurture the relationship with all health care staff.

Psychological and social aspects related to physical disabilities

Instead of thinking patients who have physical challenges as disabled, medical assistants should consider them as having special needs. People who live with physical challenges do many things others without those challenges do. They just do them differently.

Medical offices and facilities are legally required to have appropriate access for patients who use wheelchairs or other assistive devices. These include marked parking spaces, ramps and wheelchair-accessible bathrooms with large stalls and hand rails. Medical assistants can ensure these patients are comfortable and able to function well in their surroundings by organizing common areas. Psychologically, the patients will feel more at ease; as a result, it will be easier to build therapeutic relationships with them. They will see the office staff has anticipated their needs and facilitated their navigation throughout the office. Helpful office organization strategies are as follows.

- Create enough gaps between the chairs in the waiting areas and along walls for safe wheelchair access, maneuvering, and parking.

- Do not place any area rugs or throw rugs where patients walking with assistive devices or navigating with wheelchairs will encounter them.

- Eliminate metal or wooden sills in doorways. Replace them with graduated rubber coverings that provide a smoother surface for wheels to transition over.

- Remove any objects that would interfere with complete swiveling of wheelchairs.

- Position any reading materials at a height where patients in wheelchairs can reach them easily.

- Provide sturdy bars or rails along walls to help patients who have difficulty walking or have balance issues to use.

- For patients who have vision loss, provide *Braille* signs and reading materials along with large-print materials for those who have some vision. It is essential to use descriptive language when speaking with them and avoid touching without verbally alerting the patient first.

therapeutic communication. The purposeful use of verbal and nonverbal actions and interactions to build and maintain helping relationships with patients and families

Braille. A system of writing for blind people that uses raised dots to represent letters of the alphabet

- For patients who have hearing loss, offering services such as online appointment scheduling can be very helpful. Patients who have mild to moderate loss can communicate well in person but often have considerable difficulty hearing and understanding speech on the telephone, making scheduling difficult. Medical assistants speaking with these patients need to be directly in line with the patient's face when speaking, not from the side or behind her, and pronounce words clearly. This allows the individual to see lip movements as well as hear what is said. It does not help to shout. Clarity of speech is much more important in facilitating understanding. Some patients require the services of a sign-language interpreter. If requested, by federal law, the office must provide an interpreter for the individual.

- For patients who have service animals, it is important to remember these animals are not pets. The medical assistant should intervene if necessary and educate others who want to speak to, touch, or interact with these animals that they are on duty and things that distract them from their duties are inappropriate.

- Try to anticipate patients' needs and alter routines accordingly. For example, do not ask a patient whose dominant arm is in a cast to sign in. Do it for her.

Many patients with physical challenges have had them since birth. They might have endured many instances of people making tactless remarks or asking inappropriate questions. Medical assistants must be professional at all times and avoid making comments or asking questions regarding their disability unless they are essential as part of a medical evaluation or history gathering. Instead of asking, "How did that happen to you?" ask, "What can I do to make you more comfortable while you are waiting?" Being over-solicitous can come across as insincere, so it is important to balance the extremes and find the right level of attention that makes the patient feel welcome and not singled out as being different.

Developmental delays or other mental or psychological challenges

The first step when working with patients who have mental or emotional challenges is to determine how they can communicate and what level of communication they can understand. Family members and caregivers can assist with this. When communication begins and a patient becomes agitated or confused, it is crucial to remain calm. Avoid showing impatience or speaking louder, which can increase the patient's agitation. Any time the medical assistant cannot understand something the patient says, ask for clarification.

Just like patients with physical challenges, there are sometimes noticeable indications in appearance, mannerisms, or behavior that patients have developmental or psychosocial challenges. Medical assistants must advocate for these patients and treat them with respect and *empathy* at all times. They should make sure to meet their immediate needs and ask their caregivers what they can do to improve their comfort and calm their anxieties.

---

empathy. Conveyance of an objective awareness and understanding of the feelings, emotions, and behavior of patients, including trying to envision what it must be like to be in their situation

Working with patients who have a chronic or terminal illness

Individuals who have chronic or terminal illness are under an extreme amount of stress. Casual, routine opening lines like an excessively cheerful "How are you doing today?" can provoke defensive responses like, "How do you think I'm doing? I'm dying." Even if the patient doesn't say that, he might think it. Instead, medical assistants should welcome these patients warmly and respect their dignity. Treat them with kindness and caring at all times.

Medical assistants should offer support and empathy and allow the patient to set the tone of the conversation. It is crucial that the medical assistant never say they know how the patient feels. All feelings are unique to the individual, so to express this belittles the person and shows a lack of respect for their individuality and uniqueness. Medical assistants should listen carefully to the patient, maintain eye contact, and always ask how they may help. Prior to beginning medical data collection, the medical assistant can use a broad opening like, "What would you like to talk about today?" How the patient answers will help set the tone for the remainder of the interaction.

It is also important to make sure the patient has all the services he needs, such as *hospice* referrals, meal-delivery services, and home health assistance. Support groups and community services can also help; these services can provide social experiences and an outlet for dying patients and their families.

ENVIRONMENTAL AND SOCIOECONOMIC STRESSORS

A *stressor* is anything that causes anxiety or stress. Many things in the environment cause stress, as do psychological factors (grief, depression, loss, guilt). Even things that are positive (taking a vacation, having an intimate experience, graduating from college) can be stressors. Medical assistants should realize that coming to a health care facility can create a great deal of stress for a patient. This is reflected by an increase in blood pressure in the office that is not reflected in the patient's readings from home, commonly called "white-coat syndrome." This is an *objective* indication of the patient's anxiety.

Environmental stressors of life

Environmental or physical stressors include situations that cause enough stress to become obstacles to achieving goals or having positive experiences. Things in the environment (air pollution, *ultraviolet* rays from excessive sun exposure, overcrowding, language and cultural barriers, racial or ethnic discrimination) cause the body physical stress.

Events in the environment (death of a loved one, theft, vandalism, motor-vehicle crashes, physical assault, job or school problems) can also cause stress. Major disasters (fires, floods, tornadoes, earthquakes, hurricanes, war) can result in post-traumatic stress disorder (PTSD), which is a mental health condition that causes anxiety, insomnia, anger, loss of interest in daily activities, and flashbacks to the traumatizing event.

Even though a stressor might originate from the environment, it is the mind that interprets the severity of the situation and helps the person cope with it in a positive way. From there, people deal with the stressor based on their perception, experience, and resources they have available to them. When they cannot cope with the situation or do not have adequate support systems, they can develop any of a number of negative outcomes.

hospice. A service that provides care in a variety of settings for patients who have terminal illnesses that are not expected to live longer than 6 months

objective. Referring to data or information the observer can see, measure, or otherwise detect

ultraviolet. A type of radiation the sun produces

Socioeconomic stressors of life

Many people undergo a great deal of stress over financial situations. Life is expensive; sometimes it seems like an endless cycle of working and struggling to meet expenses and pay debts. Just when it seems that getting ahead financially is within reach, a sudden unexpected expense (medical bills, vehicle-repair) or a job loss eliminates the possibility of economic balance and the expenses and debt may pile up. Even people who have not had a great deal of socioeconomic stress in their lives can suddenly find themselves in a stressful situation due to retirement, changes in the economy that lead to a loss of investments, identity theft, lack of job security, involuntary job loss (getting fired), or the loss of a home or vehicle. Medical assistants encounter patients who have minimal health insurance and find the out-of-pocket costs of many diagnostic procedures, treatments, and medications far beyond what they can afford to pay.

Depression and anxiety

Depression and anxiety can result from inadequate stress management. Depression is marked by sadness, hopelessness, helplessness, little interest in life, indecisiveness, fatigue, sleep disturbances, weight changes, social withdrawal, thoughts of self-harm, and many other symptoms. It is a natural response to a major loss or trauma, and it might take some time for these feelings to pass. However, if depression becomes long-lasting or out of proportion to a triggering event, professional counseling, medication, and other therapies can help patients work toward the goal of a better balance of positive and negative emotions.

Anxiety is a feeling of apprehension, dread, uneasiness, or uncertainty as a result of a real or perceived threat. Anxiety is a normal response to many stressful life events and can actually be helpful in keeping a person's focus on something important, such as solving a problem. Anxiety can cause physical symptoms like restlessness, muscle tension, and difficulty sleeping. When anxiety becomes moderate to severe, the person cannot think clearly, loses focus, and begins feeling their pulse and breathing rates increasing. The person experiences sweating and trembling, and possibly a headache, dizziness, and nausea. If she cannot calm down, anxiety can progress to panic, at which point she loses touch with reality and cannot function.

Medical assistants work with patients who are suffering with depression or anxiety. Therapeutic communication skills (found in *Chapter 16: Communication and Customer Service*) are essential for helping these patients. In addition, it is important for medical assistants to remain calm and focus their attention on the patient. They must ensure the patient's safety and provide for basic needs, such as offering water to drink or a warm blanket. A quiet environment can help, and the patient might feel more comfortable with a friend or family member present. Avoid asking a lot of questions, but it might help to explore with the patient any strategies that have helped reduce anxiety previously.

ENRICHMENT Stress and self-esteem

The range of coping skills and defenses of different patients is variable. However, no matter what their personality types, there is one critical factor that can give the medical assistant a clue about how the patient is going to respond to stress. That factor is their level of self-esteem.

Placing little value on oneself increases patients' vulnerability to stress. When they lack the inner resources to step up to a challenge and instead become codependent, helpless, and hopeless, they can't get themselves out of the relentless cycle of stress, which leads to anxiety, depression, or both.

On the other hand, people who have high levels of self-esteem are stress-resistant. They have confidence in their ability to weather the storm and move on to the next challenge. They stop wishing for a rescue; they set new goals and rescue themselves. They are independent, responsible, and enthusiastic, even in the face of a crisis.

Any time medical assistants encounter a patient who is reporting excessive stress, they should try to gauge the patient's level of self-esteem. Most patients will need a boost in their self-esteem, which the medical assistant can accomplish in some very simple but sincere ways, such as finding or noticing something the patient is doing well and letting her know.

For example, saying something as simple as "Look at how smart you were" to a patient who highly values that quality can make all the difference in helping her regain her self-esteem.

MENTAL HEALTH SCREENINGS

In every setting where they practice, medical assistants will encounter patients who have psychological, mental, or behavioral disorders. Depression is common in patients of all ages. Suicide becomes a risk when depression worsens and patients do not receive treatment for it. Often, these psychological disorders go unnoticed in settings where patients are not specifically seeking psychiatric care or mental–health counseling. Therein lies the responsibility of all health care staff: to become knowledgeable about the signs and symptoms that require the need for psychological intervention.

Role of behavioral health in ambulatory care

In mental health or psychiatric settings, medical assistants become proficient in communicating with patients who have psychological disorders. However, in all settings, behavioral health is an essential component because it is part of holistic care—that is, caring for the entire person, body, mind, and spirit. Manifestations of disease are not simply the malfunction of one body part or system but an imbalance in the person's entire state of health and wellness. Headaches are a good example. It is common for patients to see a primary care provider for headaches. Sometimes, there is a physiologic cause. There can be serious causes, like a brain tumor, head injury, or impending stroke. But often, emotional stress can tighten the muscles in the head and neck, thus increasing blood pressure and causing the pain. The pain is real, but it stems from the patient's mental and emotional state and not from a specific physical disorder.

Mental health screening tools in ambulatory care

Mental health screening tools abound, but the most common is a 5-minute test that providers use to evaluate how a patient functions mentally. The Mini-Mental State Examination asks the patient to perform tasks in five areas: orientation, registration, attention, calculation, and language. For *orientation*, the examiner asks the patient the date or season and where her present location is. For example, the patient would reply, "It is April 23rd, and I am on the third floor of the Greenview Hospital." For *registration*, the examiner names three unrelated objects and then asks the patient to repeat them. An example is, "table, rock, canoe." For *attention and calculation*, the examiner asks the patient to begin at 100 and count backward by 7, five times. The correct response would be, "93, 86, 79, 72, 65." For *recall*, the examiner asks the patient to name the three objects they used for the orientation step. For *language*, the examiner asks the patient to name an object he points to, such as a clock; repeat a statement, such as, "Time waits for no man"; follow a three-stage command, such as, "Pick up the pencil, place it in this cup, and put the cup on the counter"; read a direction and follow it, such as, "Place your hand over your heart"; write a sentence of the patient's choosing; and copy a design, such as two overlapping squares.

Medical assistant's role in mental-health screenings

Medical assistants are observers of patients' behavior. As they perform routine tasks such as escorting the patient from the waiting room into the examination areas, weighing the patient, collecting data, and measuring vital signs, they interact with patients verbally and nonverbally. Experience in these interactions makes the medical assistant proficient at noticing words or gestures that suggest the need for a mental health screening. For example, a patient might ask the medical assistant how soon the doctor will see her, and then ask the same question again several times. Another patient might repeatedly pull on her hair. The medical assistant might ask a patient if it has gotten chilly outside and the patient replies that she is feeling better. Maybe she notices that part of a patient's blouse is unbuttoned or she is only wearing one sock. Observations like this might indicate a need for further evaluation. Medical assistants should report any unusual behaviors, mannerisms, or confused speech to the provider right away.

DEFENSE MECHANISMS

Defense mechanisms are coping strategies people use to protect themselves from negative emotions such as guilt, anxiety, fear, and shame. Individuals are generally unaware that they are using these responses to stress. Some patients use them adaptively, in a positive way, and still have the ability to change or adjust as they come to terms with the stressor. Others use them in a negative way and lack the ability to change or adjust. Developing the ability to recognize these defense mechanisms and the emotions behind them can help medical assistants tremendously in understanding patients and helping to meet their needs. Here are some common defense mechanisms medical assistants might observe.

5.3 Common defense mechanisms

DEFENSE MECHANISM	MEANING	EXAMPLE
apathy	indifference; a lack of interest, feeling, concern, or emotion	"I don't care what she puts in my evaluation, because I'm going to get a better job soon."
compensation	a method of balancing a failure or inadequacy with an accomplishment	"I ate a lot of candy yesterday, but I also ate a big green salad."
conversion	transformation of an anxiety into a physical symptom that has no cause	"I get a severe headache every time I see my ex with his new wife."
denial	avoidance of unpleasant or anxiety-provoking situations or ideas by rejecting them or ignoring their existence	"I am healthy and fit. There is no way I have cancer, so I don't need all those tests."
displacement	the redirection of emotions away from its original subject or object onto a another less threatening subject or object	"I had enough trouble handling that last patient. I don't need to deal with this malfunctioning copier right now."
dissociation	a disconnection of emotional importance from ideas or events and compartmentalizing those emotions in different parts of awareness	"I'm always getting into fights with my neighbors, which is odd because I teach an online course in conflict resolution."
identification	the attribution of characteristics of someone else to oneself or the imitation of another	"I could pass that certification test just like she just did, and I haven't even studied the material."
intellectualization	analysis of a situation with facts and not emotions	"He didn't break up with me because he didn't love me. He just had too much on his plate at work at the time."
introjection	adoption of the thoughts or feelings of others	"My dad says I should stand up for myself, so I am going to be more assertive."
physical avoidance	keeping away from any person, place, or object that evokes memories of something unpleasant	"I can't go to that hospital because that's where my father died."
projection	the transference of a person's unpleasant ideas and emotions onto someone or something else	"She leaves more charts incomplete than I do, so why am I getting this warning?"

5.3 Common defense mechanisms *continued*

DEFENSE MECHANISM	MEANING	EXAMPLE
rationalization	an explanation that makes something negative or unacceptable seem justifiable or acceptable	"My partner drinks every night to make himself less anxious about work."
reaction formation	belief in and expression of the opposite of one's true feelings	"I really hate being in the military, but I always sign some people up at recruitment events."
regression	the reversion to an earlier, more childlike, developmental behavior	"I can't do all that paperwork, and you can't make me."
repression	the elimination of unpleasant emotions, desires, or problems from the conscious mind	"They tell me I was hurt in that robbery, but I can't remember anything about it."
sarcasm	the use of words that have the opposite meaning, especially to be funny, insulting, or irritating	"You have a nice office if you like living in caves."
sublimation	rechanneling unacceptable urges or drives into something constructive or acceptable	"When I was a kid, I used to like to pull wings and legs off insects I'd catch. Now I am a biology teacher."
suppression	voluntary blocking of an unpleasant experience from one's awareness	"The doctor said I need more tests, but I'm going to take my vacation first."
undoing	cancelling out an unacceptable behavior with a symbolic gesture	"I had a big fight with my wife last night, but I'm going to buy her some flowers on my way home today.'
verbal aggression	a verbal attack on a person without addressing the original intent of the conversation	"Why would you ask me that when you can't even control your children?"

SUMMARY

Although psychology is a massive field of study, it is a science that has basic principles medical assistants can apply every day with everyone they work with in practice, staff and patients alike. Understanding the stages of development and how people grieve can be instrumental in supporting patients through these various stages. Some patients have special needs (physical and developmental challenges, chronic or terminal illnesses). Medical assistants can meet these needs with some basic guidelines and strategies for establishing communication, offering helpful resources, and making patients feel comfortable and at ease. Patients can show signs of depression or anxiety in response to life's many stressors. Medical assistants, as observers of this behavior, can initiate screenings that will help determine the need for further professional intervention. Finally, an awareness of the various defense mechanisms people use, usually subconsciously, can provide valuable clues to how well patients are dealing with environmental and socioeconomic stressors.

CHAPTER 6

Body Structures and Organ Systems

OVERVIEW

The medical assistant needs a thorough working knowledge of anatomy and physiology, including the positioning of the body structures. This chapter will review body organization, body *systems* and their functions, how body systems interact with each other, and proper terminology used in referring to the structures and their locations within the body.

BODY STRUCTURES AND ORGAN SYSTEMS

Cells are the smallest living unit within the body. Most cells and cellular structures are microscopic. Cells that are similar and organized the same are called tissues. When two or more tissue types work together, they make up an *organ*. Tissues and organs are macroscopic (can be seen with the naked eye). Body systems are organs that work together to perform complicated tasks.

Objectives

Upon completion of this chapter, you should be able to:

- Describe anatomical position and recognize directional terms used for locating different structures (anterior, posterior, lateral, distal, proximal).

- List major structures and functions of each of the body systems, including organs and their locations.

- Describe how major body systems interact with one another.

- Define homeostasis.

6.1 Structure of organ systems

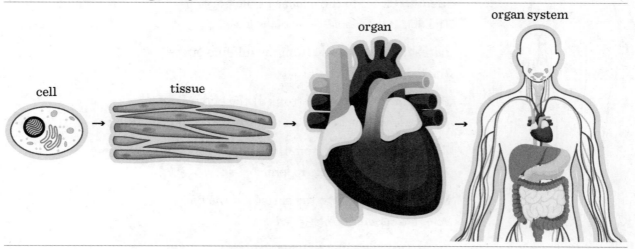

cell → tissue → organ → organ system

system. Multiple organs working together to perform a complex function

organ. Body tissues that work together to perform a specific function

ANATOMICAL STRUCTURES, LOCATIONS, AND POSITIONS

It is important to be familiar with tissues, organs, and body systems in order to communicate and provide optimal care to patients. Each of these divisions of the body has specific duties and locations, which medical assistants should easily recognize. The human body can be studied according to each structure and how it functions.

ANATOMICAL POSITION AND DIRECTIONAL TERMS

When health care personnel refer to a patient's body or body systems, *anatomical position* is used, regardless of how the patient is actually positioned. By using this universal reference point, there is no question in documentation or description of the body. Anatomical position is described as the body standing flat-footed, with toes forward, legs straight, arms at the sides, and the head and palms facing forward.

Directional terms are also commonly used in a medical office. Proper use and interpretation of these terms ensures accurate communication and documentation.

6.2 Anatomical position

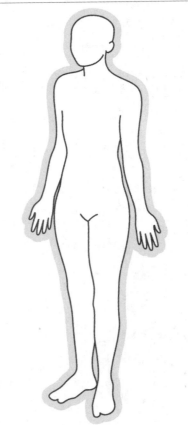

Superior (cranial): Above or closer to the head.
The esophagus is *superior* to the stomach.

Inferior (caudal): Below or closer to the feet.
The bladder is *inferior* to the kidneys.

Anterior (ventral): Toward the front of the body.
The sternum is *anterior* to the spine.

Posterior (dorsal): Toward the back of the body.
The sacrum is *posterior* to the pubis symphysis.

Medial: Closer to the *midline* of the body.
The tibia is the *medial* bone of the lower leg.

Lateral: Further away from the midline of the body.
The radius is *lateral* to the ulna.

Proximal: Closer to the trunk of the body.
The *proximal* femur articulates with the pelvis to form the hip joint.

Distal: Farther away from the trunk.
The *distal* humerus helps to form the elbow.

Superficial: Closer to the surface of the body.
Veins are *superficial* to arteries.

Deep: Farther from the body's surface.
Arteries are *deeper* than veins.

anatomical position. Standing erect, arms at the sides of the body with eyes and palms facing forward, legs parallel with toes pointing forward

midline. Divides the body into equal halves from head to feet

Planes of the body

Three main planes are used to describe sections of the body and are also frequently used with various radiographic studies. It is important to be familiar with these planes and the correct usage of these terms when discussing or documenting locations.

Sagittal plane: Divides the body into left and right sides. Midsagittal refers to an equal division of left and right sides, running along the midline of the body.

Transverse plane: Divides the body into upper and lower sections, not necessarily equally.

Frontal plane: Also called coronal plane, divides the body into anterior and posterior sections.

BODY CAVITIES

The human body can be studied according to each body of five cavities and their internal organs.

Cranial cavity: Within the bony cranium, houses the meninges (brain)

Spinal cavity: A continuation of the cranial cavity as it travels down the midline of the back

Thoracic cavity: Within the chest, houses the lungs, heart, and major vessels

Abdominal cavity: Within the abdomen, houses several major organs

Pelvic cavity: Inferior to the abdominal cavity, houses the bladder

6.3 Planes of the body

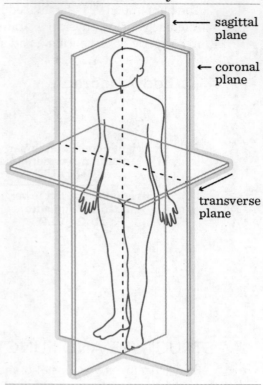

sagittal plane
coronal plane
transverse plane

6.4 Body cavities

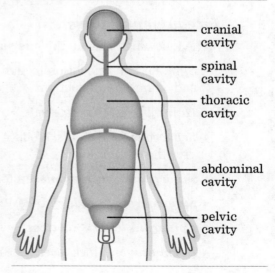

cranial cavity
spinal cavity
thoracic cavity
abdominal cavity
pelvic cavity

BODY QUADRANTS AND REGIONS

The human body can be divided into quadrants or nine regions, either of which is helpful as reference during physical examination of internal organs. Being familiar with each quadrant assists in correctly documenting a patient's chief complaint.

6.5 Body quadrants   **6.6 Nine body regions**

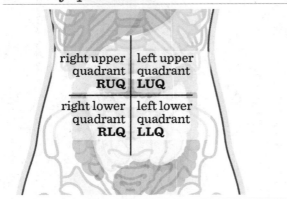

STRUCTURE AND FUNCTION OF MAJOR BODY SYSTEMS

Body systems are groups of organs working together to perform highly complex tasks. When body systems are performing efficiently, the body achieves *homeostasis*. When there is a disruption in the function of a body system, the result can be minor or significant, from a headache to organ failure. The following section reviews the components and functions of each body system.

Integumentary system

The following make up the integumentary system.

- *Skin:* Responsible for protection, temperature regulation, sensation, excretion, and vitamin D production.

- *Hair follicles:* Generate hair.

- *Sebaceous (oil) glands:* Produce sebum to keep skin and hair soft, and prevent bacteria from growing on the skin.

- *Fingernails and toenails:* Protect the ends of fingers and toes.

- *Sudoriferous (sweat) glands:* Produce sweat to aid in cooling the body.

- *Epidermis layer:* Outermost layer of epithelial tissue, covers the external surface of the body.

- *Dermis layer:* Thick layer beneath the dermis that contains arteries, veins, nerves.

- *Subcutaneous layer:* Loose, connective tissue composed of adipose tissue and lipocytes.

homeostasis. A balanced, stable state within the body

The largest organ of the integumentary system is the skin. Hair, nails, and glands are considered accessory organs of this system. The skin has several important functions, which the accessory organs also aid in.

Protection: The skin is the body's first defense against illness and injury. It also prevents exposure of the body's internal structures from dehydration and UV exposure.

Temperature regulation: The skin plays a significant role in the body's ability to maintain and regulate its temperature. When a person is hot or cold, superficial blood vessels in the skin dilate or constrict to control the flow of blood to the surface of the skin, aiding in warming or cooling.

Excretion: Perspiring aids in cooling the body but also results in the loss of water and minerals.

Sensation: The skin is loaded with nerve receptors to detect sensations (heat, cold, pain).

Vitamin D production: The body needs vitamin D in order to absorb calcium (needed for bone strength). Vitamin D comes from sun exposure to the skin.

6.7 Integumentary system

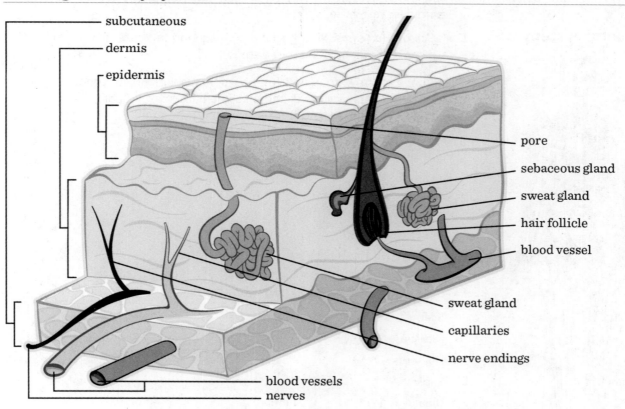

Skeletal system

The skeletal system includes the following.

- *Axial skeleton:* The adult axial skeleton has 80 bones including the skull, vertebrae, and ribs.

- *Appendicular skeleton:* The adult appendicular skeleton has 126 bones including arms, legs, and pelvic girdle.

- *Ligament:* Attaches bone to bone for joint stability.

The skeletal system's purpose is to give the body structure and posture, as well as protect the soft internal organs from injury. The skeletal system also plays a key role by serving as attachment points for muscles in the body. This symbiotic relationship between bones and muscles often results in the systems being referenced as one (the musculoskeletal system). Bones of the skeletal system are classified by their shape.

- *Long bones:* Have epiphysis, diaphysis, and medullary cavity containing yellow bone marrow. The ends of long bones are covered by articular cartilage to allow joint movement without causing friction. Examples: femur, humerus, tibia, fibula, ulna, radius

- *Short bones:* Found in the wrists and ankles, typically small and round. Examples: carpals, tarsals

- *Flat bones:* Majority of surface area is flat or slightly curved. Examples: skull, ribs

- *Irregular bones:* Unusual shape that is typically related to their function. Examples: vertebrae, pelvis

- *Sesamoid bones:* Small, round bones found in joints that are held in place by tendons. Example: patella

Red bone marrow, found within bones, is responsible for producing new blood cells. This process is known as hematopoiesis. Bones also store calcium, which is essential for proper cell function.

6.8 Skeletal system

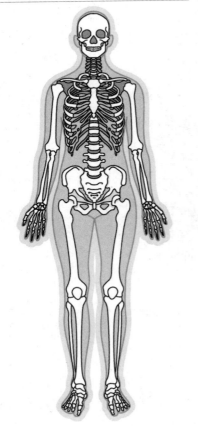

6.9 Bones by body section

BONES OF THE UPPER EXTREMITIES	BONES OF THE LOWER EXTREMITIES	BONES OF THE AXIAL SKELETON
Scapula	Pelvic girdle	Skull
Clavicle	Femur	Cervical vertebrae
Humerus	Patella	Thoracic vertebrae
Radius	Tibia	Lumbar vertebrae
Ulna	Fibula	Sacrum
Carpals	Tarsals	Coccyx
Metacarpals	Metatarsals	Ribs
Phalanges	Phalanges	

Muscular system

The muscular system is made up of the following.

- *Skeletal muscle:* Responsible for body movement, and is also called voluntary muscle or striated muscle.

- *Smooth muscle:* Found within the walls of hollow organs, blood vessels, and in the iris of the eye. Also called involuntary muscle.

- *Cardiac muscle:* Found only in the heart, cross-fibered to allow the heart to contract from the top and bottom in order to pump blood.

- *Tendon:* Ends of skeletal muscles that attach the muscle to a bone.

The muscles of the body are responsible for movement, both voluntary (like walking) and involuntary (like digestion). The heart is also a muscle made of specialized fibers that allow it to function as a pump. The muscles and skeleton work together to provide posture, movement, and other essential body functions.

Immune and lymphatic systems

The lymphatic system includes the following.

- *Lymph nodes:* Small, glandular structures concentrated in the neck, axilla, and groin, which produce and store lymphocytes, and are home to macrophages that filter lymph.

- *Lymph nodules:* Masses of lymphoid tissue comprised of macrophages and lymphocytes. Lymph nodules are not encapsulated like lymph nodes.

- *Thymus:* Located posterior to the sternum. The thymus is large in children and atrophies (shrinks) after adolescence. It is responsible for the production and maturation of T-cells.

- *Spleen:* Largest lymphoid organ, located in the upper-left abdominal quadrant. It is home to macrophages that filter the blood.

- *Interstitial fluid:* Tissue fluid found between cells. Once collected and filtered, it's called lymph.

6.10 Types of muscle tissue

cardiac muscle

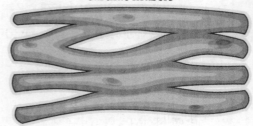

skeletal muscle

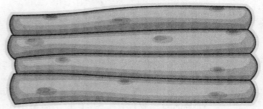

smooth muscle

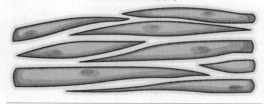

6.11 Lymphatic system

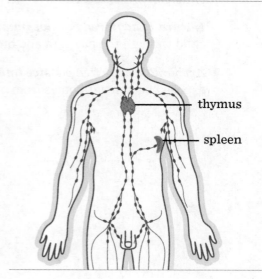

thymus

spleen

The immune system relies greatly on the lymphatic system to prevent infections in the body. When a pathogen is detected, the lymphatic system begins activating the body's defenses. A major component of these defenses are B-cells and T-cells.

Antigen: Foreign substance within the body.

Antibody: Protein the body creates in response to specific antigens.

Immunoglobulins: Antibodies.

B-cells: Type of lymphocyte that can recognize antigens and responds by turning into plasma cells. These plasma cells then create antibodies against specific antigens.

T-cells: Type of lymphocyte that can recognize antigens and attaches to them to attack the invading cells directly.

Monocytes: Engulf and destroy pathogens that have been coagulated with antibodies.

Creating immunity, or the ability to resist pathogens, is an essential function of the immune system. People are born with some immunity and develop more over time. Some immunity occurs from being exposed to pathogens and other types of immunity are developed through immunizations.

There are four primary types of immunity.

Naturally acquired active immunity: This occurs when a person has an infectious disease and then develops antibodies against the pathogen that caused the disease. The antibodies have a memory that prevents future infections by the same pathogen.

Artificially acquired active immunity: This type of immunity is the result of administering a vaccination. The antibodies are activated by the vaccine and develop memory to recognize the pathogen in the future.

Naturally acquired passive immunity: This is a short-lasting immunity passed from mother to child through the placenta and breast milk.

Artificially acquired passive immunity: Also a short-lasting immunity, this is created by giving an exposed person antibodies from a person who has previously had the disease.

Cardiovascular system

Heart: Located within the central part of the chest (mediastinum), and functions as a pump to move blood throughout the body.

Artery/Arteriole: Thick-walled vessels that carry blood away from the heart. They propel blood with each contraction of the heart and are associated with various pulse points on the body. Smaller branches are arterioles

Vein/Venule: Vessels that carry blood toward the heart. They are thinner-walled than arteries and contain valves to prevent backflow. Smaller branches are venules.

Capillary: The smallest blood vessels, which connect arterioles to venules. They aid in the exchange of oxygen and nutrients between blood and body cells.

Endocardium: Innermost layer of cells that lines the atria, ventricles, and heart valves.

Myocardium: Muscular layer of the heart.

Pericardium: Outermost layer of the heart. A membrane that surrounds the heart and secretes pericardial fluid.

The structures of the cardiovascular system work together to pump blood throughout the body. Blood carries essential oxygen and nutrients to cells and aids in eliminating cell waste. Blood travels to the heart to be pumped to the lungs for oxygen and then back to the heart for travel to the rest of the body. The average adult heart beats 60 to 80 times per minute while at rest.

The primary organ of the cardiovascular system is the heart. The heart is a muscle made up of three layers—the epicardium (outermost layer), myocardium (middle layer, thickest) and endocardium (inner layer, part of the electrical conduction system).

The heart contains four inner chambers. The right and left atria are the top chambers of the heart. The right atrium receives deoxygenated blood from the superior and inferior vena cava. The left atrium receives oxygenated blood from the pulmonary veins (the only veins in the body that carry oxygenated blood). The right and left ventricles are the bottom chambers of the heart. The right ventricle receives blood from right atrium and sends deoxygenated blood through the pulmonary valve to the pulmonary artery and then to the lungs where gas exchange occurs. The left ventricle receives blood from the left atrium and sends the oxygenated blood through the aortic valve to the aorta, which then branches off into smaller arteries that carry the blood to the body.

6.12 Cardiovascular system

heart

6.13 Anatomy of the heart

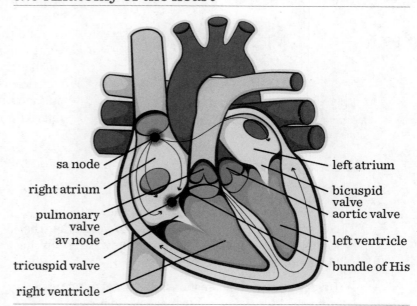

sa node
right atrium
pulmonary valve
av node
tricuspid valve
right ventricle
left atrium
bicuspid valve
aortic valve
left ventricle
bundle of His

Between the right atrium and right ventricle is the tricuspid valve. Between the left atrium and left ventricle is the bicuspid (mitral) valve. The purpose of these valves is to prevent the backflow of blood into the atria when the ventricles contract.

6.14 Pulmonary and systemic circuits

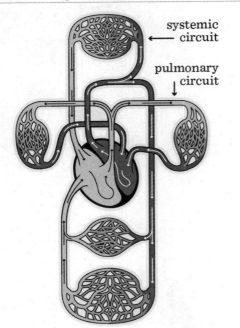

systemic circuit

pulmonary circuit

Circulation of the blood occurs through two pathways—systemic and pulmonary circulation. Systemic circulation consists of arteries, arterioles, capillaries, venules, and veins in the body as a whole. Pulmonary circulation consists of arteries, arterioles, capillaries, venules, and veins going to, within, and coming from the lungs.

The heart contains its own electrical conduction system in order to keep the cardiac muscle contracting and blood flowing. This electricity can be mapped and analyzed to detect heart issues using an electrocardiogram (EKG).

The electrical impulse is generated by the sinoatrial (SA) node, also called the pacemaker of the heart. From the SA node, the impulse travels to the atrioventricular node, also called the gatekeeper. From there, the impulse travels to the bundle of His and through the bundle branches located in the ventricular septum. Finally, the electrical impulse reaches the Purkinje fibers. These fibers cause the ventricles to contract and pump blood into the pulmonary artery and aorta. This entire process is referred to as the cardiac cycle.

Urinary system

The parts of the urinary system are:

- **Kidneys:** Located on either side of the vertebral column at the level of the top lumbar vertebrae. The kidneys are responsible for removing waste from the blood and producing urine.

- **Ureters:** Long tubes responsible for carrying urine from the kidneys to the urinary bladder.

- **Urinary bladder:** Small muscular sac located within the pelvic cavity that is responsible for storing urine.

6.15 Urinary system

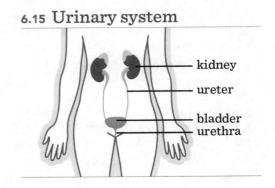

kidney

ureter

bladder
urethra

- **Urethra:** Tube responsible for carrying urine from the urinary bladder to the outside of the body. Longer in males due to pelvic shape and position of the prostate.

The urinary system is primarily responsible for filtering blood in order to remove waste products. This waste is then prepared for elimination by combining with water to form urine. Urine is produced in the kidneys and then stored in the urinary bladder to await elimination.

National Healthcareer Association

Gastrointestinal system

The gastrointestinal system is also known as the gastrointestinal tract. It begins with the mouth or oral cavity. Digestion plays a vital role in the body's ability to maintain homeostasis. Water and nutrients are essential for proper function of body systems, as well as organ, tissue, and cellular function. The primary organs of the digestive system collectively make up the alimentary canal. There are also accessory organs of the digestive system that aid in various digestive functions.

The following are part of the gastrointestinal system.

- *Mouth (oral cavity):* Responsible for initiating digestion, both mechanical (chewing) and chemical (saliva).

- *Pharynx:* Throat or the passageway for food between the oral cavity and the esophagus (also part of the respiratory system).

- *Esophagus:* Muscular tube connecting the mouth to the stomach. Uses wave-like contractions called peristalsis to propel food into the stomach.

- *Stomach:* Located below the diaphragm in the left upper quadrant (LUQ) of the abdominal cavity. Receives food from esophagus and continues breakdown using gastric juices. Propels food to small intestine. Contains *rugae.*

- *Small intestine:* Takes up most of the space within the abdominal cavity. Primarily responsible for absorption of nutrients. Divided into sections:

  ○ Duodenum

  ○ Jejunum

  ○ Ileum

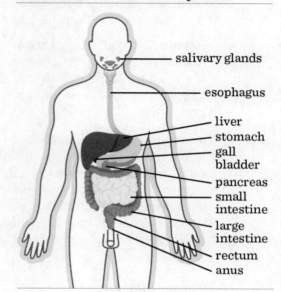

6.16 Gastrointestinal system

- salivary glands
- esophagus
- liver
- stomach
- gall bladder
- pancreas
- small intestine
- large intestine
- rectum
- anus

- *Large intestine:* Also called the colon, absorption is completed here, and feces is formed from solid waste products. Divided into sections:

  ○ Cecum: connects to ileum; where the appendix is located

  ○ Ascending colon

  ○ Transverse colon

  ○ Descending colon

  ○ Sigmoid colon

- *Rectum:* The end of the colon that stores feces until defecation.

- *Anus:* The end of the rectum, opens to the outside of the body to allow for elimination of feces.

- *Liver:* Large organ located in the right upper quadrant (RUQ) of the abdomen. Produces bile needed to break down fats.

- *Gall bladder:* Located inferior to the liver. Stores bile and connects to duodenum.

- *Pancreas:* Posterior to the stomach, and connects to duodenum. Produces enzymes that aid with digestion.

---

rugae. Folds within the lining of the stomach that aid in digestion and moving food into the duodenum

Respiratory system

The following are part of the respiratory system.

- *Nose:* Made of bones, cartilage, and skin. Contains small hairs called cilia to prevent large particles from entering.

- *Pharynx:* During respiration, air enters through the nose and mouth into the pharynx. The pharynx is also part of the digestive system.

- *Larynx:* Superior to the trachea. The larynx produces a person's voice.

- *Trachea:* Also called the windpipe, extends from larynx and branches into bronchi. Lined with cilia.

- *Lungs:* Two cone shaped organs located in the chest. Contain bronchi, alveoli, and many blood vessels. The right lung is larger and divided into three lobes. The left lung has two lobes. Both lungs are surrounded by a membrane called pleura.

The respiratory system functions by moving air in and out of the lungs, called respiration or breathing. The respiratory and cardiovascular systems work together to help deliver oxygen to the body via the blood, and eliminate carbon dioxide. The exchange of oxygen and carbon dioxide within the lungs is external respiration, and the exchange within the hemoglobin of a red blood cell is internal respiration.

Nervous system

The nervous system contains the following.

- *Brain:* Coordinates most body activities, and is the control center for the body as well as thought, emotion, and judgment. The brain is divided into four lobes: frontal, parietal, occipital, and temporal.

- *Spinal cord:* Provides a pathway for nerve impulses travelling to and from the brain, and extends from the base of the brain to the lumbar vertebrae through the vertebral column.

- *Peripheral nerves:* Includes 12 pairs of cranial nerves and 31 pairs of spinal nerves branching off from the spinal cord. Carries nerve signals between the body and the brain.

- *Neuron:* Functional unit of the nervous system.

- *Dendrites:* Has multiple branching structures.

- *Nucleus:* Directs cellular activities.

- *Cytoplasm:* Produces neurotransmitters and energy for the neuron.

- *Axon:* Stores neurotransmitters.

6.17 Respiratory system

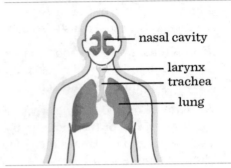

nasal cavity
larynx
trachea
lung

6.18 Nervous system

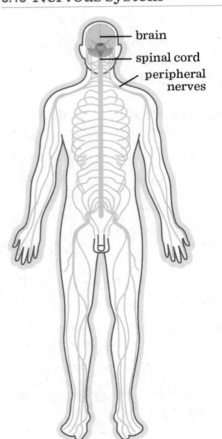

brain
spinal cord
peripheral nerves

The nervous system controls all other body systems and is divided into two main sections; the central nervous system (CNS) and peripheral nervous system (PNS). The CNS includes the brain and spinal cord. The PNS is made of peripheral nerves found throughout the body.

The PNS is broken down further into two separate branches—the somatic nervous system and autonomic nervous system. The somatic nervous system controls the body's voluntary (skeletal) muscles. Afferent nerve cells, called neurons, carry information about the body's environment to the CNS. Efferent neurons carry responses from the CNS to the body to initiate action

For example, if a person were to touch a hot stove, afferent neurons would carry the heat and pain sensations to the brain. The brain would process and respond using efferent neurons to signal the arm muscles to move the person's hand away from the source of the pain. The autonomic nervous system controls the body's automatic functions like breathing and digestion. Sympathetic branch controls the "fight or flight" response to stress. The parasympathetic branch returns the body to resting state after stress has been resolved and is responsible for maintaining homeostasis.

A neuron is able to generate an electrical impulse when stimulated. The nervous system contains multiple neurotransmitters.

Endocrine system

The endocrine system is made up of organs and glands that produce, store, and release hormones. Hormones are chemicals used by the body to increase or decrease activity of the hormone's specific target cells. This aids the body in maintaining homeostasis. There are two types of glands within the system: exocrine and endocrine. Exocrine glands release hormones into a duct for delivery to the target cells. Endocrine glands release hormones directly into the blood stream.

6.19 Endocrine system

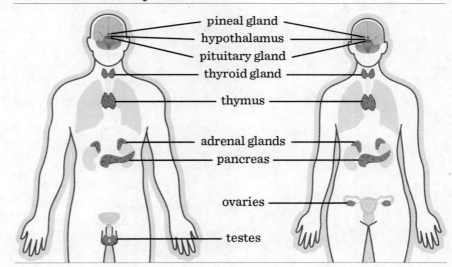

- pineal gland
- hypothalamus
- pituitary gland
- thyroid gland
- thymus
- adrenal glands
- pancreas
- ovaries
- testes

6.20 Organs of the endocrine system

ORGAN/STRUCTURE	HORMONE	FUNCTION
Adrenal glands	Cortex: Aldosterone	Regulates electrolytes and fluid volume
	Cortex: Cortisol	Regulates carbohydrates
	Medulla: Epinephrine	Fight-or-flight response
	Medulla: Norepinephrine	Vasoconstrictor
Hypothalamus	Produces: Antidiuretic hormone	Stimulates reabsorption of water in kidneys
	Produces: Oxytocin	Stimulates uterine contractions during labor and release of breast milk
Ovaries	Estrogen	Development of secondary sex characteristics in females, regulates menses
	Progesterone	Prepares the body for pregnancy
Pancreas	Alpha cells: Glucagon	Increases blood sugar
	Beta cells: Insulin	Decreases blood sugar
Parathyroid gland	Parathyroid hormone	Regulates calcium
Pineal gland	Melatonin	Regulates onset of puberty, biological clock
Pituitary gland, Anterior	Growth hormone	Stimulates body growth
	Melanocyte-stimulating hormone	Stimulates skin pigment
	Adrenocorticotropic hormone	Regulates adrenal cortex
	Thyroid-stimulating hormone	Regulates thyroid gland
	Follicle-stimulating hormone	Stimulates growth of ova and sperm
	Luteinizing hormone	Stimulates ovulation (females) and testosterone production (males)
	Prolactin	
Pituitary gland, Posterior	Releases: Antidiuretic hormone	Stimulates reabsorption of water by the kidneys
	Releases: Oxytocin	Stimulates uterine contractions during labor and release of breast milk
Testes	Testosterone	Sperm production, secondary sex characteristics in males
Thymus	Thymosin	Development of cells in the immune system
Thyroid gland	T_3 and T_4	Cellular metabolism
	Calcitonin	Increases bone calcium

Reproductive system

The male and female reproductive systems work together to achieve fertilization and produce offspring. They each contain structures and functions to aid in this process.

The following are part of the male reproductive system.

- *Testes:* Produce sperm and testosterone. Located below the pelvic cavity on the outside of the body, within the scrotum.

- *Scrotum:* A pouch of skin that houses the testes.

- *Penis:* External cylinder-shaped organ that moves urine and semen out of the body.

- *Epididymis:* Coiled tube located superior to each teste, responsible for maturation of sperm cells.

- *Vas deferens:* Connects the epididymis to the urethra.

- *Seminal vesicles:* Sac-like organs that secrete seminal fluid. This fluid stimulates muscle contractions in the female reproductive organs to aid in propelling sperm forward.

6.21 Male reproductive system

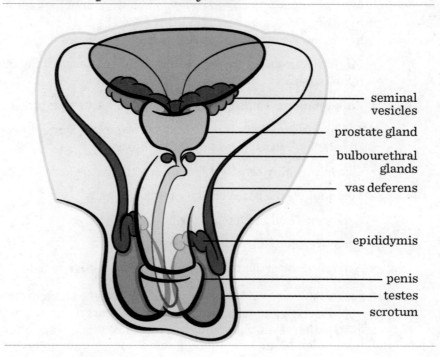

seminal vesicles

prostate gland

bulbourethral glands

vas deferens

epididymis

penis

testes

scrotum

- *Prostate gland:* Surrounds the proximal urethra, contracts during ejaculation to aid in forward movement of sperm. Secretes fluid that protects sperm within the vagina.

- *Bulbourethral glands (Cowper's glands):* Inferior to the prostate gland, secrete fluid to lubricate the end of the penis to prepare for intercourse.

- *Androgens:* Group of male sex hormones.

- *Testosterone:* Most abundant and biologically active of male sex hormones.

The female reproductive system includes the following.

- *Ovaries:* Pair of oval-shaped organs located within the pelvic cavity. Produce ova, estrogen, and progesterone.

- *Fallopian tubes:* Muscular tubes with proximal opening near each ovary, connects distally to uterus. Receives egg during ovulation.

- *Uterus:* Hollow muscular organ, lies low in pelvic cavity. Receives fertilized egg, which implants into uterine wall for fetal development. In a nonpregnant female, the uterine lining sloughs off monthly, causing menstruation. The lower portion of the uterus is the cervix, which creates a barrier between the uterus and vagina and dilates during childbirth.

- *Vagina:* Muscular tube extending from the uterus to the outside of the body. Expands during intercourse and childbirth.

- *Labia majora:* Folds of skin and adipose tissue that protect other external female genitalia.

- *Labia minora:* Folds of skin within the labia majora, pinkish in color due to high blood circulation, forms a hood over the clitoris.

- *Clitoris:* Highly sensitive female erectile tissue located anterior to the urethra.

- *Perineum:* Area between the vagina and anus.

- *Estrogen:* Group of female sex hormones.

- *Progesterone:* Hormone secreted by ovaries.

- *Estradiol:* Most abundant and biologically active female hormone.

Females have a reproductive cycle, which refers to a monthly fluctuation of hormones that aids in reproduction and prepares the uterus for carrying a child. When fertilization does not occur, menstruation takes place and the process begins again.

6.22 Female reproductive system

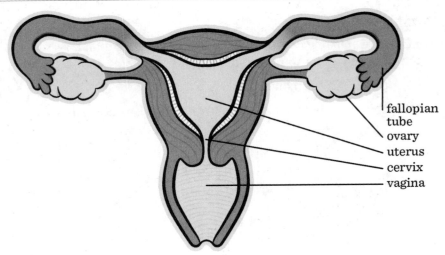

fallopian
tube
ovary
uterus
cervix
vagina

INTERACTIONS BETWEEN ORGAN SYSTEMS

When organs work together, they are referred to as systems. Body systems are responsible for all vital functions, including maintaining homeostasis.

Homeostasis

Homeostasis is achieved when the body's systems and biological processes maintain stability. The body has built-in regulatory processes that react to external environmental changes in order to sustain balance. The nervous system and endocrine system are primarily responsible for achieving and maintaining homeostasis, but all body systems play a role.

Organ systems rely on each other in the achievement of homeostasis. When there is a disease or disorder within one body system, it will have an effect on other systems and their ability to keep the body operating properly.

SUMMARY

The study of the body and its functions is a complex and fascinating subject. By understanding the organization system of the body, the structures and groups within the body, and how those groups rely on each other to maintain overall health, a medical assistant will have a strong foundation of knowledge. A thorough knowledge of anatomy and physiology will serve medical assistants throughout all phases of their careers and ensure confidence and competency within their scope of practice.

CHAPTER 7

Pathophysiology and Disease Processes

OVERVIEW

Pathophysiology describes a physiological process associated with disease or injury. Throughout the career of a medical assistant, numerous diseases, illnesses, and injuries will be encountered. Medical assistants working in all specialties must be able to recognize and understand the basic components of the disease process. To effectively assist providers, as well as care for and educate patients, a foundational knowledge of common diseases and disorders is necessary. This chapter will review the most common of these disorders, their signs and symptoms, treatment options, and possible prognoses.

Objectives

Upon completion of this chapter, you should be able to:

- List signs, symptoms, and etiology of common diseases, conditions, and injuries.
- List common diagnostic measures and treatment modalities.
- Discuss the incidence, prevalence, and risk factors of common diseases.
- List common risk factors that lead to high mortality and morbidity.
- Define epidemic and pandemics, and describe best methods for preventing them.

PATHOPHYSIOLOGY AND DISEASE PROCESSES

Each body system has unique challenges in maintaining homeostasis and overall state of health. These challenges are collectively referred to as pathophysiology. One of the reasons medicine has become so specialized is to allow providers the ability to focus on specific body systems and treatments for the various associated pathologies—in essence becoming experts in their chosen specialty. For medical assistants, recognizing common signs, symptoms, and *etiology* of various disease processes and injuries, as well as the most common and effective treatment of these, creates reliability and trust with providers and patients. The following tables list common diseases, conditions, and injuries by body system.

pathophysiology. The study of physical manifestations of illnesses and disease

etiology. The cause, set of causes, or manner of causation of a disease or condition

7.1 Endocrine system

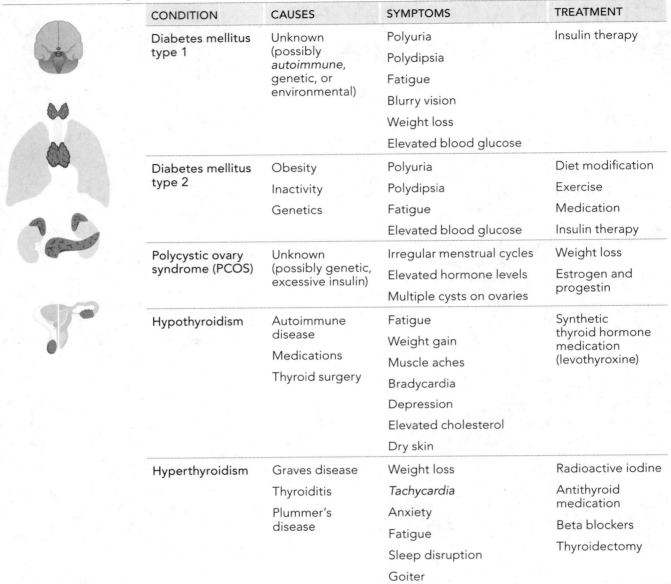

CONDITION	CAUSES	SYMPTOMS	TREATMENT
Diabetes mellitus type 1	Unknown (possibly *autoimmune*, genetic, or environmental)	Polyuria Polydipsia Fatigue Blurry vision Weight loss Elevated blood glucose	Insulin therapy
Diabetes mellitus type 2	Obesity Inactivity Genetics	Polyuria Polydipsia Fatigue Elevated blood glucose	Diet modification Exercise Medication Insulin therapy
Polycystic ovary syndrome (PCOS)	Unknown (possibly genetic, excessive insulin)	Irregular menstrual cycles Elevated hormone levels Multiple cysts on ovaries	Weight loss Estrogen and progestin
Hypothyroidism	Autoimmune disease Medications Thyroid surgery	Fatigue Weight gain Muscle aches Bradycardia Depression Elevated cholesterol Dry skin	Synthetic thyroid hormone medication (levothyroxine)
Hyperthyroidism	Graves disease Thyroiditis Plummer's disease	Weight loss *Tachycardia* Anxiety Fatigue Sleep disruption Goiter	Radioactive iodine Antithyroid medication Beta blockers Thyroidectomy

autoimmune. A condition of or related to the immune response of an organism against substances naturally present in the body

tachycardia. Heart rate greater than 100/min

7.2 Integumentary system

CONDITION	CAUSES/RISK FACTORS	SYMPTOMS	TREATMENT
Basal cell carcinoma (BCC)	Light/fair skin Sun exposure	New growth or sore that does not heal	*Curettage* and *electrodessication* *Mohs surgery* Cryosurgery Laser therapy
Squamous cell carcinoma	Light/fair skin Sun exposure Less common than BCC	Spreads to surrounding tissue Most common on face and head	Curettage and electrodessication Mohs surgery Cryosurgery Laser therapy
Malignant melanoma	Light/fair skin Sun exposure	Itchy/bleeding mole New mole Mole with changes	Depends on stage of lesion Surgery Lymph node biopsy Chemotherapy Radiation therapy Immunotherapy
Acne vulgaris	Surge of sex hormones during puberty Excess sebum on skin surface	Black heads, white heads (comedos) Papules, pustules	Regular cleansing of affected area OTC benzoyl peroxide products Prescription medication (topical or oral)
Alopecia	Often hereditary Hormone changes Chemotherapy Stress Burns Fungal skin infections	Loss or lack of hair anywhere on the body, typically on the scalp Can include eyebrows and eyelashes	No cure Hair transplants and medications can slow progression

curettage. The removal of tissue or growths from a body cavity, such as the uterus, by scraping with a curette

electrodessication. The drying of tissue by a high-frequency electric current applied with a needle-shaped electrode (also called fulguration)

Mohs surgery. A method of excising skin cancers and microscopically examining each layer until the entire tumor is removed

7.2 Integumentary system *continued*

CONDITION	CAUSES/RISK FACTORS	SYMPTOMS	TREATMENT
Cellulitis	Staphylococcal and streptococcal bacterial infections	Red, tight skin Pain in inflamed area Fever	Oral/topical antibiotics Hospitalization if at risk for developing systemic infection
Dermatitis	Multiple causative agents Contact with irritants	Inflammation of skin resulting in rash and pruritus	Treatment is based on cause Corticosteroid creams Oral steroids
Eczema	Unknown (possible allergy or inflammatory condition)	Chronic dermatitis with vesicular eruptions developing into itchy, red, scaly rash	Topical or systemic steroids *NSAIDs* for discomfort
Folliculitis	Shaving or repeated rubbing of shaved area Bacteria or fungi	Red, itchy hair follicles (pimple appearance)	Regular cleansing of affected area Topical antibiotics Electric shaver instead of razor
Herpes simplex	Contact with herpes simplex virus	Type I: painful blisters on lips, mouth, and face Type II: similar lesions, located in genital area	No cure Antiviral medication to decrease frequency of outbreaks
Impetigo	Staphylococcal and streptococcal bacteria	Itchy, oozing skin lesions with honey-like appearing crust	Antibiotics Frequent cleansing of area
Pediculosis	Parasitic lice infestation	Skin itching Nits (eggs) in hair, particularly near roots	Prescription or OTC lice treatments/shampoos
Psoriasis	Inherited autoimmune disorder	Silvery, scaly, severely itchy skin lesions Can cause systemic symptoms such as joint pain and inflammation (psoriatic arthritis)	Oral NSAIDs Topical creams containing vitamins A and D Hydrocortisone cream UV treatments
Ringworm	Contact with causative fungus	Flat, circular lesions (dry/scaly or moist/crusty)	Topical and oral antifungal medication
Rosacea	Dilation of small facial blood vessels Cause of dilation is unknown	Redness Acne-like eruptions on face	Topical cortisones Antibiotics Vascular laser therapy

NSAID. Non-steroidal anti-inflammatory medication

7.3 Musculoskeletal system

CONDITION	CAUSES/RISK FACTORS	SYMPTOMS	TREATMENT
Osteoarthritis	Inflammatory processes Metabolic disorders	Joint stiffness and pain Fluid surrounding the joint Grating sound with joint movement	NSAIDs Intra-articular injections Arthroscopy Joint replacement surgery
Rheumatoid arthritis	Autoimmune	Destruction of the joint capsule causing scar tissue to form Visible joint deformity Loss of joint mobility	NSAIDs Exercise Heat and cold therapies Cortisone injections Surgery to remove scar tissue
Bursitis	Overuse Joint trauma Bacterial infection	Joint pain and swelling	Rest Pain medication Steroid injection Aspiration of joint fluid Antibiotics
Ewing's sarcoma family of tumors	Unknown Age 10 to 20 years old Male sex	Fever Pain at tumor site Fractures Bruising	Surgery Chemotherapy Radiation therapy Bone marrow transplant Stem cell transplant
Gout	Deposits of uric acid crystals accumulate in joint spaces	Joint pain Common in big toe and knee joints Stiffness Swelling	Dietary changes (avoidance of rich, fatty foods) Pain medication Medications to aid in elimination of uric acid in kidneys during urine formation
Kyphosis	Growth retardation or improper development of growth plates Aging and degenerative disk disease contribute to adult onset	Visible upper back curvature (humpback)	Exercise Back bracing Harrington rod Spinal fusion in extreme cases

7.3 Musculoskeletal system *continued*

CONDITION	CAUSES/RISK FACTORS	SYMPTOMS	TREATMENT
Lordosis	Injury Poor posture Wearing high heels (inward positioning of back when balancing on balls of feet)	Inward curvature of the lower back (swayback)	Corrective shoes Exercise
Osteogenesis imperfecta (brittle bone disease)	Hereditary	Dental issues Fractures at birth Loose joints Muscle weakness Respiratory issues Blue sclera of the eye Triangle-shaped face Small stature Spinal curvature	Fracture repair Surgery with metal rodding Physical therapy Bracing
Osteoporosis	Hormone deficiencies Sedentary lifestyle Lack of vitamin D Corticosteroid use (long-term) Smoking	Fractures Most common in the spine, wrists, hips Loss of height Can result in kyphosis	Medications Hormone replacement therapy Exercise Supplements
Osteosarcoma	Unknown	Pain in affected bones (usually legs) Swelling with development of tumor growth	Surgery Chemotherapy and radiation Amputation of affected limb
Paget's disease	Hereditary Viral	Bone pain and deformity Fractures Excessive bone destruction	Surgery Medication Physical therapy
Scoliosis	Possibly genetic Can begin prenatally during formation of vertebrae Muscle weakness	Bent appearing spine (laterally) Back pain	Back bracing Physical therapy Surgery with rod placement

7.3 Musculoskeletal system *continued*

CONDITION	CAUSES/RISK FACTORS	SYMPTOMS	TREATMENT
Fibromyalgia	Unknown Exacerbated by sleep deprivation, emotional distress, depression	Fatigue Point tenderness and trigger points Chronic facial pain Sleep disturbances	Antidepressants NSAIDs Physical therapy Trigger point injections
Muscular dystrophy	Hereditary	Muscle weakness leading to eventual paralysis of muscle groups	Physical therapy Bracing Ambulatory devices Medications
Myasthenia gravis	Autoimmune	Double vision Muscle weakness Dysphagia Difficulty chewing Difficulty breathing	Avoiding excessive stress Rest Eye patch Medication
Tendonitis	Sports- or activity-related	Pain in joints Limited range of motion in joint	Rest Ice NSAIDs
Tetanus	Toxin produced by Clostridium tetani	Muscle spasm in jaw and neck *Dyspnea* Fever Irritability Sweating and drooling	Antitoxin and antibiotic medications

dyspnea. Difficulty breathing

7.4 Cardiovascular system

CONDITION	CAUSES/RISK FACTORS	SYMPTOMS	TREATMENT
Hypertension	Narrowing of arteries Increased arterial pressure Risk factors: obesity, smoking, stimulant use, kidney disease, high sodium intake, excessive alcohol consumption	Excessive sweating Fatigue Muscle cramps Headaches Dizziness	Treatment of underlying cause Lifestyle modifications: diet, exercise, stress management, smoking cessation Antihypertensive medication
Angina	Coronary artery narrowing Atherosclerosis	Pain/tightness in chest	Sublingual nitroglycerin Treatment of underlying condition
Coronary artery disease (atherosclerosis)	Buildup of fat and cholesterol in arteries Risk factors: high-fat diet, high LDL levels, smoking, obesity, sedentary lifestyle	Usually no symptoms prior to heart attack	Lipid-lowering medications Low-fat diet Exercise Smoking cessation Coronary artery bypass grafting in severe cases
Myocardial infarction (heart attack)	Coronary artery blockage Atherosclerosis Blood clot	Squeezing chest pain that can radiate to shoulder/arm/neck/jaw Shortness of breath *Diaphoresis* Dizziness Nausea	Aspirin CPR if unconscious Defibrillation Anticoagulant medication Immediate emergency protocol
Aneurysm	Atherosclerosis Smoking High-cholesterol diet Obesity	Usually none Possible back pain Tachycardia Dizziness	Surgery

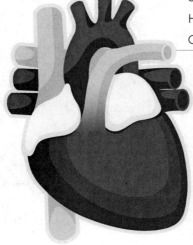

diaphoresis. Profuse sweating

7.4 Cardiovascular system *continued*

CONDITION	CAUSES/RISK FACTORS	SYMPTOMS	TREATMENT
Congestive heart failure (CHF)	Smoking Obesity Sedentary lifestyle High-cholesterol diet Hypertension	Shortness of breath Wheezing *Peripheral edema* in legs Irregular heartbeat	Medications to address tachycardia Diuretic medication to treat edema Antihypertensive medications
Mitral valve prolapse	Usually unknown Hereditary or related to nervous system disorders	Mild cases usually have no symptoms Severe cases can have shortness of breath and palpitations	None for mild cases Medication to treat symptoms Surgery to repair
Thrombophlebitis	Prolonged periods of inactivity Hormone replacement therapy Cancer Paralysis Thrombophlebitis	Pain in affected area Redness Swelling	Heat Compression stockings Anticoagulant medication Surgery

7.5 Lymphatic/immune system

CONDITION	CAUSES	SYMPTOMS	TREATMENT
Acquired immunodeficiency syndrome (AIDS)	HIV virus	Low T-cell counts Fever Diaphoresis Susceptibility to frequent infection Weight loss	Antiretroviral medication to slow progression Treatment of secondary infections with antibiotics No cure
Lymphedema	Parasitic infection Trauma Surgical removal of lymph nodes	Persistent tissue swelling	Compression stockings Lymphedema pump Surgery
Mononucleosis	Epstein-Barr virus Cytomegalovirus	Extreme fatigue Sore throat Fever	Supportive care

peripheral edema. Accumulation of fluid causing swelling in tissues, usually in the lower extremities

7.5 Lymphatic/immune system *continued*

CONDITION	CAUSES	SYMPTOMS	TREATMENT
Systemic lupus erythematosus	Medications Bacterial infections Autoimmune	Fatigue Body pain Butterfly rash on face Headaches Nausea Hair loss Weight loss Anemia Shortness of breath	NSAIDs (steroids, topical creams)
Celiac disease	Genetic defect Lack of enzyme that breaks down gluten Consumption of gluten triggers autoimmune reaction	Weight loss Bloating Loose stools Eventual systemic organ wasting due to lack of nutrients Malabsorption	Gluten-free diet

7.6 Respiratory system

CONDITION	CAUSES	SYMPTOMS	TREATMENT
Asthma	Allergens Pollutants Dust mites Cigarette smoke	Wheezing Coughing Feeling of tightness in chest	Avoiding allergens/irritants Rescue inhaler for bronchodilation Anti-inflammatory steroid inhalers Leukotriene-receptor antagonists Steroid injection for an acute episode
Atelectasis	Cystic fibrosis COPD Pleurisy Lung cancer Spontaneous	Dyspnea Cyanosis Diaphoresis Pain	Thoracentesis Chest percussion Deep breathing exercises Intermittent positive-pressure breathing

7.6 Respiratory system *continued*

CONDITION	CAUSES	SYMPTOMS	TREATMENT
Bronchitis	Viral Environmental pollutants Cigarette smoke	Yellow-gray or green productive cough Chest tightness Dyspnea Fever	Cough medicine Humidifier Inhalers Antibiotics in some cases
Chronic obstructive pulmonary disease (COPD)	Smoking Environmental pollutants	Dyspnea *Hypoxia* Fatigue Cough	Smoking cessation Inhalers Lung transplant in extreme cases
Emphysema	Damage to the alveoli caused by cigarette smoke Pollutants Specific types of dust	Shortness of breath Chronic cough Fatigue	Smoking cessation Avoiding cold environments Antibiotics for secondary lung infections
Influenza	Respiratory virus	Fever Muscle pain Fatigue Sore throat *Rhinorrhea*	Symptomatic OTC analgesics for aches and fever Antiviral medication
Legionnaires' disease	Legionella bacteria that grow in standing water	Dyspnea Cough Headache Fever	Antibiotics Respiratory medications Oxygen Fever medication (antipyretic)
Pneumonia	Bacterial Viral Parasitic	Thick, colored sputum Dyspnea Fever Cough	Rest Antibiotics OTC analgesics
Pulmonary edema	Congestive heart failure Myocardial infarction Heart valve disorders Drowning Injury	*Orthopnea* Dyspnea Wheeze Productive cough Weight gain Pallor	Oxygen therapy Diuretics

hypoxia. Lacking oxygen in the body
rhinorrhea. Runny nose
orthopnea. Difficulty breathing in any position other than standing or sitting

7.6 Respiratory system *continued*

CONDITION	CAUSES	SYMPTOMS	TREATMENT
Pulmonary embolism	Blood clot blocking an artery in the lung	Dyspnea Chest pain Cough Fainting Rapid onset of shortness of breath Diaphoresis	Circulation support (compression hose) Rest Anticoagulant medication Surgically implanted filter
Severe acute respiratory syndrome (SARS)	Viral	Fever Headache Dry cough	Rest Antiviral medication
Tuberculosis (TB)	Bacterial	Chronic cough Weight loss Fatigue Night sweats Painful or difficult breathing	Isolation if symptomatic Medication therapy for 6 to 12 months

7.7 Nervous system

CONDITION	CAUSES	SYMPTOMS	TREATMENT
Alzheimer's disease	Degenerative brain disease Possibly genetic or environmental	Confusion Memory loss Impaired judgment Personality change Worsens over time	Physical activity Socialization Medication to slow the progression No cure
Bell's palsy	Unknown cause	Weakness or paralysis of facial muscles Facial numbness and drooping Headache	NSAIDs Pain relievers Usually self-resolving
Seizures	Birth trauma Infections Brain injury Head trauma Drug withdrawal	Uncontrolled muscle contractions Loss of consciousness Visual disturbances	Medication Brain surgery

7.7 Nervous system *continued*

CONDITION	CAUSES	SYMPTOMS	TREATMENT
Meningitis	Bacterial, viral, fungal infection causing inflammation of the meninges	Stiff neck Headache Fever Vomiting	Appropriate medications for type Bacterial can be fatal
Multiple sclerosis (MS)	Viral Genetic Immune system dysfunction	Loss of ability to speak, walk Double vision Loss of balance Weakness in arms/legs	Supportive Medications to slow progression No cure
Parkinson's disease	Lack of neurotransmitters Brain tumors Drugs Head trauma	Arm/leg muscle and joint stiffness Lack of coordination Tremor	Supportive Medications to slow progression No cure
Stroke	Blockage of artery in neck or brain	Paralysis Confusion Memory impairment Some symptoms can be permanent	Physical therapy Occupational therapy Speech therapy
Migraine headache	Hormones Stress Dietary Familial	Dull to throbbing head pain Sensitivity to light, sound Nausea, vomiting Visual aura	Medications Alternative methods (acupuncture, biofeedback, magnesium)

7.8 Reproductive system

CONDITION	CAUSES/RISK FACTORS	SYMPTOMS	TREATMENT
Benign prostatic hyperplasia (BPH)	Increased age Increased level of dihydrotestosterone	Feeling of full bladder after urinating Weak urine flow Needing to urinate often	Alpha blockers Minimally invasive surgical procedures Transurethral resection of the prostate (TURP)
Hydrocele	Failure of inguinal ring to close properly in development Injury or swelling of the scrotum	Few symptoms Pain Increased size of scrotum	Surgery if symptomatic

7.8 Reproductive system *continued*

CONDITION	CAUSES/RISK FACTORS	SYMPTOMS	TREATMENT
Prostate cancer	Unknown Genetics	Pain Erectile dysfunction Dysuria	Hormone therapy Radiation therapy Surgery Cryosurgery Chemotherapy
Sexually transmitted infections	Unprotected contact with infected tissue or fluids	Varies depending on infection/disease Pelvic or penile pain Sores Itching or discharge Dysuria Body rash Infertility	Varies depending on infection/disease Medication Cryosurgery Immunizations
Endometriosis	Unknown	Most have no symptoms Pelvic pain, especially during menses Painful urination and defecation Infertility issues	NSAIDs Gonadotropin-releasing hormone agonists Oral contraceptives Progestins Surgical intervention
Pelvic inflammatory disease	Untreated STDs/STIs Multiple sexual partners Frequent douching	Lower abdominal pain Back pain Fever Rapid pulse Vaginal discharge Pain during sexual intercourse	Antibiotic treatment Surgical intervention to treat scarring
Cervical cancer	Particular strains of human papillomavirus (HPV)	Abnormal vaginal bleeding Lower abdominal or pelvic pain Abnormal vaginal discharge Pain during sexual intercourse	Surgical intervention (partial or complete hysterectomy, removal of lymph nodes in affected regions) Chemotherapy Radiation therapy

7.9 Urinary system

CONDITION	CAUSES	SYMPTOMS	TREATMENT
Acute kidney failure	Burns Dehydration Hemorrhage Low blood pressure Trauma	Little to no urine production Swelling in extremities Mental confusion Coma Seizures Nose bleeds	Increase dietary protein Fluid and potassium intake regulation Dialysis
Chronic kidney disease	Diabetes Hypertension Kidney stones Polycystic kidney disease	Headache Seizures Confusion Fatigue Anemia Abnormal heart or lung sounds	Antibiotics Blood transfusion Control of blood pressure Dialysis Kidney transplant
Incontinence	Nervous system disorders Urinary tract infection (UTI) Bladder cancer Prostate disorders	Involuntary urination	Medication Surgical removal of the prostate Kegel exercises Surgery
Polycystic kidney disease	Enlarged kidneys due to cysts Inherited	Hypertension Fatigue Anemia Heart murmurs	Medication Draining of cysts Surgical removal of kidney
Pyelonephritis	Bladder infection that spreads to kidneys	Fatigue Fever Painful urination Cloudy or bloody urine	Antibiotics
Renal calculi	Highly concentrated urine UTI Gout	Severe back or abdominal pain Fever Nausea Urgency	Medication Surgery *Lithotripsy*

lithotripsy. Destruction of kidney stones using shock waves

7.10 Digestive system

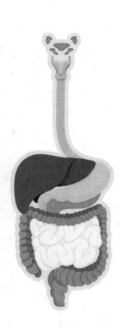

PATHOLOGY	CAUSES	SYMPTOMS	TREATMENT
Appendicitis	*Idiopathic* inflammation of the appendix	RLQ pain Loss of appetite Nausea	Antibiotics Appendectomy
Cirrhosis	Scarring of liver Can be autoimmune Medication Alcohol Hepatitis B or C	Anemia Fatigue Fever Enlarged liver Jaundice Weight loss	Avoid alcohol consumption Antibiotics Diuretics
Cholelithiasis (gallstones)	Insoluble cholesterol and bile salt	Can be asymptomatic Radiating right upper quadrant pain Fever Nausea, vomiting	Laparoscopic cholecystectomy Lithotripsy
Colitis (inflammation of the large intestine)	Viral or bacterial infection	Diarrhea Abdominal pain Bloating	Treatment of underlying cause Surgery
Constipation (difficulty eliminating feces)	Inactivity Lack of fiber and water in diet Medications	Bloating Abdominal pain Hard feces	Increased dietary fiber and water Physical activity
Crohn's disease	Inflammatory bowel disease Autoimmune	Fever Joint pain Tender gums Abnormal abdominal sounds Constipation or diarrhea Intestinal bleeding	Dietary changes Antibiotics Surgery
Diverticulitis (abnormal out-pouching of intestinal wall)	Bacterial Viral Parasitic	Constipation or diarrhea Bloody stools Abdominal pain Nausea	High-fiber diet Antibiotics

idiopathic. Of unknown origin

7.10 Digestive system *continued*

PATHOLOGY	CAUSES	SYMPTOMS	TREATMENT
Diverticulitis (abnormal out-pouching of intestinal wall)	Bacterial Viral Parasitic	Constipation or diarrhea Bloody stools Abdominal pain Nausea	High-fiber diet Antibiotics
Hemorrhoids (varicose vein of the rectum or anus)	Constipation Straining during bowel movements Pelvic pressure during pregnancy, childbirth	Itching, pain in anal area Blood with bowel movements Visible protrusion from the anus	High-fiber diet Stool softeners Surgical removal
Hiatal hernia (part of stomach protrudes through diaphragm into chest cavity)	Unknown causes Smoking Obesity	Heartburn Chest pain Excessive burping Nausea, vomiting	Weight reduction Medication Surgical repair
Stomach ulcer	Bacterial infection Smoking Medication	Nausea, vomiting Abdominal pain	Antibiotics Antacid medication Surgery

7.11 Common injuries

INJURY	CAUSE	SYMPTOMS	DIAGNOSIS	TREATMENT
Anterior cruciate ligament (ACL) tear	Plant and twist motion of the foot and knee	Pain Swelling Knee buckling	Physical exam Radiographic confirmation (typically MRI)	*RICE* Surgical repair Allograft Physical therapy
Concussion	Head impact	Nausea Loss of balance Disorientation Headache	Physical exam Neurologic testing CT of the brain	Rest Treatment of symptoms
Muscle strain	Overexertion of a muscle not properly warmed up for activity level	Pain Swelling "Tight" feeling	Physical exam MRI	RICE Avoiding physical strain to the area

RICE. The treatment for many musculoskeletal system injuries (Rest, Ice, Compression, Elevation)

7.11 Common injuries *continued*

INJURY	CAUSE	SYMPTOMS	DIAGNOSIS	TREATMENT
Epicondylitis (tennis elbow)	Overuse of elbow causing tiny ligament tears	Swelling Tenderness Grip weakness	Physical exam X-ray MRI	Rest Ice NSAIDs Forearm strap Extended break from aggravating activity
Rotator cuff tear	Repetitive stress of the shoulder joint	Pain Weakness Inability to raise arm over head	Physical exam X-ray MRI	Rest NSAIDs Cortisone injection to shoulder joint Surgery
Bone fracture	Impact injury resulting in bone cracking or breaking Stress fractures: overuse or repetitive stress	Pain Swelling Loss of function	Physical exam X-ray CT if plain films are not clear	Immobilization with internal or external device (cast, splint, pins, plates, screws)
Joint dislocation (subluxations)	Impact injury removing bones from proper joint alignment	Pain Loss of sensation Immobility	Physical exam X-ray MRI CT	Realignment of bones Immobilization Physical therapy to strengthen surrounding muscles Surgery for repeated incidences

GAME **Body systems**

Identify the body system affected by each medical condition. The systems are cardiovascular, digestive, endocrine, integumentary, lymphatic/immune, musculoskeletal, nervous, reproductive, respiratory, and urinary.

CONDITION	BODY SYSTEM	CONDITION	BODY SYSTEM
1. Acne		10. Hemorrhoids	
2. AIDS		11. Meningitis	
3. Aneurysm		12. Parkinson's disease	
4. Arthritis		13. Pneumonia	
5. Chronic kidney disease		14. Psoriasis	
6. Crohn's disease		15. Pyelonephritis	
7. Diabetes mellitus		16. Thrombophlebitis	
8. Endometriosis		17. Tuberculosis	
9. Gout		18. Pleurisy	

Key: 1. Integumentary; 2. Lymphatic/immune; 3. Cardiovascular; 4. Musculoskeletal; 5. Urinary; 6. Digestive; 7. Endocrine; 8. Reproductive; 9. Musculoskeletal; 10. Digestive; 11. Nervous; 12. Nervous; 13. Respiratory; 14. Integumentary; 15. Urinary; 16. Cardiovascular; 17. Respiratory; 18. Respiratory

DIAGNOSTIC MEASURES AND TREATMENT MODALITIES

To best assess and diagnose the pathophysiologic effects of a disease on the body, providers use a variety of diagnostic testing in conjunction with the patient's medical history and a thorough physical examination. Common tests include blood work, urinalysis, and diagnostic imaging (x-ray, ultrasound). When using an imaging modality that has radiation, there is some risk involved; however, it is generally considered minimal. It is the provider's responsibility to determine that the benefits of a radiologic procedure outweigh any risks involved. In addition, many diagnostic imaging procedures use alternate methods of image production that do not use radiation.

Diagnostic imaging studies that use radiation include x-rays, computed tomography (CT), angiography, mammography, and nuclear medicine studies. Diagnostic imaging that does not use radiation or radiologic waves include magnetic resonance imaging (MRI), which uses an electromagnetic field to produce images, and ultrasound, which uses sound waves.

The use of contrast material is also common with diagnostic imaging. Many body structures appear dark on imaging studies (radiolucent) due to their lack of density. Contrast aids in making those structures more radiopaque (lighter/brighter); thereby making them easier for the radiologist to visualize on a radiograph.

Contrast materials include air, barium, gadolinium, and iodine. These contrast substances can be administered orally, through injection, or intravenously.

Nuclear medicine is a type of diagnostic imaging that involves the administration of radioactive isotopes that will collect in areas of high metabolic activity. Examples of nuclear imaging include SPECT scan (used to assess brain damage following a stroke), PET scan (used to diagnose brain related disorders), and MUGA scan (used to evaluate the condition of the heart muscle).

INCIDENCE, PREVALENCE, AND RISK FACTORS

Incidence refers to the occurrence of new diseases or cases in a specific population over a distinct time period. Some conditions occur more often than others and more commonly in specific populations. Incidence of injuries can be classified into groups of people who participate in specific activities. For example, the number of college athletes who suffer from ACL injuries will likely be higher than the number of kindergarten teachers who do.

Prevalence refers to the proportion of a population who have a particular disease over a specific period of time. Prevalence includes all cases while incidence is limited to only new cases. In some demographic areas, there might be a higher prevalence of some diseases due to infectious reservoirs within the community. A medical assistant will often see trends in the types of conditions being treated due to environmental or seasonal changes.

Risk factors are characteristics that make a person more likely to suffer a disease or injury. These can be modifiable or nonmodifiable. For example, a high-fat diet is a risk factor for developing heart disease and is modifiable. A family history of breast cancer is considered a nonmodifiable risk factor.

7.12 Incidence vs. prevalence

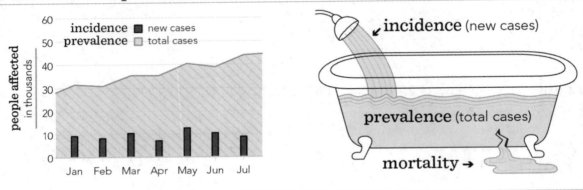

RISK FACTORS LEADING TO HIGH MORTALITY AND MORBIDITY

There are some risk factors that are out of a person's control. For example, heredity can put people at higher risk for developing diseases that their family members have also had. However, there are also many high-risk activities that contribute to the likelihood of a person becoming ill or suffering an injury.

Determinants of health

A wide range of factors influence a person's and a population's health status; these are known as determinants of health. The relationship between biology and genetics, behavior, availability of health resources, social standards, and policy/lawmaker involvement have the largest effect on the health of a population.

---

incidence. The rate of new (or newly diagnosed) cases of a disease or injury

prevalence. The number of active cases of a disease or injury

Morbidity vs. mortality

Morbidity refers to the measure of sickness or disease within a specific population or area. Mortality is the measure of deaths in an area or a population.

These two measures often go hand-in-hand because morbidity can lead to mortality. These rates are measured and tracked by the Centers for Disease Control (CDC) as well as the World Health Organization (WHO) to identify global health trends and render aid to affected areas. Documentation by the medical assistant and other health care staff is crucial in assuring the statistics are accurately reported.

Common comorbid diseases

Comorbidities are diseases or conditions in one person at the same time. Often these comorbidities are chronic in nature. Multiple health issues occurring simultaneously can make diagnosis and treatment more difficult. Obesity, heart disease, and diabetes mellitus are common comorbid conditions.

Upstream management in population health

Upstream management refers to health care organizations becoming increasingly involved in the health of its population, even when patients are not in the clinic or hospitals. Community outreach programs, education, and involvement of health care organizations in the community have shown to increase the overall health of populations, thereby reducing the number of recurring health conditions and lowering health care costs. The medical assistant plays a key role in patient education and can enhance patient compliance. The goal of upstream management is to assist patients in staying healthy and to keep them out of health care facilities by improving their understanding of contributing health factors.

ENDEMIC, EPIDEMIC, AND PANDEMIC

Endemic disease is an illness that is constantly present within a community. An epidemic is when an infectious disease spreads rapidly to a large number of people. A pandemic is a world-wide outbreak of a disease.

An epidemic can turn into a pandemic if measures are not taken to keep the illness under control. There is no absolute way to prevent an epidemic or pandemic from occurring, but vaccines help reduce the number of people at risk. Cough protocols, handwashing, and the use of hand sanitizer also aid in preventing the spread of disease and illness. Medical assistants are often involved in educating patients on these disease prevention measures. The CDC and WHO monitor disease outbreaks very closely to control the spread of illness before it reaches pandemic levels. WHO researches potential causative agents and is responsible for the development of vaccines.

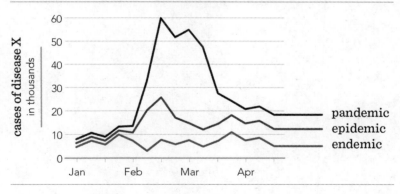

7.13 **Endemic vs. epidemic vs. pandemic**

SUMMARY

Disease, illness, and injury are threats faced by people every day in every community. The accurate diagnosis of conditions, effective treatment and management, and—most importantly—disease prevention are the cornerstones for quality medicine and health care. All health care workers commit to the safe and reliable treatment of sick and injured patients. A strong foundational knowledge of disease, risk factors, and disease prevention will aid a medical assistant throughout their career and make them an invaluable part of any health care team.

CHAPTER 8
Microbiology

OVERVIEW

Microbiology involves the study of a variety of small life forms, often at the cellular level. To understand how this science applies to everyday practice, medical assistants should have a basic knowledge of cell structure and an elemental ability to distinguish harmless microscopic life forms from harmful ones. Patients will have many different types of *infections* and infestations, so it is important to understand which types of *pathogens* cause which diseases, as well as the steps people can take to prevent acquiring and spreading these diseases.

Objectives

Upon completion of this chapter, you should be able to:

- Locate and describe the functions of a cell's organelles.
- List major categories of micro-organisms and give examples of diseases each causes.
- Differentiate between pathogens and nonpathogens.
- List infectious agents that cause disease and describe the chain of infection and conditions for growth.

MICROBIOLOGY

Microbiology is the study of living forms only visible under a microscope. Micro-organisms are everywhere and usually cause no problems; in fact, some are actually helpful. However, under conditions such as an impairment of immunity (resistance to disease), micro-organisms—especially those that are inherently harmful—can cause serious infections. Primarily, the medical assistant needs to be aware of the harmful micro-organisms to help prevent their transmission, treat infections, and instruct patients about them.

CELL STRUCTURE

To understand how micro-organisms affect the human body, it is important to understand the structure of living cells. Understanding cell structure requires a basic knowledge of chemistry, which is the study of what makes up matter and how it changes. At the body's lowest level of organization—its chemical level—are the same elements that form everything in the environment. For example, oxygen is an element made of oxygen atoms. When the atoms of the elements oxygen and hydrogen bond in various proportions, they form a compound: water.

Chemical compounds react and combine to form millions of cells, which are the basic units of life. There are many types of body cells, each with a specific purpose and function. The basic structural components of most human cells are the cell membrane, cytoplasm, nuclear membrane, and nucleus. These and other organelles (the structures within or on a cell that perform a specific function) make up the various types of cells that form the human body as a whole.

8.1 Water molecule

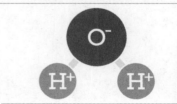

infection. The invasion and proliferation of pathogens in body tissues
pathogen. Disease-causing micro-organism.

Organelles

Cell membrane

The cell membrane is the thin, outermost structure of human cells. It is selectively permeable, which means that it lets some substances in and out but blocks the passage of others. In bacterial cells, the cell membrane lies within the cell wall.

Cell wall

The cell wall is the outmost layer of the cell that maintains its shape and protects it. Human cells do not have a cell wall, but bacteria cells do. Each bacterium has a cell wall that is either gram-positive or gram-negative, which is important when providers select a medication to treat the particular bacterial infection. A specific antibiotic targets bacteria according to its cell-wall structure but does not damage human cells because they do not contain cell walls.

Nucleus

The nucleus is a round structure that is inside the cell, usually near its center. It is the largest organelle in the cell, and it controls the cell's functions. The nucleus contains chromosomes, which are the thread-like structures made of the person's deoxyribonucleic acid (DNA), the compound that contains the body's *genetic* information.

8.2 Anatomy of a cell

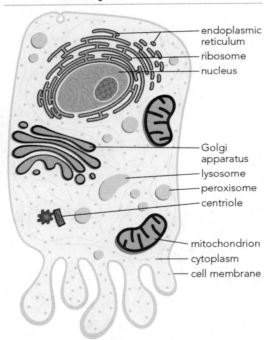

endoplasmic reticulum
ribosome
nucleus
Golgi apparatus
lysosome
peroxisome
centriole
mitochondrion
cytoplasm
cell membrane

Nuclear membrane

The nuclear membrane, or nuclear envelope, is the structure that surrounds the nucleus. It contains pores that allow larger compounds to move in and out of the cell's nucleus.

Cytoplasm

Cytoplasm is the inside of the cell that contains other organelles, such as mitochondria, that perform the functions of the cells. The components of cytoplasm are water, proteins, *ions*, and nutrients.

Ribosome

A ribosome is an organelle that contributes to protein synthesis, which is the building of proteins from their basic components, the amino acids. The ribosomes support the protein chains as ribonucleic acid (RNA) builds them.

genetic. Involving genes, the parts of a cell that control or influence the appearance, growth, and other characteristics of a living thing

ion. An atom or group of atoms that has a positive or negative electric charge

Endoplasmic reticulum

The endoplasmic reticulum provides networks of passageways for moving various substances within the cytoplasm. Where it has ribosomes on its surface area, it is the rough endoplasmic reticulum; otherwise, it is the smooth endoplasmic reticulum.

Mitochondrion

A mitochondrion is an organelle that gives the cells energy. Cells might have one or more mitochondria, depending on how much energy the particular cell needs to perform its specific functions.

Lysosome

The function of the lysosome organelle within the cell is digestion.

Centriole

A centriole is a cylindrical-shaped organelle that plays a role in cell division, with each pair in the cell making sure to divide the chromosomes equally to the cells that result from the reproduction process.

Golgi apparatus

The Golgi apparatus synthesizes carbohydrates and sorts the proteins the ribosome is supporting. It also has some storage functions prior to preparing some substances for removal from the cells.

Peroxisome

A peroxisome is an organelle in the cytoplasm that contains enzymes.

Flagellum

A flagellum is a tail-like appendage that allows the cell to move in a swimming-like motion. A sperm cell has a flagellum to help it move toward egg cells.

Cilia

Cilia are hair-like projections that help move substances through various tracts and paths in the body. Some mucous membranes, such as those in the respiratory tract, have cilia.

Q: What type of cell in the human body has a flagellum?

A: A sperm cell has a flagellum, a tail-like appendage that helps it swim toward egg cells.

ORGANISMS AND TYPES OF MICRO-ORGANISMS

Organisms are any living things. Micro-organisms are tiny (often one-celled) living things. Medical assistants should be aware of the various categories of micro-organisms that typically cause infections and other disorders.

Common categories of micro-organisms

Here are the most common categories of micro-organisms. Others, such as algae, are not major causes of common diseases.

Bacteria

A bacterium is a single-cell micro-organism that reproduces rapidly and causes many different infections. It can survive without other living tissue. Bacteria have various classifications according to their shape, cell-wall structures, ability to retain some chemical stains, and whether they can grow with (aerobic) or without (anaerobic) air. Common shapes of bacteria are coccus (round), spirillum (spiral-shaped), vibrio (shaped like a comma), and bacillus (rod-shaped). There are also distinct groups of bacteria, such as rickettsiae, that live and grow only inside of other living things, such as insects. People acquire these bacteria from insect bites.

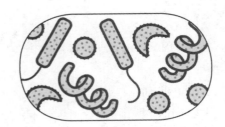

Antibiotics are medications that kill bacteria, so they are a major component of treatment plans for bacterial infections. However, with overuse of antibiotic therapy over many years, some bacteria have developed resistance to antibiotics and are now difficult to kill. Examples are methicillin-resistant *Staphylococcus aureus* and vancomycin-resistant enterococci.

Bacteria and some other pathogens have a specific naming convention. The first word conveys the micro-organism's genus, which is a biologic classification between the family and the species. The second word is its species. Examples are *Staphylococcus aureus*, *Pseudomonas aeruginosa*, and *Escherichia coli*. Thus *Staphylococcus epidermis* is a bacterium that belongs to a group (genus) of other staphylococcal bacteria, and its species is epidermis.

Q: What term describes bacteria that can live without air?

A: Anaerobic bacteria do not need air to grow.

Viruses

A virus is a tiny micro-organism that causes many infections and diseases. Viruses require living tissue to survive and grow; so unlike bacteria, they are actually *parasites*. Because viruses need living tissue to reproduce, it can be challenging for laboratory technicians to grow or test them.

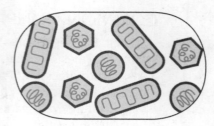

Viruses are complex. When they invade, they attach to host cells in the person. Their genetic material then takes control of the host cells, destroying them and infecting nearby cells. Some viruses attack immediately, while others lie dormant and attack later. Viruses tend to change (mutate) during replication (reproduction), which makes it difficult to build adequate immunity to them. Some are difficult or impossible to kill with medications. Some antiviral drugs exist, but they have various degrees of effectiveness against some viruses. Common viruses include the human immunodeficiency virus (HIV), influenza viruses, and human papilloma virus (HPV).

Fungi

A fungus is a micro-organism that grows on or in animals and plants. The single-cell fungi are yeasts; multi-cell varieties are spore-producing molds. Most fungi do not normally cause disease. Those that do tend to cause superficial infections like athlete's foot and vaginal yeast infections. People who have a weakened *immune system*, however, are at risk for much more serious internal fungal infections.

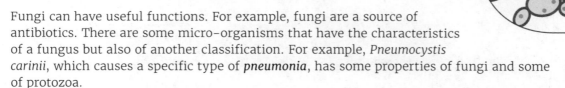

Fungi can have useful functions. For example, fungi are a source of antibiotics. There are some micro-organisms that have the characteristics of a fungus but also of another classification. For example, *Pneumocystis carinii*, which causes a specific type of *pneumonia*, has some properties of fungi and some of protozoa.

Protozoa

A protozoon is a single-cell parasite that can be microscopic or large enough to see without a microscope. Protozoa thrive in damp environments and in bodies of standing water, such as ponds and lakes. They replicate rapidly inside a living host. An example of a disease-causing protozoon is *Entamoeba histolytica*, an ameba that causes dysentery, a severe type of diarrhea.

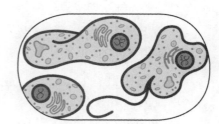

Multicellular parasites

Although this category does not fit the definition of microbiology, these organisms cause infections and infestations. Examples are lice, bed bugs, scabies, and pinworms.

parasite. An organism that lives in, on, or at the expense of another organism without contributing to the host's survival

immune system. The organs and structures that regulate the body's immunity, or resistance to disease

pneumonia. Inflammation of the lungs

COMMON NONPATHOGENS AND PATHOGENS

Some micro-organisms are helpful or do not cause disease under normal circumstances. These are nonpathogens. For example, the bacteria in the *gastrointestinal tract*, such as *Lactobacillus acidophilus*, assist with digestion. Probiotics (micro-organisms that promote health) have become popular dietary supplements. They are live micro-organisms (usually bacteria) that are similar to the beneficial micro-organisms in the gastrointestinal tract. Proponents make claims about the health benefits of using these often costly supplements, and there is some evidence probiotics are helpful with digestive disorders and in preventing the diarrhea that easily results from antibiotic therapy. However, the validity of other health claims is still uncertain, as is the safety of probiotics in supplement form. Remind patients that probiotics are available in much less costly products (yogurt, sauerkraut, kimchi [Korean-style fermented vegetables]).

Some micro-organisms are not so helpful. These are pathogens, the micro-organisms that cause infectious disease and infestations. Everyone is at risk for the infections and infestations pathogens cause, but those whose immunity is low, such as patients receiving *chemotherapy* to treat cancer and those who have *acquired immunodeficiency syndrome (AIDS)*, are at especially high risk. Infection can also result when micro-organisms usually present in the body, its normal flora, "overgrow" for any of a variety of reasons. The following tables list disease-causing pathogens by classification.

8.3 Common disease-causing viruses

PATHOGEN	DISEASE	TRANSMISSION
adenovirus	*pharyngitis*	*droplet*, direct *contact*
Epstein-Barr	mononucleosis	contact with saliva
hepatitis A	hepatitis A	fecal-oral
hepatitis B	hepatitis B	*bloodborne*, sexual
hepatitis C	hepatitis C	bloodborne
herpes simplex	cold sores, genital herpes	contact with blister fluid, sexual
human immunodeficiency	AIDS	bloodborne, sexual
human papillomavirus	genital warts	sexual
influenza	influenza	*airborne*, droplet
measles	measles	airborne, droplet
molluscipoxvirus	molluscum contagiosum warts	contact

gastrointestinal tract. The organs and structures of the digestive tract, from the mouth to the anus

chemotherapy. Course of treatment with drugs that destroy or inhibit the growth and division of malignant (cancerous) cells; any chemical agents that treat disease, but in common usage generally means cancer treatment

acquired immunodeficiency syndrome (AIDS). The most advanced stage of infection with the human immunodeficiency virus and resulting in low resistance to disease

pharyngitis. Inflammation of the pharynx, the back of the throat between the mouth and the nasal cavities

droplet. Referring to the transmission of diseases from an infected person propelling pathogens through the air on particles larger than 5 microns in size to a susceptible person's eyes, nose, or mouth. Droplet transmission is usually limited to a distance of 1 meter or 3 feet.

contact. Referring to the transmission of diseases by the physical transfer of pathogens from a contaminated object to a susceptible host's body surface

bloodborne. Referring to direct contact through nonintact skin or mucous membranes with blood, body fluids, or tissue from an infected person

airborne. Referring to the transmission of diseases from an infected person propelling pathogens through the air on particles smaller than 5 microns in size to a susceptible person's eyes, nose, or mouth. Airborne particles are transmitted as aerosols and can be suspended in the air for long periods of time.

8.3 Common disease-causing viruses *continued*

PATHOGEN	DISEASE	TRANSMISSION
mumps	mumps	airborne, droplet
parvovirus	fifth disease	droplet, bloodborne
rabies	rabies	*vector* (infected animal)
rhinoviruses	common cold	droplet, contact, *fomites*
rotavirus	rotavirus	fecal-oral
rubella	German measles	airborne, droplet
varicella-zoster	chickenpox, shingles	airborne, droplet, contact with blister fluid
Variola major	smallpox	contact, fomites

8.4 Common disease-causing multicellular parasites

PATHOGEN	DISEASE	TRANSMISSION
Ascaris lumbricoides	roundworm	contact with contaminated soil
Cimex parasites	bed bugs	contact with infested bedding or furniture
Diphyllobothrium latum	tapeworm	foodborne (raw, infected fish)
Enterobius vermicularis	pinworms	fecal-oral
Pediculus humanus capitis	pediculosis (head lice)	contact with infested hair
Phthirus pubis	pubic lice ("crabs")	contact with infested pubic hair
Sarcoptes scabiei	scabies	contact

8.5 Common disease-causing fungi

PATHOGEN	DISEASE	TRANSMISSION
Aspergillus fumigatus	aspergillosis	airborne
Candida albicans	candidiasis (thrush, vaginal yeast infection)	overgrowth of normal flora, not usually sexual
Cryptococcus neoformans	cryptococcosis	contact with poultry droppings
Trichophyton rubrum, Trichophyton tonsurans (dermatophytes)	ringworm	contact
Histoplasma capsulatum	histoplasmosis	airborne
Pneumocystis jirovecii, Pneumocystis carinii	Pneumocystis pneumonia	airborne

vector. A living thing that carries pathogens

fomite. Any nonliving object or substance capable of carrying infectious organisms

8.6 Common disease-causing protozoa

PATHOGEN	DISEASE	TRANSMISSION
Entamoeba histolytica	amebiasis	fecal-oral
Giardia intestinalis (Giardia lamblia)	giardiasis	fecal-oral
Plasmodium parasites	malaria	vector (mosquito)
Toxoplasma gondii	toxoplasmosis	foodborne, vector (animal), transplacental (pregnant patient to fetus)
Trichinella spiralis	trichinosis	foodborne (undercooked pork)
Trichomonas vaginalis	trichomoniasis	sexual

8.7 Common disease-causing bacteria

PATHOGEN	DISEASE	TRANSMISSION
Bacillus anthracis	anthrax	vector, contact with or eating undercooked meat from infected animals, spore inhalation
Bordetella pertussis	whooping cough	airborne
Borrelia burgdorferi	Lyme disease	vector (tick)
Campylobacter jejuni	food poisoning	contaminated food and fluids
Chlamydia trachomatis	chlamydia	sexual
Clostridium botulinum	botulism	foodborne
Clostridium difficile	colitis	fecal-oral
Clostridium perfringens	gas gangrene	contact (wounds)
Clostridium tetani	tetanus	contact through a deep cut
Corynebacterium diphtheriae	diphtheria	droplet
Escherichia coli	diarrhea	foodborne
Group B streptococcus	meningitis	droplet
Haemophilus influenzae	pneumonia, epiglottitis meningitis	droplet
Helicobacter pylori	peptic ulcer disease	fecal-oral, oral-anal, possibly others
Legionella pneumophila	Legionnaires' disease	water aerosol
Listeria monocytogenes	meningitis	droplet
Mycobacterium leprae	leprosy	airborne, droplet
Mycobacterium tuberculosis	tuberculosis	airborne, droplet
Mycoplasma pneumoniae	pneumonia	droplet
Neisseria gonorrhoeae	gonorrhea	sexual
Neisseria meningitidis	meningitis	droplet

8.7 Common disease-causing bacteria *continued*

PATHOGEN	DISEASE	TRANSMISSION
Pseudomonas aeruginosa	"hot tub rash"	contaminated water
Rickettsia prowazekii	typhus	vector (tick)
Rickettsia rickettsii	Rocky Mountain spotted fever	vector (tick)
Shigella sonnei	shigellosis	fecal-oral
Staphylococcus aureus	boils, septicemia, pneumonia	contact
Streptococcus pneumoniae	pneumonia	airborne, droplet, contact
Streptococcus pyogenes	strep throat	droplet
	rheumatic fever, septicemia	
Treponema pallidum	syphilis	sexual
Vibrio cholerae	cholera	fecal-oral, contaminated water
Yersinia pestis	plague	vector (fleas, rodents)

Q: What term describes the usual environment of micro-organisms in the human body?

A: The micro-organisms usually present in the body are the normal flora. Infection can result when the micro-organisms overgrow for various reasons.

TRANSMISSION OF INFECTIOUS AGENTS

Infectious agents

Infectious agents are pathogens that cause disease, infection, or infestation. Antimicrobial medications (those that kill or halt the growth of pathogens) can cure or resolve many of these infections. But pathogens—particularly viruses like HIV and herpes simplex—are difficult, if not impossible, to eradicate completely.

The means of transmission of pathogens varies. Some, like HIV and the hepatitis B virus, are bloodborne, meaning they can only be acquired by direct contact between the infected person's blood, tissue, or other body fluids and the other person's nonintact skin or mucous membranes. It is important to understand that a person cannot "catch" a bloodborne virus by casual contact with the infected person or by breathing the same air. However, pregnant patients can transmit some pathogens to the fetus. Cytomegalovirus is an example.

Other pathogens, such as the viruses that cause influenza, spread through the air. A person can acquire those viruses by breathing air an infected person exhales. Still others, such as herpes simplex, can survive on inanimate surfaces or objects (countertops, water bottles) or in food. Contact with the contaminated surface or object spreads the infection. These pathogen–carrying objects are fomites. There are also pathogens (the parasite that causes malaria, and the virus that causes the West Nile virus) that require a vector, such as an insect, to transmit the infection.

Chain of infection

Transmission of a pathogen depends on connecting the following links in the chain of infection.

- Infectious agent

- Reservoir host

- Portal of exit

- Mode of transmission

- Portal of entry

- Susceptible host

Effective infection control breaks this chain, thus preventing the cycle from continuing. Hand hygiene breaks the chain at its first link: the infectious agent.

Killing the agent or removing it from hands helps prevent its transmission to the reservoir host, where it would otherwise infect the host and multiply to later infect others. When it gets that far, it has to have a way to exit the reservoir host. Depending on the pathogen, that could be via blood, body fluids, feces, breath, eyes, ears, nose, mouth, or wounds. The means of transmission is either direct (via contact with the infected person or body fluids and secretions) or indirect (via contaminated objects, vectors, and fomites). Indirect transmission is only possible for pathogens that can survive outside of the reservoir host. Once the infectious agent has a portal of entry—a way to get into the body of the susceptible host—infection flourishes.

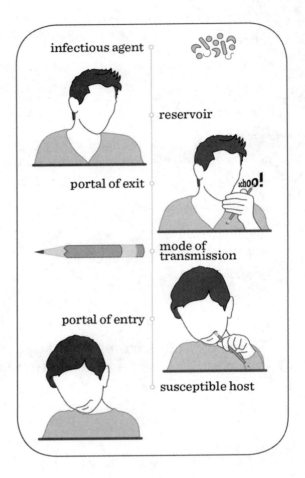

Q: What intervention breaks the chain of infection at its first link?

A: Hand hygiene breaks the chain of infection at its first link: the infectious agent. Killing an infectious agent or removing it from hands interrupts its progression so it cannot reach the second link, the reservoir host.

Conditions for growth

Many factors contribute to the growth of infections, with environmental factors playing a major role. In general, many pathogens multiply easily in moist, dark conditions. Insects that carry pathogens generally require specific environmental conditions. An example is how standing water in a warm climate "breeds" mosquitoes. Poor food safety and handling also increases the risk of infection, especially when food is not stored at safe temperatures via refrigeration or freezing, or when food processing or restaurant workers do not follow hygienic practices such as handwashing and gloving. Another example is handling feces, such as by health care workers or infant day care center employees. Hand hygiene and gloving are absolutely essential for preventing the transmission of *enteral* pathogens.

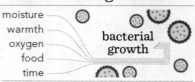

8.8 Conditions for bacterial growth

moisture
warmth
oxygen   bacterial growth
food
time

SUMMARY

A working knowledge of microbiology is a powerful tool for preventing infection and saving lives. Pathogens live to infect, and all health care professionals can use this knowledge to stop pathogens before they can get to a human host. Understanding cell structure and how micro-organisms can invade the body's cells supplies the basis for infection control. Knowing how specific types of pathogens spread and the diseases they cause prepares medical assistants for helping patients—especially those whose immune systems are not fully functioning—to protect themselves against the diseases these tiny pathogens can cause.

---

enteral. Within or by way of the gastrointestinal tract

CHAPTER 9

General Patient Care

OVERVIEW

Medical assistants in ambulatory care provide quality patient care, interact effectively with patients, ensure safety, and assist the provider as necessary. This chapter focuses on those particular areas, highlighting critical knowledge to know and apply in the health care setting.

GENERAL PATIENT CARE

A medical assistant who works in the clinical area of the office must complete several activities prior to the provider examining the patient. Although patient encounters are individualized, the medical assistant follows a consistent intake procedure to ensure patient safety and preparedness for the examination.

PATIENT IDENTIFICATION

The first step in ensuring safety is proper patient identification. The Joint Commission stresses the need to use two methods of identification to validate that care and treatment are delivered to the correct patient. The most common method is to have patients state their full name and date of birth. Avoid stating the patient's name and then asking them to confirm it. A patient could respond to the wrong name, especially in a time of crisis, stress, or illness.

Refer to the study guide addendum on the NHA website for details on CLSI guidelines for patient identification specific to specimen collection.

Objectives

Upon completion of this chapter, you should be able to:

- Positively identify patients following the Joint Commission's National Patient Safety Goals.
- Explain the medical assistant's role in preparing the examination and procedure room.
- Ensure patient safety within the clinical setting and make appropriate adjustments related to the patient's specific needs.
- Complete a comprehensive clinical intake process, including the purpose of the visit.
- List methods and techniques for measuring vital signs.
- Explain methods for obtaining anthropometric measurements.
- Identify, document, and report abnormal vital signs to the appropriate provider.
- Assist the provider with general physical and specialty examinations.
- Prepare patients for procedures.
- List appropriate steps for preparing and administering medications.
- State safe techniques for administering optic, otic, and topical medications.
- List methods that can be used for performing an ear and eye irrigation.
- Identify and respond to emergency or priority situations.
- State procedures for administering first aid and basic wound care.
- List the role of the medical assistant when CPR needs to be administered.
- Assist providers with patients who have minor and traumatic injuries.
- Assist providers with surgical interventions.
- Explain steps for removing staples and sutures.
- Review a provider's discharge instructions or plan of care with patients.
- Follow guidelines for sending orders for prescriptions and refills by telephone, fax, or e-mail.
- Document patient care in the patient's record.
- Perform basic functions in an EHR or EMR.

PREPARING EXAMINATION AND PROCEDURE ROOMS

At the end of each day, disinfect the work area and stock the exam rooms. Upon arriving to work the next day, recheck the rooms for cleanliness and adequacy of supplies. Anticipating items that might be needed for a visit and preparing the room in advance demonstrates a well-run, organized facility. Doing these things each day enhances patient confidence and assists in operational efficiency.

Review schedule to determine reason for visit

The daily schedule typically identifies the patient's name and the reason for the visit. This helps determine how to approach the patient and how to prepare for the visit. If a patient is being seen because a family member is concerned about a progressing Alzheimer's disease, the medical assistant might ask a family member to accompany the patient to the room. Take time to get familiar with the patient by further reviewing the medical record in advance. This allows for an enhanced understanding of the patient's history and concerns while interacting with the patient.

Clean and disinfect the room

Surfaces, including counters and exam tables, should be cleaned at the beginning and end of each day, and between patients to reduce the risk of transmitting infectious agents. The most common solutions used to disinfect surfaces are a sodium hypochlorite solution (which is a 1:10 dilution of household bleach to water) or a commercial chemical surface disinfectant.

Pull appropriate equipment and supplies for visit

Stock routine items such as *personal protective equipment (PPE)*, sharps and biohazard waste containers, exam gowns, and table paper in each of the examination rooms. Also add other items that might be used for the visit. For instance, if a patient is visiting for a history of chest pain, have the EKG machine in the room or nearby with all the supplies necessary to run the tracing. Do not perform testing prior to the provider reviewing the medical record or examining the patient and prescribing the test.

ENSURE PATIENT SAFETY IN THE CLINICAL SETTING

The importance of physical safety in the ambulatory care setting cannot be understated. Take every effort to maximize the safety of patients and staff to prevent injury and avoid litigation. Plan for other considerations, such as fires and natural disasters, to protect human life. This involves preparing emergency policies and evacuation plans, and having emergency equipment easily accessible.

Safety concerns

Avoid cluttered hallways, spills, items on the floor, furniture with sharp corners, restricted doorways, and dimly lit areas in a medical facility. Using floor signs, cleaning spills immediately, strategically arranging furniture, and avoiding loitering in hallways assist in accident prevention. The medical assistant is responsible for helping maintain safety in the office. Resolve safety concerns promptly or report them to the proper authority. Contractors often maintain most of the external environment, but the medical assistant should report sidewalk cracks, loose handrails, snow, or ice to their immediate supervisor.

---

personal protective equipment (PPE). Barrier equipment used to prevent exposure to blood and other body fluids (gloves, goggles, masks)

Safety adjustments for specific populations

Pay particular attention to safety for pediatric patients, older adult patients, and those who have specific needs. Children are prone to injuries by falling on sharp objects, choking on items in a waiting room, or touching electrical sockets. When preparing the patient prior to being seen by the provider, take precautions to avoid a child falling from the examination table. Maintain visual and physical contact with patients until they are returned to their parent or guardian.

Older adult patients or patients who have disabilities can need assistance with walking or getting onto an examination table. Some patients might also need supervision while waiting to be seen. Bathrooms should be equipped with emergency alert buttons; if they aren't available and there is a safety concern, someone should be with or near the patient.

Regardless of patient age or condition, always be alert for potential hazards and take measures to maximize patient safety.

COMPREHENSIVE CLINICAL INTAKE

Upon escorting the patient to the examination room, obtain initial information so the provider can deliver care. An effective medical assistant uses therapeutic communication techniques during the intake process.

Interviewing techniques

Therapeutic communication begins with *active listening*. This allows the medical assistant to fully understand what the patient is communicating verbally and nonverbally. Interviewing also involves asking *open-ended questions* to elicit a more detailed response without leading a patient toward an intended response. *Restatement*, *reflection*, and *clarification* are also valuable tools to use during the interview process.

Medical assistants must also be aware of the *nonverbal communication* they are presenting. For instance, the medical assistant might be trying to ask questions and write at the same time. This can be interpreted as the medical assistant being in a hurry or disinterested in what the patient has to say. Nonverbal communication is left to the interpretation of the receiver. Awareness of posture and gestures, and use of good nonverbal communication facilitate effective therapeutic interactions. Make eye contact with the patient during the interview process. Entering patient information into a computer without looking away from the screen can appear as though the medical assistant is disengaged. This can lead to reluctance by the patient to be completely forthcoming regarding their medical condition.

active listening. Using techniques that allow the receiver to fully understand the message being communicated

open-ended questions. Questions that lead to further explanation (vs. a yes or no response)

restatement. Repeating or paraphrasing information relayed by the sender to confirm accuracy

reflection. When the receiver focuses on the main idea of the message but incorporates feelings the sender might be exhibiting or possibly feeling

clarification. Summarizing the information relayed by the sender to clear up any confusion

nonverbal communication. Gestures and actions that leave interpretation up to the receiver

Rapport and empathy

The patient needs to be able to trust the medical assistant to communicate honestly. Providing privacy, showing interest, and respecting the diversity and individuality of each patient facilitates a trusting relationship. Empathy is an effective tool in communication and establishing a rapport, whereas *sympathy* leads to poor therapeutic communication and health professional burn-out.

Parts of the intake process

The intake process is also referred to as "rooming" patients. It is the process of gathering initial information. Depending on the type of visit, the amount of information collected varies, but all patients should have a chief complaint and medication review at each visit.

Obtaining the chief complaint

A *chief complaint* is *subjective information* and best documented in the medical record in the patient's own words. This is likely the first piece of information the medical assistant records that identifies the reason for the visit. "Please tell me why you are coming in today" and "What brings you to the office today?" are open-ended questions that elicit the chief complaint.

Performing a drug reconciliation

Routinely ask patients to bring all medications or a current list to the office for appointments. This helps the medical assistant compare medications being taken to those in the medical record, and assists in ensuring patients are following the correct instructions.

Medication reconciliation is a formal process necessary at every office visit. Comparing the patient's list of medications to the medical record is a safety measure that reduces the risk of improper prescription, medication interactions, and adverse reactions.

---

sympathy. Feeling compassion, sorrow, or pity for the hardships that another person encounters

chief complaint. Reason for the office visit

subjective information. Information that is personal or what someone is feeling

Documenting allergy status

A patient can be quick to identify an *allergy* if any unusual reaction to a substance occurs. Ask what allergies the patient has and what kind of reaction occurred to help the provider determine if an allergic reaction is likely to occur in the future. Document the allergy status in the medical record. Avoid exposing a patient to a substance that can lead to an allergic reaction or life-threatening *anaphylaxis*. Most electronic formats offer safety measures of alerting the provider if a prescription that causes a reaction is prescribed. In a paper chart, the allergy should be flagged in several areas.

Completing personal and family history

A personal and family history is completed prior to the first office visit. This document contains information reported by the patient as a starting point for the provider collecting the patient's *objective information*. First go over the form to ensure that it is complete, and then answer any questions the patient has. This documentation identifies any predispositions to diseases and conditions, and forms an overall picture of the patient's health based on past events. Although this extensive history is usually only completed once, routinely review it when a patient visits and determine whether changes or updates need to be included. Many clinics request the patient update their medical history form annually.

Preventive services/screenings

Screenings are often performed during routine physical exams. Among those are *audiometry*, *visual acuity testing*, routine urinalysis, *anthropometric measurements*, and *vital signs*. Infants and small children should have a growth chart completed once measurements have been taken, and may also be screened to check developmental progress through a *Denver Developmental Screening Test*. Teenagers have *scoliosis* screenings, while older adults can have *Mini-Mental State Examinations* to evaluate for dementia. Be aware of patients' developmental stages and prepare to complete these relatively simple but important screening exams.

allergy. Adverse reaction caused by an antigen-antibody response

anaphylaxis. Life-threatening allergic reaction that leads to circulatory collapse, shock, and death if left untreated

objective information. Information collected that is observed by someone other than the patient

audiometry. Test to determine level of hearing

visual acuity testing. Use of tools such as a Snellen chart to screen for visual impairments

anthropometric measurements. Screening tests that include height and weight (as well as head circumference in infants)

vital signs. Also known as cardinal signs; includes temperature, heart rate, respirations, and blood pressure measurements; used to evaluate homeostasis

Denver Developmental Screening Test. A series of activities used to determine the developmental stage of children

scoliosis. Abnormal lateral curvature of the spine

Mini-Mental State Examination. A tool used to determine the level of awareness of current events and recall of past events to screen for orientation or dementia

MEASURING VITAL SIGNS

Vital signs are key indicators of homeostasis. Alterations in these values could indicate an imbalance, which could be a precursor of illness or disease. Factors such as stress, food or liquid intake, medical conditions, age, and physical activity can affect vital signs. It is extremely important to be proficient in obtaining vital signs as well as knowledge of normal and abnormal values to effectively communicate with the provider and deliver education to patients. Accurate charting serves as a key communication tool among health care professionals.

Temperature

Measuring temperature is actually determining the relationship of heat production and heat loss in the body, also referred to as metabolism. The most common cause of *pyrexia*, or fever, is infection. Fever is the body's natural defense to fight invasive organisms and is therefore a normal reaction to illness. Patients who have a fever can present with chills, anorexia, malaise, thirst, and a generalized aching.

Temperature is measured orally via a digital thermometer, aurally using a tympanic thermometer, or temporally using a temporal artery scanner. Axillary and rectal temperatures determine skin and core temperature but are not commonly performed.

Ingesting hot or cold liquids prior to taking an oral temperature and cerumen in the ear when taking a tympanic temperature can result in inaccurate results. Normal oral, tympanic, and temporal temperatures are 98.6° F (37° C). Axillary temperature will be 1° F cooler on average, while rectal temperatures average 1° F higher.

Take into consideration temperature results, patient history, and clinical appearance.

Heart rate

Heart rate is a reflection of pulse and is best palpated when an artery can be pushed against a bone. The second and third fingers should be used to palpate the pulse. Pulse sites are chosen based on the particular circumstance.

- The radial pulse, located on the thumb side of the wrist, is the most common site for taking an adult pulse.

- The brachial pulse, inside the upper arm, is the most common for children.

- The carotid, located in the neck just below the jaw bone, is most common for use in emergency procedures.

pyrexia. Raised body temperature; fever

Other locations reflect circulation distal to the pulse site. For instance, a strong femoral pulse demonstrates circulation being sent to the lower extremity. If a pedal pulse is absent, circulation to the toes is affected.

In addition to *palpation*, pulse can be determined through *auscultation*. The apical pulse is counted by listening to the heart beat at the apex of the heart. Auscultation is also incorporated when taking a blood pressure.

Pulse is evaluated on rate, rhythm or regularity, and volume or strength. A pulse can be described as 70/min (rate), regular (rhythm), and thready (strength). Thready reflects a pulse as difficult to detect or faint. Bounding describes a pulse as being very strong.

Pulse rates depend on the patient condition and age. Time of day, activity level, and medications can also affect heart rate. Average heart rates tend to slow with age, as identified in the following chart.

9.1 Pulse sites

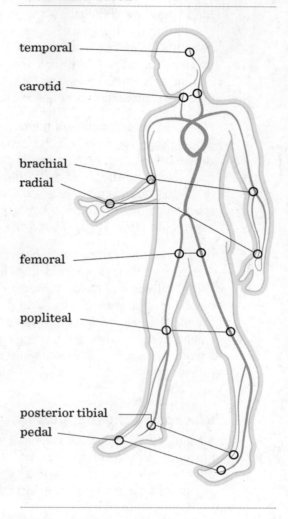

9.2 Average heart rate by age

AGE	AVERAGE HEART RATE
Newborn (birth to 1 month)	120 to 160/min
Infant (1 to 12 months)	80 to 140/min
Toddler (1 to 3 years)	80 to 130/min
Preschool (3 to 5 years)	80 to 120/min
School-age (6 to 15 years)	70 to 100/min
Adult (older than 15 years)	60 to 100/min

Respiration

Respirations are evaluated on rate, rhythm, and depth. Respiratory rate also decreases with age, and is affected by health conditions or environmental factors. Respiratory rhythm is the breathing pattern, and depth describes how much air is inhaled. For example, a patient might have a rate of 28/min with an irregular rhythm and shallow depth. This would indicate some form of respiratory distress, as all three notations are abnormal.

One respiration includes an inhale and exhale. The normal respiratory rate in a newborn averages 30 to 50/min compared to an adult rate of 12 to 20/min. When observing the chest, the respiratory rate is counted, but when incorporating auscultation, the medical assistant may hear abnormal sounds that include *wheezing*, *rales*, or *rhonchi*. All of these are abnormal and the provider should be notified.

palpation. The act of touching

auscultation. Listening, usually with a stethoscope

wheezing. A whistling sound heard on expiration that is the body's attempt to expel trapped air

rales. Clicking or crackling sounds heard on inspiration that can sound moist or dry

rhonchi. Common rattling snoring sounds often associated with chronic lung diseases

Blood pressure

Blood pressure is the single most important vital sign in identifying the force of the blood circulating through the arteries. Obtaining accurate blood pressure can significantly affect the patient's treatment or additional diagnostic tests. Equipment used to manually determine blood pressure includes a *sphygmomanometer*, blood pressure cuff, and stethoscope. Electronic equipment can interpret blood pressure without auscultation. However, it is important to be able to accurately determine blood pressure both manually and electronically.

Measured in millimeters of mercury (mm Hg), the *systolic pressure* is recorded when the first sharp tapping sound is heard, which is when the blood begins to surge into the artery that has been occluded by the inflation of the blood pressure cuff. The *diastolic pressure* is noted when the last sound disappears completely and the blood is flowing freely. These two readings are phase I and V of the *Korotkoff sounds*, or distinct sounds that are heard throughout the cardiac cycle. In phase II, there is a swishing sound as more blood flows through the artery. In phase III, sharp tapping sounds are noted as even more blood is surging. In phase IV, the sound changes to a soft tapping sound which begins to muffle.

Blood pressure readings vary based on age, internal conditions, and external influences. Genetics also play a role in a predisposition to developing hypertension. Blood pressure tends to rise with aging. Infants and children average blood pressures between 60/30 to 100/80 mm Hg. For adults, blood pressure lower than 120/80 mm Hg is considered normal, and systolic readings between 120 and 129 mm Hg are considered elevated. Readings in the ranges of 130 to 139/80 to 89 are considered stage 1 hypertension, and readings greater than 140/90 are considered stage 2 hypertension. Refer to the study guide addendum on the NHA website for details on updated ACC/AHA blood pressure guidelines.

Pulse oximetry (oxygen saturation)

Although usually not considered a vital sign, pulse oximetry is a valuable tool and a simple procedure to ascertain the percentage of oxygen saturation in the blood. Many pulse oximeters also display the heart rate. A patient experiencing symptoms associated with lung conditions such as pneumonia, asthma, or bronchitis are candidates for this noninvasive assessment.

A probe is attached to the finger that incorporates an infrared light to obtain the reading. Nail polish blocks light and interferes with the results, and should be removed prior to the test. Alternatively, the probe could be clipped to the earlobe instead of the finger if necessary. A pulse oximeter reading of 95% or higher is considered a normal result.

Pain scale

Pain is subjective and therefore difficult to interpret. Observe the patient to gather clues about the level of pain, such as facial grimacing or holding body parts. However, asking the patient to rate pain on a scale of 1 to 10 (with 10 being the worst pain) is a means of assessing what the patient is experiencing. Ask additional questions to determine the location, onset, and characteristics of the pain, and whether methods used for relief have been effective.

---

sphygmomanometer. Instrument used to measure blood pressure that has a graduated scale for determining systolic and diastolic pressure by increasing and gradually releasing the pressure in the cuff

systolic pressure. The first sound heard during a blood pressure reading

diastolic pressure. The last sound heard during the blood pressure reading

Korotkoff sounds. The five phases of articular relaxation that are audible while obtaining a manual blood pressure

ABNORMAL SIGNS AND SYMPTOMS

The medical assistant is responsible for obtaining assessment results and communicating abnormalities to the provider. Expect to perform most of these skills during the intake process.

9.3 Skills performed during client intake

SKILL/ACTIVITY	POPULATION AFFECTED	WHEN/HOW OFTEN
Chief complaint/history	All patients	Every visit
Height	All patients	As part of a complete physical exam, scoliosis exam, or if growth concerns are present
Weight	All patients	Every visit
Head circumference	Children 3 years and younger	As part of a complete physical exam or if growth concerns are present
Temperature	All patients	Every visit
Heart rate	All patients	Every visit
Respirations	All patients	Every visit
Blood pressure	Adults (children and infants vary)	Every visit
Pulse oximetry	Patients who have chronic lung disease or respiratory symptoms	As needed based on symptoms and condition
Visual acuity (Snellen chart)	Children (adults vary)	As part of a complete physical exam and some adult screening tests for work-related hire
EKG	Adults (uncommon for children in ambulatory care)	As part of a complete physical in middle-aged adults or if experiencing chest pains
Urinalysis	All patients	Part of a maternity visit, complete physical exam, or when abnormal urinary symptoms are present

The usual process for obtaining intake information is to first record the chief complaint and weight. Take vital signs in the order they are charted: temperature, heart rate, respirations, and blood pressure. Other skills tests are completed based on the reason for the visit and the particular patient.

Clearly document intake information in the medical record and alert the provider of any abnormal results prior to them seeing the patient.

ANTHROPOMETRIC MEASUREMENTS

Anthropometric measurements can play a significant role in assisting the provider with making a diagnosis. Measuring height and weight can be a sensitive issue with patients. Be alert to these concerns and display empathy while ensuring accuracy when obtaining measurements.

Height

Height is a part of a routine physical to track normal development, monitor conditions such as scoliosis or osteoporosis, and assist in determining BMI. Patients should stand erect looking forward without shoes. The leveling bar on the wall or scale needs to sit squarely on the top of the head to get an accurate reading.

If measurements are obtained in inches, the medical assistant might need to convert inches to feet and inches for charting. Measurements can also be recording in centimeters depending on the provider's preference.

To convert height from inches to feet and inches, divide inches by 12.

Example: 62 inches = 62/12 = 5 feet 2 inches

Weight

Obtaining a patient's weight is necessary at each office visit. Medications are often determined based on weight. BMI, predisposition to medical conditions, and the monitoring of eating disorders and weight management are among the reasons weight is obtained. Patients are often embarrassed about their weight and resistant to having it measured. Obtain weight in a private area and avoid stating the measured weight loud enough for others to hear. Completing the task in a timely, efficient manner reduces patient anxiety regarding this part of the visit. Make sure the scale is balanced and review the record to determine a baseline weight prior to asking the patient to stand on the scale. Take special precautions to protect the patient from injury. Assist the patient on and off the scale and monitor stability as needed. Weight is measured in pounds or kilograms.

1 kg = 2.2 lb

To covert pounds to kilograms, divide the weight in pounds by 2.2.

To convert kilograms to pounds, multiply the weight in kilograms by 2.2.

CHALLENGE Measurement conversion

Practice conversion by calculating the correct answers.

1. 20 lb = kg	3. 260 lb = kg	5. 65 in = ft in
2. 65 kg = lb	4. 5 kg = lb	6. 4 ft 5 in = in

Key: 1. 9.09 kg; 2. 143 lb; 3. 118.2 kg; 4. 11 lb; 5. 5 ft 5 in; 6. 53 in

Body mass index

Body mass index (BMI) is not an indicator of health or a means to deliver a diagnosis. Rather, it is a tool to screen patients and classify results into weight categories. This classification then can be used to correlate risk factors or predisposition for conditions such as heart disease or diabetes. BMI is calculated using the following formula.

$$\frac{weight\ in\ kg}{height\ in\ m^2} = BMI$$

or

$$\frac{weight\ in\ lb}{height\ in\ inches^2} \times 703 = BMI$$

A BMI of 18.5 to 24.9 is considered normal. Results less than 18.5 classify an individual as underweight. Greater than 24.9 leads to a classification of overweight, with obesity being 30.0 and greater. The medical assistant may be responsible for calculating BMI using graphs or using a computer program.

9.4 BMI chart

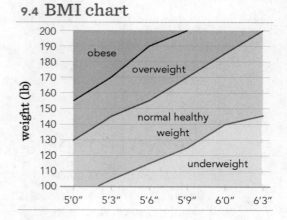

Pediatric measurements

Pediatric measurements monitor growth. Height, weight, and head circumference are completed during a routine physical exam. If there are no concerns about growth, then weight is typically the only anthropometric measurement obtained at each office visit.

It can be challenging to measure a child's growth patterns due to lack of cooperation from the child. The medical assistant can need to ask a parent to hold an infant in place to get an accurate height. Another option is giving the child something to hold or distracting them while the measurements are obtained.

If the child is unable to stand erect, lay the child or infant flat on a paper-covered table. Place a mark at the top of the head and at the heel of the flexed foot. Record this measurement in centimeters or inches.

Weight is more accurate if the infant is able to lie down or sit in an infant scale. Infant scales measure in pounds and ounces and therefore are more accurate. Weigh infants without clothing or a diaper. Using a tape measure, measure head circumference at the widest area, which is usually right across the eyebrows, measuring in inches or centimeters. Repeat the height and head circumference twice to confirm the results.

Growth charts

Pediatric measurements are important in the physical assessment of infants and children up to 3 years of age. These measurements are plotted on a growth chart to provide a visual representation of growth. This alerts the provider to potential concerns. The growth chart also provides a tangible piece of data to have conversations with parents and guardians regarding concerns such as obesity or malnutrition.

Considerations related to age, health status, and disability

The medical assistant must be aware of normal growth and development as well as the patient's physical and medical status in determining the best method to obtain anthropometric measurements. For example, an infant cannot stand on an adult scale, an adult who is unstable might need assistance to get on the scale, and some patients might need a scale that has bars for stability. Patients who have vision and hearing impairments need additional assistance in other instances.

As a last resort, the medical assistant might need to record the measurements as reported by the patient or caretaker. If this is done, make a note in the chart to explain how the measurement was obtained. Regardless of the method, take care to maximize patient safety and obtain an accurate measurement.

ASSISTING PROVIDERS WITH EXAMINATIONS AND PROCEDURES

General physical exams

The medical assistant is responsible for preparing the patient for the examination and assisting the provider as necessary. A medical assistant uses critical thinking skills in determining how to properly prepare the patient for the exam, what equipment needs to be prepared, and what supplies are needed.

Positioning and draping requirements

The medical assistant prepares patients for examinations and procedures based on the reason for the visit. Patients are not usually placed in specific examination positions until the exam is conducted. However, advance preparation that includes patient instructions and appropriate disrobing saves time when the provider is ready to perform the procedure.

Positioning is based on the reason for the visit and the general physical condition of the patient. A patient who is experiencing orthopnea might need adjustments in the usual positioning for a particular exam. A patient who is unstable might need to wait to get on the examination table until the provider is present. Protecting patient privacy through proper draping is also important. Provide a gown, cape, or drape if disrobing is required.

9.5 Patient positions for physical exams

Fowler's	Semi-Fowler's	Sims' (lateral)	Knee-chest
DESCRIPTION	DESCRIPTION	DESCRIPTION	DESCRIPTION
Sitting position with the back of the exam table raised to a 90° angle	Seated leaning against the back of a table that has been raised to a 45° angle	Laying on the left side with the left leg slightly flexed and the right leg flexed at a 90° angle	Prone and bent at the waist resting on the knees with the arms above the head
EXAMINATION TYPE	EXAMINATION TYPE	Can involve a pillow placed between the knees	EXAMINATION TYPE
Exams involving the eyes, ears, nose, throat, chest	Exams involving the chest	EXAMINATION TYPE	Gynecological or rectal exams
	Exams that should be administered in a supine position but the patient is unable to lay flat	Exams involving the rectum, enemas	Treatments of spinal adjustments
	Exams for patients experiencing shortness of breath		

9.5 Patient positions for physical exams *continued*

Jack-knife

DESCRIPTION
Lying over an exam table that is lifted in the middle

EXAMINATION TYPE
Rectal exams or instrumentation (flexible sigmoidoscopy)

Lithotomy

DESCRIPTION
Lying flat on the table with buttocks at the end of the table and feet resting in stirrups

EXAMINATION TYPE
Female pelvic exams

Dorsal recumbent

DESCRIPTION
Lying flat on the back with the knees bent

EXAMINATION TYPE
Catheterizations

Genital examination of younger children, adolescents

Prone

DESCRIPTION
Lying flat on the abdomen with the arms above the head

EXAMINATION TYPE
Exams involving the back of the body including the bottoms of the feet

Supine

DESCRIPTION
Lying flat on the back with the arms down to the side

EXAMINATION TYPE
Exams involving the front of the body

Administration of CPR

Trendelenburg/ modified Trendelenburg

DESCRIPTION
Legs elevated above the head to force circulation to vital organs

EXAMINATION TYPE
Shock (requires a specific table)

Instruments and equipment necessary for a general physical exam

A routine physical exam generally progresses from the head to the feet. Instruments such as an ophthalmoscope, otoscope, and stethoscope are routinely used.

GAME Instruments for physical exams

Match the instrument with the body part used during the assessment.

Instrument:
1. Sphygmomanometer
2. Ophthalmoscope
3. Otoscope
4. Stethoscope
5. Reflex Hammer
6. Tuning Fork
7. Temporal Thermometer
8. Speculum

Body part:
A. Heart/lungs/abdomen
B. Knees
C. Head
D. Arm
E. Nose
F. Eyes
G. Forehead
H. Ears

Key: 1. D, 2. F, 3. H, 4. A, 5. B, 6. C, 7. G, 8. E

Assisting the provider during an exam

The provider might be able to conduct the examination without assistance. Sometimes the medical assistant is needed as a chaperone, especially during female examinations. Holding an uncooperative child can be necessary so that an examination can be safely performed. The medical assistant can also serve as the nonsterile circulating staff for procedures such as suturing, which can include setting up and adding items to a sterile field. During a pelvic examination, the medical assistant might need to hand the provider instruments and receive specimens obtained during the examination.

Collaborative relationship with providers

It is important for the medical assistant to learn the nuances of the providers they frequently work with. Something as simple as remembering what size sterile gloves the provider prefers assists with the efficiency of the examination and the patient's confidence in the skills and abilities of the health care team. The medical assistant should feel comfortable asking the provider questions and be willing to take constructive criticism to improve techniques and processes.

Specialty examinations

Specialty exams depend on services provided by the provider and the availability to provide these services. Gynecological examinations, allergy tests, and cardiac stress tests are some of the procedures with which a medical assistant might need to assist.

Preparing patients for procedures

Prior to preparing a patient for any procedure, consider what equipment and supplies are needed and ensure the room is ready for the examination. Anticipation of patient preparation is equally important. All procedures should begin with a routine introduction; a patient interview that includes a chief complaint, review of medications, and assessment of allergies; and collection of vital signs and anthropometric measurements.

PREPARING AND ADMINISTERING MEDICATIONS AND INJECTABLES

Administering medications requires consistent diligence. Even simple errors can lead to adverse reactions. For additional details on medication administration, refer to *Chapter 3: Pharmacology*.

Checking the medication order

The name of the medication, dosage, time, and route of administration direct the medical assistant in preparing medication for administration. Consent for administration of a medication should be obtained from the patient or guardian prior to preparing the medication. Tell the patient what the medication is, what it is given for, the dosage, and the route that will be used. Checking the medication three times helps prevent medication errors. The first check is comparing the medication order to the medication. The second check occurs after the medication is prepared for administration. The third check is completed immediately prior to administering the medication to the patient.

Injection equipment and supplies

The correct syringe and needle for the route of administration and the medication are among the supplies to gather for injections. Alcohol swabs are necessary to wipe off vials or wrap around the neck of an ampule, as well as for skin preparation. A gauze pad is used to apply pressure or hold at the site after administration. An adhesive bandage should be available if there is bleeding at the site. A sharps container should be located nearby to avoid transporting contaminated needles from where the injection was administered. A biohazard container is necessary for disposal of other potentially contaminated items. A tray for transporting prepared medications and supplies from the workstation to the patient can increase efficiency. Injection is an invasive procedure and the medical assistant could be exposed to blood and body fluids, so nonsterile gloves and other appropriate PPE are required.

Needle safety

All health care professionals must abide by the OSHA Needlestick Safety and Prevention Act. This means that engineering controls must be implemented to eliminate or reduce the risk of exposure to bloodborne pathogens. Easily accessible sharps containers and self-sheathing or safety needles are examples of required controls. Never recap a used needle. Ensure that patients are prepared for the injection or ask for assistance in holding the patient still if needed to avoid accidental needle sticks.

9.6 Safety needle

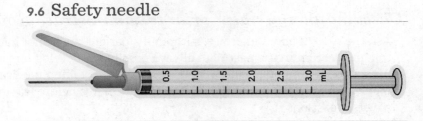

Keeping equipment sterile

Whenever invasive procedures are conducted, take precautions to maintain sterility of devices that break the protective skin layer. Needles and syringes must be sterile. Check the expiration date of solutions before preparing the medication, and evaluate the integrity of the container. The use of alcohol swabs on a vial stopper assists in preventing introduction of germs into the solution as well as keeping the needle sterile. Do not introduce the needle into the vial more than once. Each re-puncture into a vial dulls the needle and predisposes the equipment to contamination. Allowing solutions to run down a needle also increases the likelihood of contamination. Take care to not place the exposed needle on a tray or countertop. Although a clean needle may be recapped for protection prior to injection using a one-handed scoop method, this should only be done if absolutely necessary because contamination by an incidental stick is possible.

Selecting the needle gauge and length

The gauge describes the diameter of the lumen of the needle. The lower the gauge number, the wider the lumen. Gauges range from 14 to 31, with 14 being be the largest and 31 the smallest. The length indicates the distance from the hilt to the point of the needle. Needle lengths range from 3/8 to 4 inches.

The following chart provides basic uses for lengths and gauges. To select the appropriate needle, the medical assistant must be familiar with the viscosity of the medication, route selected, and location of administration. When choosing a length, also consider the size of the patient.

9.7 Needle lengths and gauges

ROUTE	NEEDLE GAUGE	NEEDLE LENGTH
Intradermal (ID)	27 to 28	3/8 inch
Subcutaneous (SC)	25 to 26	½ inch, ⅝ inch
Intramuscular (IM)	20 to 23	1 to 3 inches (depending on muscle and patient size)

Checking allergy status prior to administration of medication

Ask the patient about allergies. Although a patient might not have had an allergic or adverse reaction to a medication in the past, it is always possible to develop a reaction in subsequent treatments. Alert patients to potential adverse reactions when taking medications. After administration of any medication, ask the patient to wait 10 to 15 minutes before leaving for observation of any possible adverse reactions.

Anaphylaxis is the most severe form of an allergic reaction and tends to occur rapidly after the administration of a medication. The route affects the speed of reaction because medications enter the circulatory system based on absorption into the bloodstream. A medication that is administered intramuscularly absorbs more rapidly than an oral, subcutaneous, or intradermal medication.

Following the rights of medication administration

Incorporate several checks and balances with every medication administration to confirm the right patient, right dose, right route, and other confirmatory measures are in place prior to any medication administration. Refer to Chapter 3: Pharmacology for additional details regarding the rights of medication administration.

Administration of medications

Choose the appropriate site based on the medication to be administered, the dosage, and the route of administration. The routes of administration typically used in parenteral administration of medications are identified in the following charts. The dorsogluteal site is no longer recommended largely due to the potential complications that can occur if the sciatic nerve is damaged.

9.8 Parenteral intramuscular injection sites (IM)

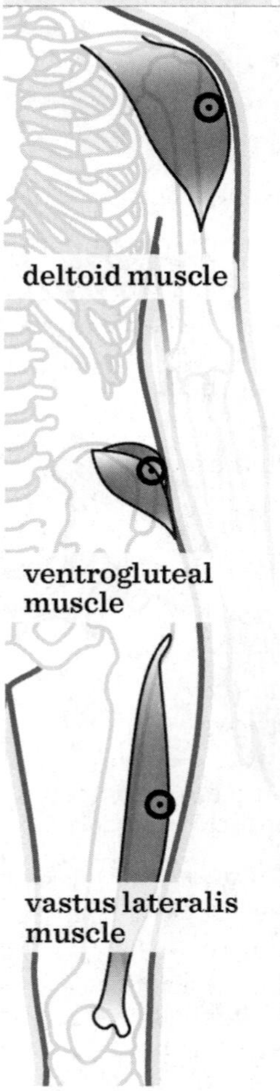

MUSCLE	LOCATION	ANGLE/ASPIRATION	NOTES
deltoid muscle	1 to 2 inches below the acromion	90° angle Do not aspirate vaccines Aspirate most other types of medications administered via this route*	Many adult and older child vaccines are administered via this route. Do not use this site for infants or children younger than 3 years old. The dose given in the deltoid should not exceed 1 mL. Depending on protocols, 2 to 3 mL can be used on adults and larger children. The site is typically massaged after medication administration.
ventrogluteal muscle	The ventrogluteal site is located by placing the heel of the hand on the greater trochanter (right hand placed on left hip and left hand placed on right hip), the middle finger is placed on the iliac crest, and the fingers are spread. Give the injection where the V is made between the index finger and middle finger.	90° angle Do not aspirate vaccines Aspirate most other types of medications administered via this route* Note: The dorsogluteal injection is no longer used, but the ventrogluteal site is a good substitute	This site is used when deep IM injections are prescribed or when larger quantities of medicines are needed. This site is good for viscous medications.
vastus lateralis muscle	Administration location in the mid to upper outer thigh	90° angle Do not aspirate vaccines Aspirate most other types of medications administered via this route*	This site is routinely used for vaccines and medication administration for infants and children younger than 3 years old.

When administering immunizations intramuscularly, aspiration prior to injection is not recommended per the CDC. For all other medication administrations, consult with the provider regarding aspiration policy.

9.9 Parenteral subcutaneous and intradermal injection sites (SQ, ID)

TYPE	LOCATION	ANGLE/ASPIRATION	NOTES
Subcutaneous	Multiple subcutaneous tissue (SC) sites are readily available for injections.	45° angle Do not aspirate for vaccines, insulin, or heparin Aspirate for most other types of medications administered via this route	When administering heparin or insulin, the site should not be massaged. When regularly used for health maintenance, the sites should be rotated. Common sites include the upper outer arm, abdomen, and thigh
Intradermal	When using the forearm, measure using one hand width from the wrist and one hand width from the elbow. Any area within the anterior forearm visible is acceptable for the injection. The upper back may be used for testing as well.	10° to 15° angle Do not aspirate	Used for testing The presence of a wheel is expected. Do not massage or apply pressure to the site. Most common site for TB testing is the mid forearm. Allergy testing usually is done on the back.

Proper administration of medications administered via other routes besides injected are equally important. Routes of administration vary based on the medication, target location, and desired absorption rate.

9.10 Other medication routes

Oral
LOCATION
In the mouth

TIPS
Solids: For multiple-dose bottles, pour pills into the lid first, then the medicine cup.

Liquids: Read liquids at the lowest point of the curve of the liquid (meniscus) and "palm" the label to prevent distortion if medication drips down the bottle

Buccal
LOCATION
Between the cheek and gums resulting in rapid absorption.

The medication bypasses the digestive system, resulting in smaller doses required for therapeutic effects.

TIPS
The medication is designed to melt while held in the cheek area. The patient should not chew or swallow the medication.

Eating, drinking, or smoking can influence the absorption rate.

Sublingual
LOCATION
Under the tongue.

Nitroglycerin tablets and spray are common forms of medication administered via this route.

Because the medication bypasses the digestive system, smaller doses are required for therapeutic effects.

TIPS
Solids: The medication melts and absorbs into the bloodstream rapidly.

Liquids: Sprays are occasionally used to deliver sublingual medications.

Eating, drinking, or smoking can influence the absorption rate

Inhalation
LOCATION
Typically used for targeted areas such as the bronchial passages

Can be delivered via a nebulizer

TIPS
For the medication to be effective, the patient must hold the medication in the lungs as long as possible.

When using inhalers or nebulizers, patients can tend to become shaky and experience some dizziness due to the medication and hyperventilation. Coaching on proper breathing techniques is important.

9.10 Other medication routes *continued*

Topical

LOCATION
Designed to react locally and systematic absorption is minimal.

TIPS
Can serve as a barrier to prevent irritants from damaging the skin or can be used to treat a local condition (acne, athlete's foot)

Typically oil- or water-based products

Monitor for skin irritation or reaction. Instruct patients to apply as prescribed.

Mucosal

LOCATION
Designed to absorb into and through mucous membranes

In addition to nasally, medications can be administered in the vagina, rectum, eye, or ear

TIPS
Can cause irritation to the mucosa.

Ensure patients understand the correct procedure for administering the medication based on the medication and route.

Transdermal

LOCATION
For continuous slow absorption of various medications

Used for smoking cessation (nicotine patches), pain medication, hormone delivery

TIPS
Avoid touching the medication when applying the patch.

Dispose of patch in a container that is not accessible to children.

Monitor skin for irritation, rotate sites

Storing medications and medication logs

Store medications according to the manufacturer directions and in their original containers. This can include specific instructions such as refrigerating or protecting from light. Controlled substances identified by the Drug Enforcement Agency (DEA) must remain locked and secured. A log book and a daily count by two people are required for controlled substances kept in the office.

Medication logs ensure that all medications are accounted for. They are required to be maintained for controlled substances administered to patients. In addition, when medications need to be destroyed due to expiration or other circumstances, two people should witness the process and their names should be documented in the disposal log.

Immunization information

Vaccines are administered to provide immunity from specific diseases that lead to morbidity or mortality. Immunizations begin as early as 1 month old with childhood vaccines and continue through adulthood with tetanus boosters and the shingles vaccine. While vaccines prevent or reduce the symptoms of various diseases, complications and adverse reactions are possible. Be aware of potential adverse reactions and gather a thorough vaccine history from the patient to ensure the patient is not allergic to any of the ingredients in the vaccine being administered.

The current recommended vaccine schedule is available on the Centers for Disease Control and Prevention website at www.cdc.gov.

EYE, EAR, AND TOPICAL MEDICATIONS

Prior to administering medications to the ears or eyes, ensure the medication is at room temperature, the patient is properly positioned, and gloves are worn during administration. The tip of the containers should not come in direct contact with the patient, as this could lead to contamination of the solution.

Apply the same principles when administering topical medications. Take precautions not to touch topical medications. In addition to contamination concerns, medications applied topically can absorb into the body and lead to adverse reactions. Use an applicator to apply topical medications.

EYE AND EAR IRRIGATION

Irrigations of the eye and ear are done for a variety of reasons. The eye can be irrigated to remove a foreign body or toxic substance. The ear can be irrigated to remove a foreign body or remove wax that prevents the provider from seeing the tympanic membrane through the otoscope. When any irrigation is conducted, the solution should be tepid or room temperature. Irrigants that are too cold can lead to dizziness or discomfort, and too hot can lead to discomfort, pain, or even burns.

Properly position the patient based on the route of irrigation. Conduct eye irrigations so that solutions do not flow down the tear duct. Irrigation of the ear is contraindicated if there is a ruptured tympanic membrane or the patient has tubes in the ears.

IDENTIFYING AND RESPONDING TO EMERGENCY/PRIORITY SITUATIONS

It is important to be prepared, alert, and ready to respond to potential threats or emergencies in the clinical setting. Emergencies such as choking, allergic reactions, and trauma require emergency first aid procedures. Any condition that leads to cardiac or respiratory failure mandates rapid implementation of life-saving measures, including calling 911 and initiating CPR.

Be aware of external and environmental emergencies as well. These include weather-related emergencies (tornadoes, hurricanes, fires) and human-related threats such as assault with deadly weapons. All employees should annually review and be knowledgeable of the emergency evacuation and response plans. In addition, if any updates are made to the plans, the employees must be notified of the revisions.

Emergency action plan

The emergency action plan can include *triage* to deliver immediate care to patients who have life-threatening conditions. Action plans should identify when and who should contact emergency medical services during a crisis situation. Emergency equipment (*automatic external defibrillator [AED]*, vital sign equipment, bandages, dressings) are often needed for physical emergencies and should be readily accessible. All staff should know the location of fire extinguishers and emergency evacuation routes. In the event of an emergency situation, the medical assistant or other available health care staff should stay with the patients until a provider or emergency services personnel are available to take over and be responsible for delivering emergency care when necessary. In addition, the medical assistant is often the member of the health care team who is responsible for making sure all needed equipment and supplies are ready for the provider during an emergent situation.

triage. Ranking based on the most critical to the least critical

automatic external defibrillator (AED). An external device attached to the chest with which to shock the heart if in asystole or arrhythmia in hopes of restarting or re-establishing a normal heart rhythm

FIRST AID AND BASIC WOUND CARE

The goal of providing care in an emergency is to stabilize the patient and prevent further injury. When administering first aid, the use of PPE is imperative.

Types of tissue injuries

Wounds can be open (the skin is broken) or closed (there is no break in the skin). For any open wound, the tetanus immunization status must be obtained for the provider to determine the appropriate treatment. The following are some common types of injuries in the clinical setting.

9.11 Common tissue injuries

Abrasion

DESCRIPTION
Scrape or rub

Superficial wound often affecting the knees, elbows

EMERGENCY PROCEDURES
Apply pressure if bleeding.

Clean and/or flush to remove debris.

Apply bandage.

Incision

DESCRIPTION
Open injury typically caused by a sharp object causing a straight cut

Bleeding can be profuse

EMERGENCY PROCEDURES
Apply pressure until bleeding is controlled.

Clean gently. (Rigorous cleaning can reinitiate bleeding.)

Apply bandage.

Laceration

DESCRIPTION
Open injury that is jagged in nature and caused by a sharp object

Bleeding can be profuse

EMERGENCY PROCEDURES
Apply pressure until bleeding is controlled.

Clean gently. (Rigorous cleaning can reinitiate bleeding.)

Apply bandage.

Puncture

DESCRIPTION
Open wound that is caused by an instrument that delivers a stab

Usually small with limited bleeding

EMERGENCY PROCEDURES
Apply pressure if bleeding.

Clean and/or flush to remove debris.

Apply bandage.

Contusion

DESCRIPTION
Closed injury, also known as a bruise

Caused by a blunt-force trauma

Ranges in severity based on the trauma received and the location

EMERGENCY PROCEDURES
Apply cold pack or ice.

Elevate limb if affected.

Observe for signs of increased intracranial pressure if the head is contused. (This would require immediate emergency care.)

Concussion

DESCRIPTION
Closed head trauma in which the brain has been jolted or shaken

EMERGENCY PROCEDURES
Measure vital signs.

Observation

Provider assessment and possible computed tomography scan (CT).

Types of limb injuries

Mild to moderate injuries to the extremities are common in an ambulatory care setting. Medical assistants need to be familiar with the more common types of injuries to the limbs to assist the provider with these patient conditions. The following are some common types of injuries occurring to the limbs.

9.12 Common limb injuries

Strain	Sprain	Fracture
DESCRIPTION	**DESCRIPTION**	**DESCRIPTION**
Injury due to excessive overstretching of a muscle or tendon	Injury due to tearing of a tendon, ligament or cartilage of a joint	Break in bone
		Open fracture: skin is broken
		Closed fracture: no break in skin
EMERGENCY PROCEDURES	**EMERGENCY PROCEDURES**	**EMERGENCY PROCEDURES**
Rest, ice, compression, elevation (RICE)	RICE	Control bleeding.
		Immobilize area.
		Apply ice.
		Check for a pulse below the fracture site.
		Treat for shock.

Other types of emergencies

In the event of a medical emergency, the medical assistant must be prepared to react and respond appropriately while assisting the provider with treatments or medication administration. General guidelines for identifying and responding to each emergency are listed in the following table.

9.13 Other common emergencies

Anaphylaxis	Acute abdominal pain	Bleeding emergencies	Eye and ear injuries
DESCRIPTION	**DESCRIPTION**	**DESCRIPTION**	**DESCRIPTION**
Severe allergic reaction in which there is circulatory shutdown and respiratory distress, which results in shock	General symptom that can be life-threatening	Can occur internally or externally	Foreign bodies are the most common cause
		The amount of bleeding depends on the blood supply in the location of the injury and the vessel that was torn or cut. Arterial bleeding is more of a medical crisis than capillary bleeding.	Trauma is another cause
	EMERGENCY PROCEDURES		Characterized by pain, decrease or sensitivity in hearing or vision
	Obtain detailed chief complaint, keep the patient NPO, have an emesis basis available, keep the patient warm but do not apply heat to the abdomen, monitor vital signs and observe for signs of shock.		
EMERGENCY PROCEDURES			**EMERGENCY PROCEDURES**
Extreme emergency: provide basic life support, administer oxygen and epinephrine based on provider order, call 911.	Describing the severity, quadrant, or abdominal region assists in diagnosing the condition.	**EMERGENCY PROCEDURES** Apply pressure, elevate the site if possible, apply ice, limit movement, keep the patient quiet, monitor vital signs and observe for signs of shock.	Prevent further trauma by limiting contact. Cover the eye or ear to decrease sensitivity. Administer eye and ear irrigations based on provider direction.

9.13 Other common emergencies *continued*

Burns

DESCRIPTION

Severity is based on location, extent of body surface affected, and degree of tissue involvement.

Classified as first-degree (first layer of tissue; sunburn), second degree (involve subcutaneous tissue and will blister), and third-degree (involve muscle and possibly bone; appear dry and charred)

Can be electrical, chemical, or thermal

EMERGENCY PROCEDURES

Remove the patient from the source.

Flush profusely with cool water.

Do not remove clothing (unless chemical burn).

Monitor vital signs and observe for shock.

Assess body area affected using the Rule of Nines.

Choking

DESCRIPTION

Caused by obstruction of the airway

Patient is unable to breathe or speak and displays the characteristic sign of holding the hands to the neck.

EMERGENCY PROCEDURES

Ask the patient, "Are you choking?"

Do nothing if the patient can speak or cough.

If patient is unable to breathe or talk, perform the Heimlich maneuver.

If the patient is unconscious, perform CPR, looking for a foreign body in the mouth and removing it if visible.

Diabetic emergencies

DESCRIPTION

Diabetic coma (hyperglycemia) characterized by malaise, dry mouth, polydipsia, polyuria, nausea, vomiting, dyspnea.

Insulin shock (hypoglycemia) characterized by sweating, anxiety, irritability, tachycardia, headache, hunger

Can lead to seizures, coma, death if left untreated.

EMERGENCY PROCEDURES

Administer glucose for insulin shock.

Administer insulin for diabetic coma.

When in doubt, give glucose. Monitor vital signs.

Call 911 if rapid improvement is not noted.

Seizures

DESCRIPTION

Can result from trauma or alterations in metabolism such as with fever

Can be idiopathic in nature

Can range from generalized (grand mal) to short staring episode (petit mal)

EMERGENCY PROCEDURES

Assist the patient to a lying position.

Protect from injury.

Tilt the head to the side to prevent aspiration.

Time the seizure.

Stay with the patient and observe.

If seizures continue (status epilepticus), call 911.

Stroke

DESCRIPTION

Results from hypoxia in the brain usually due to a blood clot, or rupture or occlusion of a blood vessel

Patient can be *aphasic* or *dysphasic*; experience weakness or paralysis on one side of the body, or drooping of the mouth; lose consciousness

EMERGENCY PROCEDURES

Protect the patient.

Keep the patient NPO.

Obtain vital signs.

Collect as much medical history as possible.

Administer oxygen.

Call 911.

9.14 Rule of Nines

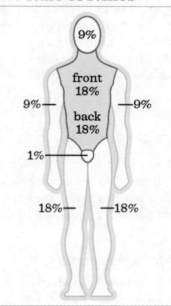

aphasia. Inability to speak

dysphasia. Difficulty speaking

Wound care follow-up

Wounds can be open or closed, intentional through surgical intervention, or accidental through trauma. Wounds heal based on location, mode of injury, available blood supply, and the patient's general health status.

The medical assistant is often responsible for patient education regarding the healing process of a wound. Making sure the patient understands the importance of notifying the provider if infection is suspected is a crucial part of this education.

Signs of infection

Typical signs of infection include the following.

- Redness and swelling at or around the site
- Feeling hot to touch
- Drainage (other than clear)
- Foul odor from the site
- Fever
- Malaise
- Red streaks extending from the wound (lymphangitis)

Changing a sterile dressing

In preparation for a dressing change, the medical assistant should wash their hands using proper hand hygiene prior to donning sterile or non-sterile gloves. The use of sterile gloves is uncommon but should be considered if contact with underlying tissues is anticipated. For dressings that are stuck to the wound, soak the dressing in sterile saline or sterile water prior to removal. Always take precautions to prevent further contamination of the wound when conducting a dressing change.

Remember that dressings are sterile and bandages are nonsterile. Dressings cover wounds and bandages cover dressings. When changing a dressing, discard all waste contaminated with body fluids in a biohazard container. When applying medications to the wound, use an applicator and avoid touching the tube or container to the wound. Do not re-insert an applicator into a medication container once used. Open dressing packages without touching the contents. When grasping a dressing, touch only the edges that will not come in contact with the wound. Once the wound is covered, a bandage or tape can be applied.

PERFORMING CPR

There is no way of knowing when emergency cardiopulmonary resuscitation (CPR) will be needed. The medical assistant should be certified in CPR and familiar with how to use an AED. Provider-level training is offered through the American Red Cross and the American Heart Association. Regular renewal of certification is mandatory for credentialed medical assistants.

Safety concerns

It is not uncommon to cause fractured ribs during CPR. However, this can be minimized with proper hand positioning and technique. An adrenalin reaction to emergencies causes excessive forceful breathing. This can lead to a ruptured lung in an infant. The ultimate goal is to restore circulation and breathing while minimizing complications.

The medical assistant must also take precautions to protect him or herself when administering CPR. The use of disposable gloves and CPR mouth barriers prevent exposure to body fluids and should be accessible to all health care staff.

Breathing emergencies

Patients who have compromised pulmonary function due to respiratory diseases are prone to dyspnea and apnea. Antigen-antibody reactions can lead to anaphylaxis and respiratory emergencies. Additionally, airway obstructions due to disease or foreign bodies can lead to respiratory distress. In a patient who has normal lung function, a high carbon dioxide level causes breathing. In a patient who has a pulmonary disease, a low oxygen level is the stimulus for breathing. Patients who have chronic lung disease have adapted to a high carbon dioxide level; and if they receive too much oxygen to treat the respiratory distress, they can develop apnea. Therefore, providers use oxygen cautiously based on the patient's underlying condition. Based on a provider's instructions, the medical assistant can be responsible for administering medications or breathing treatments via nebulizer to patients experiencing dyspnea.

One-rescuer vs. two-rescuer CPR

Health care professionals should remain up to date with their CPR and first aid certifications. It is important to understand how to perform CPR as a single rescuer. Ascertain responsiveness, activate emergency medical systems (EMS), and check the carotid artery for a pulse. If no pulse is present, then the patient receives CPR at a rate of 100 to 120 chest compressions per minute with a ratio of 30 compressions to 2 breaths. The count remains the same with two rescuers, but alternating roles can decrease fatigue in performing chest compressions.

AED

Because most patients who go into cardiac arrest initially experience ventricular fibrillation, the AED is useful to convert the patient back to sinus rhythm. This device provides automatic voice instruction on the process to follow when the chest leads are connected and an interpretation of cardiac rhythm is analyzed. It is important to follow the commands and to also place the defibrillator directly on the pads which are placed on dry skin. Avoid touching metal during defibrillation or placing the defibrillator over jewelry.

ASSISTING WITH MINOR AND TRAUMATIC INJURIES

When a patient presents to the office with minor or traumatic injuries, the medical assistant is responsible for obtaining a chief complaint, collecting vital signs, and assisting the provider as necessary. This can include cleaning wounds, preparing sterile fields for minor surgical interventions, bandaging wounds, administering injections, instructing patients on the signs of infections, providing wound care, and scheduling follow-up appointments.

ASSISTING WITH SURGICAL INTERVENTIONS

A medical assistant assists both the patient and the provider in regards to surgical interventions:

- Preparing the surgical area and assisting the provider during the procedure

- Providing education and support to the patient

The goal of surgical intervention is to deliver a treatment and prevent further damage. Skills in assisting with sterile procedures are important to avoid complications as well as efficiently and effectively deliver the necessary treatment.

Explaining the procedure and obtaining consent

The provider is responsible for obtaining consent for surgical procedures. However, the medical assistant needs to have the forms ready for the provider, serve as a witness on the form, and be available to answer basic questions or defer questions to the provider. No surgical interventions should be completed without the expressed written consent of the patient, parent, or guardian.

Pre- and post-surgical instructions

Planned surgical procedures commonly performed in a provider's office include mole removals, ingrown toenail removals, or wart removals. Unplanned surgical procedures include foreign body removal or wound suturing.

Planned surgical procedures are often easier to instruct the patient for as far as what to expect and how to prepare. Although the time is limited in an emergency situation, make an effort to allay fears by informing the patient on what to expect.

Postsurgical instructions include when to return for follow-up, contact information in case of complications, signs of infection, and how to care for the wound. Patients are often anxious and have a difficult time remembering instructions following a trauma, so written information should be reviewed and sent with the patient.

Setting up for the procedure

When setting up for the procedure, avoid contamination of the sterilized items or sterile field. When opening sterile packets or a Mayo stand cover, open the flaps away from you first and then open the closest flap. At least 1 inch around the sterile field is considered nonsterile, so do not place items in this area. Basic principles in maintaining a sterile field include the following.

- Open packages so that they can easily drop onto the sterile field or be grasped by the provider without touching the outer wrapper.

- Lip the bottle of liquids prior to pouring into sterile containers.

- Do not leave a sterile field unattended, reach over a sterile field, or turn your back to a sterile field.

- Medication vials should be cleaned with alcohol prior to holding with two hands for the provider to inject the needle into.

Minor surgery procedures

Minor surgical procedures are often completed in the ambulatory care setting. The medical assistant is responsible for preparing the patient for the procedure, obtaining a brief history including documentation of allergies, and collecting vital signs. Postprocedure responsibilities include ensuring the patient has follow-up appointments and instructions. Many clinics require the medical assistant to communicate with the patient via phone within 24 hr of the procedure to check on progress. Some common procedures are listed in the following table.

9.15 Common surgery procedures

Mole or cyst removal

DESCRIPTION

Moles that change color, size, or texture should be evaluated for signs of cancer.

Cysts are collections of fluid that can be infectious.

SUPPLIES AND EQUIPMENT

Local anesthetic (xylocaine), scalpel or punch device, suture supplies

TIPS

Obtain a detailed history regarding the change in the mole(s).

Obtain a family history regarding melanoma.

All specimens should be sent to the laboratory for evaluation.

Instruct the patient to monitor the wound for infection and return for follow-up suture removal and care.

Colposcopy/hysteroscopy

DESCRIPTION

Using an instrument to inspect the vaginal area and cervix or the uterus and deliver treatments or perform diagnostic testing

Cryosurgery, conization, or biopsies may be included.

SUPPLIES AND EQUIPMENT

Colposcope/hysteroscope; exam table with stirrups

TIPS

The patient will be in the lithotomy position and will experience discomfort and pressure.

Provide patient instructions.

Assist the provider as needed.

All specimens should be properly collected and prepared for transport to the laboratory.

This procedure should not be performed while the patient is having menses.

Toenail removal/Ingrown toenail treatment

DESCRIPTION

A toenail removal can be partial or complete.

The provider removes a toenail spur that is causing an ingrown toenail.

The procedure is completed after local anesthetic or digital block.

SUPPLIES AND EQUIPMENT

Sterile scissors and forceps or hemostats, anesthetic (xylocaine), bandaging materials

TIPS

The patient will experience throbbing or discomfort after the anesthetic wears off. Soaking in warm salt water facilitates healing and reduces discomfort.

Provide patient instructions.

Assist the provider as needed.

Bandage the wound.

Cryosurgery

DESCRIPTION

The process of exposing tissues to extreme cold temperatures to destroy cells

May be performed for conditions such as warts or cervical dysplasia

SUPPLIES AND EQUIPMENT

Canister with liquid nitrogen, cryoprobe

TIPS

Provide patient support and instructions. (The patient should expect to have discomfort as the tissue warms.)

Assist with procedure.

Endoscopy

DESCRIPTION

A small tube with a light and camera is inserted into the upper or lower gastrointestinal system or through a small incision to access a body cavity for inspection or minor procedures such as biopsies.

Typically done in a specialty office

SUPPLIES AND EQUIPMENT

Gastroscope, laparoscope, hysteroscope (depends on area of inspection) with cables and light sources

TIPS

Inspect equipment prior to and after use.

Assist with patient positioning and support.

Avoid touching skin with the light source, which could be very hot.

Package specimens and prepare for transport.

Electrosurgery or electrocauterization

DESCRIPTION

A pulse of electrical current is sent through tissue to cauterize (or burn) tissue.

Used to minimize or stop bleeding, destroy small polyps, or break scar tissue

SUPPLIES AND EQUIPMENT

Electrocautery unit with foot pedal, grounding cable, and pad

TIPS

Inspect pad and cable prior to usage.

Avoid placing the pad on areas with excessive hair, over bony parts, or over pacemakers or metal implants

Note the condition of the area after treatment.

STAPLE AND SUTURE REMOVAL

Under the direction of the provider, medical assistants can remove sutures or staples. Prior to removal, a thorough inspection of the wound to approximate the edges and the absence or presence of drainage is necessary. Wounds that have crusting blood or exudate will usually need soaking with saline prior to removal of the sutures or staples.

Equipment for suture removal includes stitch or suture scissors and forceps. A staple removal device is used to remove staples. Remove every other suture or staple while observing the site. If at any time there is gaping, stop and notify the provider. Account for the total number of staples and sutures that were used to close the wound. When cutting sutures, cut close to the knot and pull the suture out with forceps by grabbing the knot and pulling, observing to ensure the entire suture was removed.

Butterfly closures can be used to provide reinforcement of the wound after removal of the sutures or staples depending on the condition and location of the wound.

REVIEWING DISCHARGE INSTRUCTIONS WITH PATIENTS

When patients are under stress, they often do not comprehend all instructions from the provider. Provide written instructions whenever possible. Review all instructions with the patient and answer questions prior to their departure.

Reviewing discharge instructions or plan of care

Discharge instructions or the plan of care after any visit in the ambulatory care setting includes the following.

- *Activity restrictions:* This includes bathing and exercising.
- *Diet restrictions:* It is unlikely to have dietary restrictions following minor ambulatory surgery. However, in cases of abdominal pain, diarrhea, or vomiting, a liquid diet with progress as tolerated may be recommended.
- *Wound care:* This includes instructions such as changing the dressing, applying medications to the wound, and observing for signs of infection.
- *Medications:* If the patient has prescriptions for medications such as antibiotics, instruct the patient on how and when to take the medication, how it should be stored, and possible side effects.
- *Follow-up appointments:* This includes when to return to the office and how to contact the office if an unexpected event occurs.

Setting up referrals

The primary care provider might need to elicit an opinion from a specialist, or the patient might need to be referred for procedures or treatments not available in the office. Ensure that the referral process is handled as smoothly and efficiently as possible. Obtain the necessary information from the patient (available days and times, contact numbers) and confirm insurance information. In addition, determine what preparations are needed for the appointment and provide that information to the patient.

Precertification of procedures

For some insurance providers (especially managed care plans) to cover expenses associated with diagnostic or therapeutic procedures, *precertification* may be required. It is always advisable to have the patient contact their insurance provider to confirm coverage, but the medical assistant might also need to provide referral information to the insurance provider for approval prior to scheduling the appointment.

Participating providers

Some diagnostic procedures, such as a chest x-ray, do not require precertification. However, patients might receive a greater coverage of expenses if they seek services from a provider who participates with their insurance plan. The medical assistant should be familiar with the insurance plan and inquire about participation with the plan when scheduling an appointment. If the patient can schedule the appointment on their own, educate them to confirm that the provider is participating in the insurance plan to maximize coverage.

Following up with the patient

With the implementation of the Affordable Care Act, the medical assistant often acts as the patient navigator or case manager. This means that the care is all-encompassing and delivery is not simply at the office level. It is important to have a follow-up conversation with the patient to see if they kept their referral appointment. If treatments were carried out in the office, a follow-up call can ensure that the patient understands and is following instructions delivered by the provider.

GUIDELINES FOR SENDING PRESCRIPTIONS AND REFILLS BY PHONE

The medical assistant cannot write or prescribe medications but is authorized to send medication prescribed by the provider to the pharmacy electronically or via phone. The medical assistant must be familiar with regulations regarding refills and controlled substances. Clear communication with the pharmacy is necessary to avoid mistakes and potential harm to the patient, which can lead to legal action against the provider and practice.

Federal and state requirements

As part of recent federal requirements, only licensed or credentialed individuals may send prescriptions electronically. To comply with this law, upon receiving the prescription for a medication, the medical assistant must be credentialed to perform this function.

The medical assistant might need to call a refill to the pharmacy. When phoning a prescription, speak clearly, provide the full name and birthdate of the patient, identify the medication being prescribed, and avoid using abbreviations that could lead to a misunderstanding of the directions.

Schedule II substances identified by the DEA may not be called to the pharmacy; the patient must deliver the physical prescription to the pharmacy. For further information on controlled substances, go to the DEA website at www.dea.gov.

---

precertification. Approval obtained by insurance providers that identifies insurance coverage for diagnostic or therapeutic activities

Parts of a prescription

To ensure a prescription is accurate, the pharmacy will only accept the prescription if all of the parts identified on the prescription are completed. The same information is relayed to the pharmacy whether the prescription is transmitted electronically or via phone.

Methods for creating and sending prescriptions

Electronic health records in the ambulatory care setting allow prescriptions to be written and transmitted to the pharmacy selected by the patient. Other methods of transmission include faxing, phoning, or providing a written prescription. All of these methods are effective and used for various circumstances. It is important to follow the policies and procedures identified by the facility.

9.16 Parts of a prescription

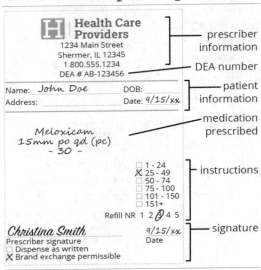

Paper vs. electronic prescriptions

The chance of human error is reduced when using electronic prescriptions. The medical assistant or the pharmacist does not need to interpret handwriting from the provider, which reduces medication errors. Medications can also be rapidly sent and ready for the patient upon arrival when electronic. In addition, the chance of medications being abused is reduced when paper prescriptions are not available in the examination area or given to patients. Be alert for patients who repeatedly contact the office stating they lost their written prescription and need another one or want the prescription called to a different pharmacy.

One of the downfalls of electronic prescriptions is the potential for network problems, which could result in a failed or delayed receipt of prescriptions. In addition, the person transmitting the prescription must be credentialed, which limits who is authorized to handle this duty.

Faxing prescriptions

Faxing is effective if a patient contacts the pharmacy for their medication and there are no refills. The pharmacy may choose to contact the provider via fax asking for authorization of refills. The medical assistant may be responsible for retrieving the fax and delivering it to the provider as well as communicating further instructions to the patient.

DOCUMENTING RELEVANT ASPECTS OF CARE IN PATIENT RECORD

The importance of documentation cannot be understated. Documentation is used for communicating among the health care team as well as in cases of legal actions. The old saying "If it isn't charted, it wasn't done" is still true. The legal system tends to side with the patient if documentation is not clearly validated within the medical record.

Documenting the chief complaint

The chief complaint is subjective information that should be described using the patient's own words. If the words are exactly as the patient relayed, put them in quotation marks. Use the chief complaint to further describe what is happening with the patient by using observations, asking questions, and collecting objective data.

> An example of a chief complaint: "I have had a headache for 2 days."

Documenting procedures

Procedural documentation includes how the patient was prepared for the procedure, the position used, the last time the patient had anything to eat or drink, the procedural process, and how the patient tolerated the procedure. Most of this information is documented by the provider, but the medical assistant documents preprocedure information (vital signs, informed consent) and postprocedure instructions.

Required components of the medical record

Whether the office uses an electronic or paper record, there are specific sections that house the various documents.

- **Demographic information:** This includes name, address, birthdate, Social Security number, phone number, and insurance information. It is important to review this section at each visit to ensure accurate information for insurance filing and billing, as well as contacting the patient.

- **Medication record:** Review and update this information at each visit. Patients should be asked to bring their medications from home and compare each of them with the medical record. Ask about over-the-counter medications and supplements as well as any allergies.

- **Progress notes:** This is where the chief complaint or *SOAP note* that describes each visit can be located.

- **Laboratory or diagnostic reports:** This section houses laboratory reports and EKG or other diagnostic tests.

Other sections (consultations, problem lists) may be included in the medical record as well. The medical assistant must be familiar with where to locate specific information related to the patient they are caring for. All of these sections should be organized in chronological order, with the most recent reports on top or listed first.

SOAP note. Method of charting commonly used in ambulatory care (subjective, objective, assessment, plan)

Medical necessity guidelines

Medical necessity is used by third-party payers (insurance companies or other entities responsible for payment of medical services) to identify that a specific procedure or test is necessary for the care or diagnosis of the patient. For insurance to cover a specific item, it would need to be deemed medically necessary. This is often seen with hospitalizations, but random tests will not be approved without validation in the medical record supporting the medical need. For instance, an EKG might not be medically necessary for a 30-year-old unless the patient is experiencing chest pain. Documentation is required to support the necessity for the test and for the insurance company to remit payment.

Diagnostic and procedural coding

Diagnostic and procedural coding is a universal language of numbers used for billing and reimbursement. Various organizations use this as a means of gathering health data for research and initiatives. Accurate coding maximizes the provider reimbursement, but knowingly upcoding (coding for more than what was performed) for a higher reimbursement can lead to fraud and legal action against the provider.

OPERATE BASIC FUNCTIONS OF AN EHR/EMR

Electronic health record (EHR) and electronic medical record (EMR) are often used interchangeably. However, the EHR can be incorporated across more than one health care organization. The EMR is used within a single organization. In essence, they are a collection of health information that has been gathered, organized, and managed in an electronic format that is accessible to people who have proper authorization.

Security information

Patients are often concerned about the security and privacy of their information, especially when stored electronically. It is important for the medical assistant to be able to answer questions patients have regarding the security of their information. Sharing such things as who has access to the information and the use of passwords and firewalls for security measures will help to allay many of the fears of accessibility to their private information.

Functions of an EMR

The EMR (sometimes referred to as a practice management system) is capable of performing multiple tasks including the following.

- *Appointments:* This includes scheduling, reminders, and confirmations.
- *Prescription services:* Prescriptions can be written and printed from the EMR or transmitted to the pharmacy.
- *Billing procedures:* Charges associated with the codes can be captured and entered in the system.
- *Insurance services:* Eligibility can be verified and referrals can be managed.
- *Laboratory and other ancillary services:* Orders can be generated from the EMR for services such as laboratory work or x-rays.
- *Patient portal:* A means of communication between the provider and patient to relay information, schedule appointments, access account information, and send e-mails.

Computerized physician order entry (CPOE)

Providers can directly document orders into the EMR. This point-of-care documentation allows for completion of the medical documentation at the time of the visit, assists in decreasing errors associated with legibility of writing, and ensures seamless communication between members of the health care team.

For additional information on CPOE regulations see the Centers for Medicare and Medicaid Services website at www.cms.gov.

Using the patient portal to communicate with patients

Most EMR systems offer the opportunity to connect with patients through the patient portal. Using this type of system helps to bridge the distance and time gap between the health care facility and the patient. Questions can be answered promptly, refills for prescriptions can be requested, results of testing can be shared, and patients can receive appointment reminders. The patient portal was designed to empower the patient to take an active role in their care. This has proven very effective as more people use this method of communication. While the patient portal is a fast and convenient method of relating information to patients, there are times when a patient should be contacted directly by someone from the office. The portal should not be the only means of patient-facility communication.

SUMMARY

Clinical care of the patient includes more than hands-on skills. It involves the ability to communicate and educate as well as perform administrative functions at the point of care, including entry into the electronic health record. As technology evolves and advances, the medical assistant will have improved equipment to use and technology for communications and charting. The medical assistant must continue to grow with the rapidly changing health care environment.

CHAPTER 10
Infection Control

OVERVIEW

The purpose of infection control is to minimize and remove a variety of disease-causing micro-organisms from the health care environment. These pathogens need to be minimized at every opportunity. Effective infection control helps to ensure the safety of patients and health care staff. As a member of the health care team, the medical assistant plays a vital role in the implementation of infection control procedures. From basic hand washing to the appropriate disposal of *biohazardous* material, the medical assistant can break the cycle of infection, resulting in fewer pathogenic transmissions.

INFECTION CONTROL

The employer has the responsibility to ensure a safe work environment. Several *Occupational Safety and Health Administration (OSHA)* measures contribute to employee safety in a health care setting, and infection control is one of them. Along with OSHA, the *Centers for Disease Control and Prevention (CDC)* provides recommendations to keep patients and workers safe according to established best practices. The CDC introduced universal precautions in the 1980s in response to the growing number of *human immunodeficiency virus (HIV)* and *hepatitis B virus (HBV)* cases. This has evolved into the current practice of standard precautions. In 2001, OSHA implemented the Bloodborne Pathogens Standard in order to provide further protection to patients and workers exposed to disease-causing micro-organisms.

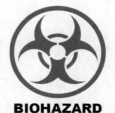

BIOHAZARD

Objectives

Upon completion of this chapter, you should be able to:

- Recognize agents that cause disease, and identify measures, strategies, and techniques used to prevent the disease.

- List six links in the chain of infection.

- Differentiate between medical and surgical asepsis.

- Describe clean vs. aseptic technique and when to use it.

- Adhere to guidelines regarding hand hygiene recommendations, and follow proper technique when washing hands.

- Perform sanitization, disinfection, and sterilization procedures.

- List steps that should be taken for biological and chemical spills.

- List the purpose of Safety Data Sheets, what is included on an SDS, and where they should be stored.

- List components of an exposure control plan.

---

biohazard. A biological or chemical substance that is dangerous to human beings and the environment

Occupational Safety and Health Administration (OSHA). Agency of the government that oversees and regulates worker safety

Centers for Disease Control and Prevention (CDC). Provides safety guidelines for medical offices and facilities

human immunodeficiency virus (HIV). A retrovirus that invades and inactivates helper T-cells of the immune system and is a cause of AIDS and AIDS-related complex

hepatitis B virus (HBV). Liver infection caused by the hepatitis B virus that is transmitted by blood, semen, or another body fluid from an infected person

OSHA requires all health care facilities to develop and annually review an effective exposure control plan specific to the organization. At a minimum, the plan must consist of the following: protections in place for jobs with exposure to infectious material, use of personal protective equipment (PPE), action plans when an exposure incident occurs, labeling of hazardous substances, immunizations offered, record-keeping, and training for employees related to the Bloodborne Pathogen Standards. The use of standard precautions greatly reduces the number of *healthcare-associated infections (HAIs)*.

Six links in the chain of infection

In order for the transmission of a pathogen to occur, the following links must be connected.

- Infectious agent

- Reservoir

- Portal of exit

- Mode of transmission

- Portal of entry

- Susceptible host

Effective infection control consists of breaking this chain, thus preventing the continuation of the cycle.

10.1 The chain of infection

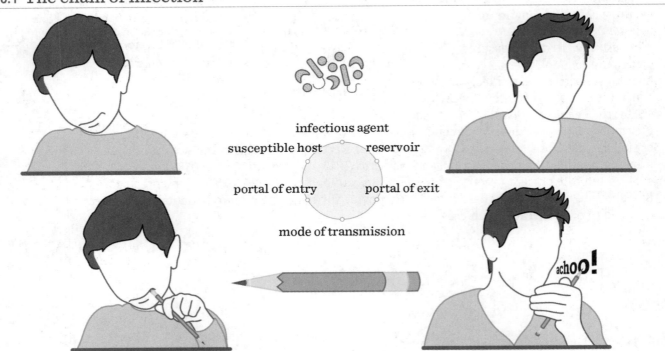

infectious agent

susceptible host   reservoir

portal of entry   portal of exit

mode of transmission

---

healthcare-associated infections (HAI). Infections acquired in a health care setting

Disease transmission and prevention

In order for the transmission of a disease to occur, there must be a pathogen or infectious agent present. These disease-causing micro-organisms are most often in the form of viruses, bacteria, fungi, or protozoa. An environment conducive to pathogen survival is known as a reservoir. In a clinical setting, the reservoir is often the patient but can also be an inanimate object such as a piece of medical equipment. The human body makes an ideal reservoir for microbial growth because of the presence of nutrients, moisture, ideal temperature, and pH levels. The portal of exit is the passageway that the pathogen uses to exit the reservoir. This can be the infected body fluids of an individual in a patient care setting. Once the pathogen exits the reservoir, a mode of transmission is necessary in order for the cycle to continue. A direct transmission takes place when there is contact with the infected person or body fluid that is carrying the pathogen. Indirect transmissions occur when there is an intermediate step between the portal of exit and portal of entry. Either fomites or vectors play a role in an indirect transmission. Once the pathogen has a means of transmission, it will need a new portal of entry to continue the infectious cycle. Pathogens often enter into a host via an open wound or through the mouth, nose, eye, intestines, urinary tract, or reproductive system. The final step in the cycle is the presence of a susceptible host. Several variables make the human body—especially of a compromised patient—the ideal susceptible host. Factors such as overall health, age, and the condition of a person's immune system all affect the chances of them becoming a host for a disease transmission. If one of the links in the infection cycle is broken, the transmission is halted. It is the responsibility of all health care professionals to take the necessary steps to break this cycle.

10.2 Agents of indirect transmission

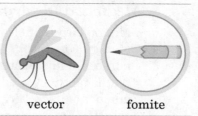

vector   fomite

Each pathogen has specific routes in which transmissions can occur. Clinical facilities issue a variety of isolation practices according to the identified pathogen. If one is not identified, the most restrictive isolation is often used.

CHALLENGE Disease transmission

Read the following scenario and answer the questions below.

Mr. Green arrives in the reception area and signs in using the clipboard and pen. He is being seen for possible influenza and is sneezing and coughing excessively. He is not covering his mouth or nose while doing so, and the medical assistant moves him into an exam room right away. Ms. Stevens immediately arrives and uses the same pen and clipboard to sign in and proceeds to wait. Ms. Stevens is immunocompromised due to a new medication therapy. Mr. Green receives an influenza diagnosis, and Ms. Stevens has an uneventful visit. However, Ms. Stevens returns within a few days with influenza symptoms.

1. Which of the following would the pen and clipboard be considered in this situation?
   A. Fomite
   B. Vector
   C. Reservoir
   D. Portal of exit

2. Which of the following would Mr. Green be considered in this situation?
   A. Fomite
   B. Vector
   C. Portal of entry
   D. Portal of exit

3. Which of the following would Ms. Stevens be considered in this situation?
   A. Portal of entry
   B. Portal of exit
   C. Reservoir
   D. Fomite

Key: 1. A; 2. D; 3. A

ASEPTIC TECHNIQUES FOR CLINICAL SITUATIONS

Asepsis is the condition of being free from infection or infectious material. Keeping the work and reception areas clean is an important step in slowing or stopping the spread of infectious agents in the clinical environment. Below are a few simple, yet effective methods to accomplish this goal.

- Clean the office daily.

- Move sick and contagious patients to an exam room or separate waiting area away from well-check patients upon arrival.

- Do not allow eating or drinking in patient areas.

- Hang reminder signs regarding good hand hygiene and other prevention methods.

Medical and surgical asepsis

Medical asepsis or clean technique is used daily in every clinical setting and consists of the removal of micro-organisms after they leave the body. The overall goal of medical asepsis is to reduce the number of micro-organisms and prohibit their growth. Handwashing is a medical aseptic technique that is routinely used to prevent the spread of infection. Medical asepsis is used to reduce the number of micro-organisms, therefore reducing the chances of disease transmission. This type of asepsis does not eliminate all possibility of pathogen presence, but it greatly reduces their numbers and their ability to multiply and cause further infections. Gloves, gowns, and masks may be used during medical asepsis, but it is done to protect the health care worker more than the patient.

Medical assistants use clean or medical aseptic technique daily. Washing hands prior to and after each patient encounter, assuring the work space is clean, using gloves when in contact with body fluids, and the proper cleaning of supplies are just a few of the examples of clean technique in action.

Surgical asepsis is the removal of all micro-organisms and must be used during invasive procedures or when there is a penetration of the patient's skin or mucous membranes. The goal of surgical asepsis is to eliminate micro-organisms from entering the body. Surgical asepsis protects the patient more than the health care worker. Supplies such as sterile gloves, gowns, and drapes are often used when a surgical aseptic technique is necessary. Antiseptic skin preparation is also required with surgical aseptic technique if the patient's skin is to be punctured.

Medical assistants need to know when to use medical vs. surgical aseptic techniques. However, there are several actions that medical assistants can take to reduce the chances of pathogen transmission. Breaking the cycle of infection be done with the simple act of covering the nose and mouth during a sneeze or avoiding patient encounters if a cold or other illness is present.

---

medical asepsis. Clean technique; the practice designed to reduce the number and transfer of pathogens; also helps in breaking the chain of infection

surgical asepsis. The complete removal of micro-organisms and their spores from the surface of an object

GUIDELINES REGARDING HAND HYGIENE

In many situations, both in clinical and nonclinical settings, good hand hygiene can be the force that stops the cycle of infection. Both clinical staff and patients benefit from this essential safety practice. Clinical staff are discouraged from wearing excess jewelry (rings, bracelets). These items can harbor pathogens and make asepsis difficult to achieve. If such items are worn, they should be removed prior to hand hygiene for the best results. Artificial nails should not be worn in a clinical setting. If visible contamination is not present on health care workers' hands, an alcohol-based sanitizer may be used.

CDC hand hygiene recommendations

Proper hand hygiene must be used in the following situations even if disposable gloves are used.

- Before and after patient contact
- After contact with contaminated surfaces
- After contact with blood or body fluids
- Before performing an aseptic procedure (blood draw, medication administration)
- Before and after contact with supplies or equipment near patients
- After contact with a contaminated body site prior to contact with a clean body site
- After glove removal

Steps for washing hands using soap and water

Start by wetting hands with clean, running warm water. Apply soap and rub hands together for at least 20 seconds, making sure to pay attention to all surfaces, including between fingers and nails. The friction that is created with this step helps to lift debris from the skin. Microbes tend to concentrate near and under the nails, so pay special attention to these areas. Rinse hands with running water, and dry with a clean towel or air-dry. If using a standard faucet, once the hands are clean and dry, use a paper towel to shut the faucet off to avoid exposing the hands to a contaminated surface.

Steps for using an alcohol-based sanitizer

If clean water and soap are not available, an alcohol-based sanitizer with a minimum of 60% alcohol can be used. When using an alcohol-based sanitizer, apply a small amount (usually dime-sized) into the palm of one hand and rub both hands together creating friction, making sure to cover all surfaces including between fingers and nails. Continue rubbing until the solution has dried. Keep in mind that sanitizers can be a good solution in specific circumstances, but they should not be used if hands are visibly dirty. In this situation, soap and water must be used to remove the debris and wash the hands.

DISINFECTION/SANITIZATION

Infection control includes not only the patient and the employee, but also ensuring that the equipment and supplies used in the clinical setting are free from disease-causing micro-organisms. The type of cleaning depends on the piece of equipment and the type of procedure it will be used in. Surgical instruments handled differently than patient assessment tools found in an exam room.

Sanitization

Sanitization is often the first step in assuring that a piece of medical equipment is as clean as possible. This process reduces the number of microbes to a lower level so that they are ready to undergo the *sterilization* or *disinfection* process. Sanitization is especially helpful if there is visible debris present on the equipment. Gloves must be worn during this process. If there are sharps needing sanitization, wear thick utility gloves to avoid injury. Follow manufacturer's instructions regarding water temperatures and types of detergent to use during this process. It is important to keep the work area separated into dirty and clean areas to avoid cross-contamination of equipment. For facilities that work with very delicate instruments, ultrasonic sanitization is used to avoid damage to the equipment. Rather than using friction to remove the debris, the sound waves loosen the debris so the object is free from excess material going into the disinfection or sterilization phase. Ultrasonic sanitization also reduces the risk of sharps exposure for the health care worker.

Disinfection

Disinfection is the process of destroying pathogens on a surface. Even though it might not destroy all of the microbial spores, it greatly reduces the spread of infection by destroying or limiting microbial activity. The solutions used in disinfection are effective when used correctly. The process can often require lengthy submissions in the chemical. Glutaraldehyde is a common disinfectant used in the clinical setting but usually requires a long submersion time in order to be fully effective. A cheaper and effective alternative is a 1:10 bleach solution. Chemical disinfectants cannot be used on patients and are reserved for medical supplies, equipment, and surroundings.

---

sanitization. Reducing the number of micro-organisms by removing debris with soap and water prior to disinfecting

sterilization. A technique for destroying pathogens and their spores on inanimate objects, using heat, water, chemicals, or gases

disinfect. To clean something (e.g., work area, equipment) using chemicals that kill pathogens but not their spores

STERILIZATION OF MEDICAL EQUIPMENT

The destruction of all pathogens and their spores can be achieved with sterilization. This step is necessary for surgical asepsis. Although medical assistants might not do it every day, it is important to understand and be able to perform sterilization of supplies and equipment used in surgical and other invasive procedures.

Sterilization of supplies and equipment

The use of dry heat, gas, chemicals, ultraviolet radiation, ionizing radiation, chemicals, or steam under pressure in an *autoclave* are all methods that can be used in the sterilization of medical equipment. Medical facilities can purchase supplies and equipment from manufacturers already sterilized and packaged, or they can establish a sterilization space in the facility. Once an item is sterilized, specific handling must occur so the item is not contaminated.

Disinfection/sterilization of endoscopes

The disinfection and sterilization of *endoscopes* is a complex process due to the nature of the procedure this device is used for and because the normal sterilization techniques will most likely damage the endoscope. Therefore, the medical assistant should review and follow the manufacturer's guidelines for cleaning the endoscope. The following is a description of the steps that are most often used to process an endoscope prior to and after patient exposure.

10.3 Sanitizing, disinfecting, and sterilizing

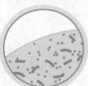
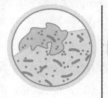

sanitization

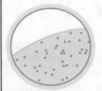

disinfection

sterilization

- *Pre-cleaning:* Done immediately after the endoscope has been removed from the patient, this consists of wiping the tube with a wet cloth and then soaking the tube in a cleaning solution.

- *Leak testing:* Use air, pressure, and water to determine if any damage to the endoscope has occurred.

- *Manual cleaning:* Use the recommended cleaning solution to manually remove debris from the internal and external surfaces of the endoscope.

- *Rinse after cleaning:* Rinse all parts of the endoscope with clean water to further reduce the chances of any debris or cleaning solution from remaining.

- *High-level disinfection (manual or automated):* Use the recommended high-level disinfectant that the manufacturer suggests for immersion and flushing of endoscope pieces.

- *Rinse after high-level disinfection:* Rinse all parts to assure no residual chemical disinfectant remains on the endoscope.

- *Drying:* Rinse all parts with alcohol and then dry with forced air. Store the endoscope vertically in a clean, dry, and dust-free environment.

autoclave. An instrument that sterilizes equipment and supplies by subjecting them to high pressure saturated steam

endoscope. A medical device consisting of a tube and optical system for observing the inside of a hollow organ, cavity, or tissue plane

DISPOSAL OF BIOHAZARDOUS MATERIALS

OSHA also requires the disposal of infectious and hazardous waste to be handled according to safety standards. The use of PPE and *Safety Data Sheets (SDSs)* provides the health care worker with the tools and resources to maintain a safe clinical work environment. The proper identification and disposal of contaminated material is another step in preventing the spread of infectious material.

OSHA guidelines for disposal of biohazardous materials

Any item that comes into contact with blood or body fluids must be disposed of properly. Needles must not be recapped, but rather placed in a *sharps container* immediately after use on a patient. Any item that has sharp edges or blades, such as a scalpel, should also be placed in a sharps container.

10.4 Biohazard waste container

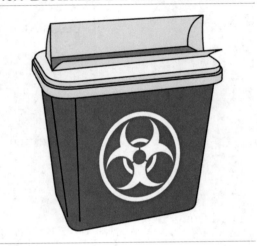

Sharps containers must be made of a puncture-proof, leak-proof material and be labeled with the biohazard symbol. Gloves, gauze, bandages, and other items that do not have sharp edges or contain needles should be placed in a biohazard bag, which is leak-proof and labeled with the biohazard symbol. When a sharps container is two-thirds full, the container should be sealed and placed in the designated area for disposal.

All biohazard waste must be identified with the biohazard symbol and must be contained. All bags used to collect infectious material must be made of an impermeable polyethylene or polypropylene material. A lid must be present on all boxes or receptacles and replaced after each use. A waste management company is often used for pick-up and disposal of biohazard material from medical facilities. These agencies also must abide by OSHA standards regarding biohazard material handling and disposal.

Personal protective equipment

Employers must provide PPE to all employees when there is a potential for exposure to blood or body fluids. It is the employee's responsibility to use the PPE when contact with blood or body fluids is anticipated. Examples of PPE include gloves, goggles, face shields, and gowns. If an employee is allergic to latex or the powder used in the gloves provided, the employer must provide hypoallergenic or powder-free gloves at no expense to the employee.

Safety Data Sheets (SDS). Documents containing necessary information regarding chemicals in the work environment

sharps container. A puncture-proof container designed specifically to safely dispose of needles, scalpels, and other sharp disposable medical instruments

Safety Data Sheets

OSHA requires that all employers provide SDSs to their employees. Any time a new chemical is brought into the work environment, SDS information must accompany the chemical. Medical assistants work with a variety of solutions ranging from mild detergents to toxic chemicals. The following information must be included on the SDS in order to communicate the hazards and actions necessary if exposure to the chemical occurs.

- *Identification:* Product identifier, manufacturer information, recommended use, restrictions on use

- *Hazard identification:* All hazards related to the chemical including label requirements

- *Composition/ingredients:* Chemical ingredients

- *First-aid measures:* Symptoms and effects from exposure including treatment necessary

- *Fire-fighting measures:* Appropriate extinguishing methods and chemical hazards from fire

- *Accidental release measures:* Emergency procedures, PPE, containment, and cleanup

- *Handling and storage:* Safe handling and appropriate storage requirements

- *Exposure controls/personal protection:* Recommended exposure limits and PPE necessary

- *Physical and chemical properties:* Chemical characteristics

- *Stability and reactivity:* Chemical stability and potential reactions

- *Toxicological information:* Measures of toxicity, acute and chronic effects, routes of exposure; also needs to include ecological, disposal, transport, and regulatory information regarding the chemical

- *Other information:* Additional information including last revision

Exposure control plan for a biological or chemical spill

It is the responsibility of the employer to have an exposure control plan in place and available for all employees. The plan should be reviewed with each employee upon hiring, annually, and after any updates. The exposure control plan covers all scenarios regarding emergency procedures specific to their practice. Included in these plans should be the steps to be followed in the event of a biological or chemical emergency. Medical professionals often recognize a looming community emergency before the public does. Whether it is the rapid transmission of an infectious disease or the response to an acute traumatic event, medical staff must be ready to respond accordingly. It is important for the medical assistant to know which health officials to notify regarding the incident. Local emergency management agencies along with various governmental agencies might need to be collaborated with in order to provide the best care and communication for the public.

SUMMARY

From handwashing to equipment sterilization, medical assistants play a vital role in successful infection control within the clinical setting. Breaking the cycle of infection is key to reducing the number of pathogenic transmissions. The main goal of infection control is to reduce and eliminate the transmission of infectious agents. By accomplishing this goal, patients, staff, and the community are safer. Each employer needs to ensure their employees are given the necessary training and tools to carry out the goal of infection control in the workplace. However, it is the employee's responsibility to take appropriate action to assure the best practices are carried out in each situation.

CHAPTER 11

Testing and Laboratory Procedures

OVERVIEW

Point-of-care testing, specimen collection, and performance of screening procedures are important aspects of the medical assisting scope of practice. Patient education and preparation, as well as proper specimen handling, are imperative to ensure accurate results. This chapter focuses on *Clinical Laboratories Improvement Amendments (CLIA)* waived laboratory testing and other screening procedures.

NONBLOOD SPECIMENS

The medical assistant must be familiar with the types and requirements of tests ordered and ensure that the patient receives complete instructions on how to collect the specimen to maximize accuracy of results. The patient should also receive the appropriate specimen containers with directions for their use.

Collection of urine specimens

Urine is the most commonly tested specimen in an ambulatory care setting. There are various means of collecting urine specimens.

Random urine: The patient urinates in a clean, nonsterile container. This specimen is used for screening purposes.

First morning specimen: The patient collects the first specimen of the morning in a clean container. This specimen is more concentrated and used for pregnancy testing, or when other analytes (protein, nitrites) need to be evaluated.

Clean-catch midstream: The patient performs perineal cleaning using moist wipes, begins to urinate, and then collects the specimen midstream in a sterile urine container. This specimen is used for cultures or when a noncontaminated specimen is desired.

Objectives

Upon completion of this chapter, you should be able to:

- Follow proper procedures for collecting nonblood specimens including urine, stool, sputum, and cultures.
- Perform point-of-care testing following CLIA regulations.
- Describe the purpose of COLA and list other organizations that perform similar services.
- Describe the purpose of a laboratory quality control program and explain the importance of running controls and calibrating laboratory equipment.
- Describe logs that are required for a laboratory quality assurance/control program and the purpose of the logs.
- Describe the parts of a lab requisition form including demographic, billing, coding, and testing sections.
- Identify requirements for matching, labeling, handling, processing, storing, transporting, and disposing of laboratory specimens.
- Recognize normal and abnormal values for common laboratory tests and describe common protocol for handling lab values that are abnormal or at critical levels.
- List and describe procedures for testing vision and hearing in the ambulatory care environment.
- List steps for performing a scratch test and intradermal allergy testing.
- Perform spirometry testing and educate patients on how to use a peak flow meter.

Clinical Laboratory Improvement Amendments (CLIA). Federal standards that regulate laboratory testing, handling, and processing

random urine. A urine specimen collected in a clean container for screening purposes; no preparation is required

clean-catch midstream. A urine specimen that is collected in the middle of the urinary stream in a sterile container after perineal cleaning

24-hour: This method uses a container with preservatives. The patient discards the first morning specimen and collects all specimens for the next 24 hr, including the first void of the second day. This type of collection is important in *quantitative* analysis of components such as protein when analyzing kidney function.

Catheterized collection: This method is used when a sterile urine sample is needed or if patients are unable to provide a specimen on their own. It involves insertion of a sterile tube (catheter) through the urethra into the bladder. This procedure is performed by the provider or nurse, with the medical assistant prepping the patient and assisting.

Collection of stool specimens

A *fecal occult blood* test requires a stool specimen collection to screen for the presence of blood, which can indicate a disease process or gastrointestinal bleeding. Correct patient instructions are imperative to ensure that false positives do not occur. Instruct the patient on medications and foods to avoid for 3 days. The patient will then collect three separate specimens on filter paper.

The tape test is used to detect pinworms, which typically affect small children. Provide parents with a slide with a piece of tape on it. The tape is placed over the child's anus before getting up in the morning and then back on the slide, which is brought to the provider for analysis.

Stool specimens can also be collected for parasites or to evaluate for bacterial infections. Specific containers are used for each of these tests. Provide the container to the patient along with instructions on collection. This ova and parasites (O&P) testing detects the presence of parasites and their eggs, either of which require treatment.

Collection of sputum specimens

Sputum specimens are collected in sterile containers. When obtaining a sputum specimen, it is important for the patient to produce a deep, productive cough. This produces a specimen from deep within the lungs rather than saliva from the mouth. Sputum specimens are best collected in the early morning before eating or drinking. Patients should avoid mouthwashes prior to sputum collection.

Collecting specimens for cultures

Specimens for cultures are always collected in sterile containers. Take precautions to avoid touching the insides of lids, swabs, or containers, which could contaminate the specimen. If the specimen is not properly collected, the identification of the causative agent will not occur and proper treatment cannot be started.

Reminders for specimen collections

- Collect the specimen at the appropriate time.
- Collect the specimen from the site of suspected infection.
- Minimize transport time to a reference lab.
- Collect the appropriate quantity.
- Use the appropriate containers and label them accordingly.

quantitative. Analysis that identifies quantity or actual number counts

fecal occult blood. Evaluation of a stool specimen for hidden blood

CLIA-WAIVED TESTING

The Food and Drug Administration (FDA) requires that all testing meet federal guidelines and determines the complexity of the tests performed in the laboratory. Ambulatory care centers typically perform Clinical Laboratories Improvement Amendments (CLIA) waived testing, which is the simplest of laboratory procedures. Medical assistants are trained in CLIA-waived testing and may perform these tests per provider request.

Point-of-care testing

Various tests related to chemistry, immunology, microbiology, and hematology are identified as CLIA-waived and easily performed in physician office laboratories. Common point-of-care tests include the following.

- *Pregnancy testing*: Urine is screened for the presence of human chorionic gonadotropin (hCG) antibodies.

- *Rapid Streptococcus testing*: Throat swabs are obtained to screen for Group A streptococcus.

- *Dipstick, tablet, or multi-stick urinalysis*: The urinalysis is a screening tool for analytes that are excreted in the urine.

- *Hemoglobin*: A machine is used to screen for the oxygen-carrying protein in whole blood, performed using capillary blood from a fingerstick (capillary puncture).

- *Spun hematocrit*: Fingerstick collection of blood in microcapillary tubes is centrifuged and evaluated for the percentage of red blood cells.

- *Blood glucose*: Whole blood is analyzed in a glucometer for a quantitative glucose level and is a screening test for diabetes, performed using capillary blood from a finger stick (capillary puncture).

- *Hemoglobin A1c*: This capillary blood test shows diabetes control over an approximate 3-month period.

- *Cholesterol testing*: Lipids are evaluated using capillary blood.

- *Helicobacter pylori*: A blood sample screens for *H. pylori*, which is the main cause of gastric ulcers.

- *Mononucleosis screening*: This screening tool tests for the presence of the Epstein-Barr virus in capillary blood.

- *Nasal smear for influenza types A and B*: This screening is a *qualitative* test for influenza antigens using a swab that is inserted into the nostril.

- *Drug testing*: Substances can be detected in urine and blood samples.

- *Fecal occult blood*: This test is performed to screen for hidden blood in the stool.

qualitative. Analysis that identifies quality or characteristics of components such as size, shape, and maturity of cells; typically reported as positive or negative

CLIA regulations

CLIA was established in 1988 to ensure quality of diagnostic testing through laboratory regulations. There are three designations for laboratory testing based on the complexity.

CLIA-waived is the most common designation for ambulatory care and is the lowest level of complexity. These tests could be performed in the home environment or easily conducted in the medical office.

Moderate- and high-complexity tests are considered nonwaived. Labs performing these tests must have a CLIA certificate and undergo inspections to ensure standards are being met. These tests are typically performed in a reference or hospital laboratory.

Some providers in the ambulatory care setting choose to view some specimens microscopically. Although this is considered a form of moderate-complexity testing, CLIA approves *provider-performed microscopy procedures* for microscopic screening of some specimens such as urine or body excretions. This allows the provider to develop a preliminary diagnosis and begin treatment as warranted.

COLA and other CLIA accreditation organizations

CLIA develops their standards and regulations with support from the Food and Drug Administration (FDA), Centers for Disease Control and Prevention (CDC), and the Centers for Medicare and Medicaid Services (CMS).

The *Commission on Office Laboratory Accreditation (COLA)* is an independent accreditor for laboratories; it focuses on meeting CLIA regulations with a goal of providing the best care to the patient. Additional accreditors approved under CLIA can be found at www.cms.gov.

Quality assurance and quality control

The importance of quality cannot be understated in maximizing accuracy and patient safety. *Quality assurance* is comprehensive and relates to policies and procedures that must be implemented for reliability of test results. *Quality control* is included in quality assurance but is more specific; it is related to test reliability and accuracy while attempting to uncover errors and eliminate them.

For example, reviewing the expiration of urine multi-sticks is a means of quality control, whereas policies related to rotating stock to put newest containers in the back of the storage area is a quality assurance measure.

Also, checking the temperature of the laboratory refrigerator and documenting it on a log is a quality control measure. The policy of checking the temperature and maintaining it between 39° and 41° F is a quality assurance measure.

---

provider-performed microscopy procedure. A CLIA term for microscopic examinations that require the expertise of a physician or mid-level provider qualified in microscopic examinations; falls under CLIA's moderate-complexity category

Commission on Office Laboratory Accreditation (COLA). An independent firm that provides accreditation for laboratories and has a goal of meeting CLIA standards

quality assurance. Policies and procedures to maximize patient safety and ensure reliability related to laboratory testing

quality control. Measures incorporated to maximize reliability and accuracy of results while recognizing and eliminating errors in testing

Quality control procedures

When testing specimens, quality control samples are tested to ensure patient samples are accurate. Quality control samples are referred to as *controls* and use a quantitative result range or qualitative descriptor.

For example, when testing hemoglobin, the control cuvette in the machine can be calibrated to be 12.6 ± 0.3. Therefore, if the result falls between 12.3 and 12.9, it is anticipated that the patient sample will be accurate when tested. When evaluating a qualitative result, if using a fecal occult slide, a control strip turns blue if the developer is effective. If this strip does not turn blue, either the developer is not working or the slide is not valid. Either way, the test will not be accurate.

11.1 Quantitative vs. qualitative

results of a urinalysis	quantitative	
	glucose	negative
	specific gravity	1.020
	pH	6.1
	protein	negative
	ketones	negative
	WBCs	negative
	bilirubin	negative
	blood	negative
	nitrate	negative
	urobilinogen	0.3
	qualitative	
	clarity	clear
	color	amber

Quality control logs

The medical assistant is responsible for monitoring the functionality of various pieces of equipment within the health care facility. This ensures that equipment is working properly and the accuracy of test results is maximized. For example, the temperature of the refrigerator is a quality control measure. In addition, when running controls on new testing kits or running a daily control, maintain logbooks to validate the test was conducted under optimal conditions and control samples were accurate prior to testing patient samples.

MATCHING SPECIMEN TO PATIENT AND COMPLETED REQUISITION

The medical assistant can complete lab requisitions based on providers' orders. Requisitions that are not accurately completed can result in a rejected specimen, which causes patient dissatisfaction and possible delays in treatments.

It is the responsibility of the medical assistant to properly label all collected specimens and ensure the specimens are matched with the correct lab requisition or order. Incorrect specimen labeling contributes to laboratory error more than any other factor. Specimen containers should be labeled with patient information at the time of collection. The labels should then be verified against the patient chart and the lab order before sending the specimen to the lab for processing.

Computerized physician order entry

Only licensed or legally authorized individuals are allowed to enter laboratory orders in the electronic record. Under the direction of a provider, only credentialed medical assistants are authorized to enter orders. In April 2015, Meaningful Use was replaced with the Medicare Access and CHIP Reinforcement Act of 2015 (MACRA), which deals with payment for health care under the direction of the CMS. The credentialing requirement will likely continue to be enforced through MACRA.

controls. Specific tools used in the laboratory with a known result, used to compare with results of a patient sample to confirm validity of the test and specimen

Parts of a laboratory requisition form

Whether the laboratory requisition form is electronic or paper, there are specific parts included in both. The first part of the requisition includes patient demographic information. If the requisition is computer-generated, this information should populate automatically. A provider's signature or authentication that the provider ordered the lab work is present on all requisitions. The specific tests need to be marked and are often organized on a laboratory requisition based on the department that will test it. The source of the specimen, as well as date and time of specimen collection, is also required on the requisition.

Demographic information

Demographic accuracy on the requisition form is important for billing purposes and patient identification. Requisitions can vary based on the organization, but typical demographic information found on a requisition includes the following.

- Patient name
- Address
- Date of birth
- Sex
- Telephone number
- Insurance information
- Provider information
- Diagnosis or indications for testing
- Order date

Billing information

Before billing the insurance company for services rendered in the laboratory, compare the insurance card to the requisition for accuracy. The guarantor, insurance plan, and ID numbers are necessary to file the insurance claim. Accurate contact information for the patient will facilitate billing when the patient is a self-pay or if the insurance company does not cover the cost of the testing.

ICD-10 coding information

Some requisitions are already populated with the appropriate ICD-10 codes. Laboratory testing is strictly coded from the provider's reason for ordering the test. To appropriately assign codes, ensure that complete diagnosis information is included on the form.

Testing information

Each test is individually checked unless a *panel* (which encompasses a variety of tests related to one body system) is ordered. An example of this is testing related to the liver, so a lipid panel or profile might be ordered. Validate that the tests on the requisition match the provider's orders in the medical record. If additional information is required, ensure that it is completed. For instance, if a pregnancy test is ordered, add the date of the last menstrual period.

panel. A group of tests that are connected to one particular body system; profile

Labeling specimens

The information included on a specimen label depends on laboratory and facility policy. However, all specimens should contain the patient's name and the date and time of collection. Other information that might be required includes the patient's date of birth, provider's name, and initials of the person collecting the specimen. Make sure to label the container of a specimen and not a lid, which could mistakenly be put on another container.

Matching specimens to the lab requisition form

The medical assistant is responsible for ensuring that the collected specimens are verified by matching them to the lab requisition. Failure to collect the appropriate specimen, properly label it, and verify that the information on specimen and requisition form match could lead to rejection of the specimen for testing. Many requisitions also include numbered identification stickers that should be adhered to all specimen containers; this is an added verification tool to ensure the specimen and requisition match.

GAME Laboratory tests

Match the laboratory tests with the department.

Laboratory tests:	Departments:
1. Fasting blood sugar	A. Hematology
2. White blood cell count	B. Chemistry
3. Culture and sensitivity	C. Urinalysis
4. Type and cross-match	D. Blood bank
5. Pap smear	E. Microbiology
6. Nitrite	F. Cytology

Key: 1. B, 2. A, 3. E, 4. D, 5. F, 6. C

PROCESSING, HANDLING, AND TRANSPORTING SPECIMENS

Medical assistants must take precautions to avoid contamination of specimens that are being prepared for transport and testing, and protect themselves from exposure to potentially infectious agents. Proper processing, handling, and transporting of specimens is also important to ensure that the test can be conducted and that the results are accurate. Handwashing is the most effective means of preventing the spread of infection, but personal protective equipment should be used based on the specimen being handled. The most common types of specimens in the ambulatory care setting are blood, urine, and swab samples.

Handling nonblood specimens

Always follow proper office procedure and reference the lab manual for proper handling of nonblood specimens. For example, when collecting and handling specimens for drug testing for employment or a court subpoena, a *chain of custody* is required to ensure that specimen tampering did not occur. A kit is usually provided for these types of tests, and a signature of everyone who has contact with the specimen is required. Also, a urine test that requires testing for bilirubin needs special handling to protect the specimen from light, which would affect the accuracy of the testing. For this particular situation, a dark container is required for the specimen.

chain of custody. A series of processes and procedures used to ensure security and accuracy

Processing nonblood specimens

Specimens might need to be processed prior to transport to maintain the integrity of the specimen. Something as simple as making sure that a swabbed specimen is moist by breaking the fluid chamber within the specimen container is a processing technique. Although somewhat unusual in ambulatory care, urine specimens for microscopic analysis can require centrifuging prior to transport with the supernatant fluid removed. Another component of processing is proper storage.

Storing nonblood specimens

Some specimens, like urine, can require refrigeration if testing is not immediately performed. This is done to avoid chemical changes or biological breakdown of the specimen. For example, urine left at room temperature for more than 2 hr will begin to have pH changes and is generally considered unfit for testing. Other specimens might need to be maintained at body temperature, such as swabs for sexually transmitted diseases. If these specimens are cooled, the organisms can be killed, affecting the results or preventing the test from being performed. The medical assistant needs to be familiar with the characteristics of the specimen being collected and refer to the lab manual for proper handling and storage.

Transporting nonblood specimens

Appropriate packaging for nonblood specimens is imperative. If the container has the potential to break or crack, padding and protection from leakage must occur. Wrapping the container in absorbent material and placing the item in a biohazard bag are added safety measures to ensure that the outside of the package does not get contaminated. Whenever specimens are transported via mail, biohazard identification on the outside of the package alerts handlers of a potentially infectious agent within the package.

Proper disposal of nonblood specimens

Specimens need to be properly disposed of to prevent spread of infection. Red biohazard waste bags are sufficient for specimen containers that are not breakable. Use sharps containers for anything that could break or splinter. A designated sink is often adequate for disposal of urine specimens. Always follow the policies and procedures outlined by the facility and adhere to OSHA standards.

RECOGNIZING, DOCUMENTING, AND REPORTING LABORATORY VALUES

When performing office laboratory testing, the medical assistant should be familiar with normal values or results. There can be times that the provider needs to be notified immediately of abnormal results to provide immediate patient care. Even if laboratory testing is not done in the office, a general knowledge of normal values of the most commonly performed laboratory tests is important to alert the provider of abnormalities and provide education to the patient.

Values for common laboratory tests

The medical assistant should be familiar with normal ranges for the most common tests conducted in the ambulatory care setting. The following chart represents some common tests and their normal values. There can be slight variances in reference ranges at various laboratories.

11.2 Common laboratory test values

TEST		EXPECTED REFERENCE RANGE	
		MALES	FEMALES
Hemoglobin (Hgb)		13 to 18 g/dL	12 to 16 g/dL
Hematocrit (Hct)		42% to 52%	36% to 48%
Fasting blood glucose (FBS)		60 to 110 mg/dL	
Total cholesterol		Less than 200 mg/dL	
Low-density lipoprotein (LDL)		Less than 130 mg/dL	
High-density lipoprotein (HDL)		Greater than 40 mg/dL	
Triglycerides		Less than 150 mg/dL	
Erythrocyte sedimentation rate (ESR)		0 to 20 mm/hr	0 to 30 mm/hr
International normalized ratio (INR)		0.8 to 1.2	
Prothrombin time (PT)		10.4 to 15.7 seconds	
Urine	pH	4.5 to 8	
	Specific gravity	1.005 to 1.030	
	Urobilinogen	0.1 to 1	
	All other values	Negative	

Procedures for normal values

With the implementation of electronic medical records (EMRs), communication of laboratory tests is expedited through the provider portal. This eliminates the need for the laboratory to deliver a hard copy of the results. However, some offices do not have a lab interface, which means the results need to be scanned or uploaded into the portal.

When providers review results, note the date of review and the action to be taken. If possible, results should be made accessible to patients for viewing in their EMR. The medical assistant might need to call the patient or mail the results. Ensure the correct address for the patient and verify identity when communicating information over the phone to maintain HIPAA compliance. Do not release any lab results to patients without the provider reviewing and signing off on them first. Miscommunication of laboratory results can have a significant, negative effect on patients.

Abnormal or critical lab values

CLIA requires rapid communication of critical laboratory values. Electronic technology allows laboratories to send electronic alerts to the provider for rapid review. If the medical assistant takes a call from the laboratory with a *critical value*, ensure accuracy of the information by repeating the test results back to the laboratory personnel. After obtaining the information, notify the provider immediately and accurately document the communication and actions taken in the medical record.

VISION AND HEARING TESTING

Screening tests are frequently conducted in ambulatory care and provide guidance for treatments or referrals. Vision and hearing screenings are affordable, as well as easily and efficiently conducted.

Vision tests performed in ambulatory care

The medical assistant performs noninvasive screenings to detect visual abnormalities of the eye (*hyperopia*, *myopia*, *presbyopia*). Using charts and having the patient identify shapes or letters assists with diagnosis.

Near vision testing

Near vision testing screens for presbyopia or hyperopia using a near vision acuity chart. Ask the patient to read printed material of various sizes 14 to 16 inches away from the eyes without corrective lenses. Test each eye separately and then both together. The level at which the patient can read the smallest printing clearly is the result.

11.3 Near vision acuity chart

10 M	Testing vision	20/500 — 24 d
9 M	is tricky. With	20/450 — 22 d
8 M	this test we can	20/400 — 20 d
7 M	get a rough idea	20/350 — 18 d
6 M	of the state of your	20/300 — 16 d
5 M	vision. Please remember	20/250 — 12 d
4 M	that this is a simple evaluation	20/200 — 10 d
3 M	and you should follow up with a vision	20/150 — 8 d
2 M	specialist. An optometrist can test your vision	20/100 — 5 d
1.6 M	in a much more precise and careful manner, using different equipment.	20/80 — 4 d
1 M	That's the kind of test you will need in order to get a prescription for glasses.	20/50 — 2.5 d

Test at 40 cm, with best correction, in a properly lit environment. Do not rush the patient.

Distance vision testing

Distance vision is easily tested by using a distance vision acuity chart to evaluate for myopia. Patients stand 20 feet from a chart at eye level and identify letters, shapes, or the direction an "E" is pointing. The eyes test separately and together, but the patient can wear corrective lenses during the test. The line at which the patient can clearly see the letters or pictures is the result. The patient can miss one item and still pass that line. Vision is recorded as a fraction, with 20/20 representing normal vision.

---

critical value. A laboratory result that is outside of the established reference range and presents potential health risks to a patient

hyperopia. Difficulty seeing things up close; farsightedness

myopia. Difficulty seeing things far away; nearsightedness

presbyopia. A gradual, age-related loss of the eyes' ability to focus actively on nearby objects

Color vision testing

Males are more commonly affected by color blindness. The most common type of color blindness is a red–green deficiency. Screening is done by testing the patient on 11 plates within an *Ishihara* book. If the patient misses four or more, there might be a color deficiency and further testing is warranted.

Visual field testing

Also known as perimetry testing, visual field testing detects eye diseases such as glaucoma. Instruct the patient to look straight ahead and respond to instructions. In an automated test, patients respond to seeing lights flash. In a manual test, patients identify when they can see hands or fingers in their peripheral vision.

Hearing tests performed in ambulatory care

Tympanometry

Tympanometry records movement of the tympanic membrane, which can be affected by increased pressure in the middle ear. Using a small ear bud, eardrum movement can be measured by changing the amount of air pressure applied. This test is valuable for determining presence of fluid and potential infections in the middle ear. A normal tympanogram produces a peak on the graph, whereas an abnormal tympanogram will produce a flat line.

Speech, tone, and word recognition information

Medical assistants can perform audiometry if patients (especially children) can respond to directions of pushing a button or raising a hand to acknowledge when various tones are heard through headphones. The level of hearing is documented in decibels and the frequency in hertz. An adult who has normal hearing should be able to hear tones at 25 decibels, and a child should be able to hear at 15 decibels.

Tuning forks are used to determine the patient's ability to hear tones transmitted through air and bone conduction. The vibrating tuning fork is placed on top of the head or on the mastoid process to test hearing.

11.4 Distance visual acuity chart

B	1	20/200
E R	2	20/100
Z Q S	3	20/70
D F C L	4	20/50
F C D P E	5	20/40
L C P Z D E	6	20/30
B E R Z Q S T	7	20/25
L R P O S T E D	8	20/20
B E R Z Q S T F	9	
L R P O S T E D	10	
L R P O S T E D G	11	

11.5 Ishihara plate

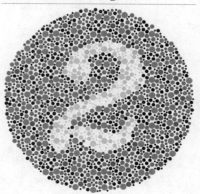

Ishihara test. A set of templates with patterns or numbers embedded within them to test for color blindness

tympanometry. The process of recording the movement of the tympanic membrane through pressure variances in the external ear canal

ALLERGY TESTING

A medical assistant who works in an allergist's office will likely perform allergy testing. Medical assistants in other ambulatory care settings can be responsible for scheduling the referral appointment and need to be aware of how the tests are performed and what the patient should expect in preparation for the testing.

Skin testing

Skin testing delivers rapid results and is minimally invasive. It is typically performed on the forearm or the back, depending on how many allergens are being tested. Skin testing needs to be conducted with provider supervision because allergic reactions and anaphylaxis are possible.

Scratch testing

A diluted allergen is applied to a scratch or prick on the surface of the skin. If a wheal occurs in the first 15 minutes, the allergist can identify the substance as a possible allergen and consider intradermal testing. Generally, the larger the wheal, the more significant the allergy.

Intradermal testing

A diluted allergen is injected intradermally, and the patient is observed. An initial wheal is expected. If the wheal becomes inflamed with induration (raised, hard area), the substance can be identified as an allergen.

RAST testing

Radioallergosorbent (RAST) testing checks blood for specific antibodies that could indicate an allergy. This test is more invasive because it requires a blood draw, but safer regarding avoiding a potential allergic reaction.

Challenge testing

Challenge testing is sometimes used to detect specific allergies, such as food allergies. It is not a first choice of testing but can be prescribed if scratch or intradermal tests are positive and the patient (usually a child) has suspected life-threatening food allergies. In food challenge tests, the patient receives increasing amounts of food suspected of causing an allergy. This must be conducted in a controlled environment where medication and treatment are available for acute allergic reactions.

radioallergosorbent test (RAST). A blood test used to detect antibodies associated with allergens

SPIROMETRY/PULMONARY FUNCTION TESTS (ELECTRONIC, MANUAL)

Noninvasive lung functioning tests can be used in the ambulatory care setting. The medical assistant is responsible for preparing the patient for the procedure, performing and documenting the procedure, and providing results to the provider for interpretation. Two of the most common noninvasive methods are spirometry and peak flow meter testing.

Peak flow testing

Instruct the patient about the proper way to perform peak flow testing. This test can be used to monitor lung function in the home, especially for patients who have chronic respiratory diseases such as asthma. The peak flow meter measures the *forced expiratory volume*, which indicates the effectiveness of airflow out of the lungs. Peak flow meters can vary in size and shape depending on the manufacturer, but most are inexpensive.

11.6 Peak flow meter

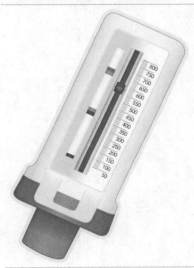

Patient instructions are the same across models.

- Wear nonrestrictive clothing.

- Begin with the marker at the bottom of the scale on the meter.

- In an upright sitting or standing position, take a deep breath and forcefully blow out of the mouth, which is secure around the mouthpiece of the machine.

- Record the number where the marker is located at the end of the test.

- Repeat the test two to three times and record the results.

Assist the patient by providing instructions, demonstrating the technique, and allowing the patient to practice several times before completing the procedure.

Spirometry testing

Spirometry is an automated test that produces a graphic result. It is conducted similar to the peak flow meter. The patient should wear loose clothing, sit in an upright or standing position, and breathe through the mouth, pursing the lips around the mouthpiece. The medical assistant will likely apply a clip to the patient's nose to avoid nose-breathing during the procedure. The patient should lift the chin slightly and extend the neck a little during the test to reduce breathing resistance.

11.7 Spirometer

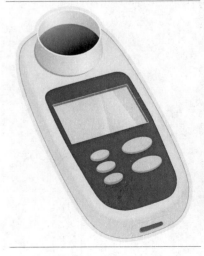

Patients require additional pretest preparation, which includes no large meals 2 hr before the test, no smoking 1 hr before the test, and discontinuing the use of bronchodilators or other breathing therapies (inhalers, nebulizers) for at least 6 hr before the test.

forced expiratory volume. The amount of air that can be forcibly exhaled

SUMMARY

The medical assistant performs many diagnostic screening and laboratory tests. A thorough knowledge of the tests and proper specimen handling requirements, as well as skill in assisting with or performing these tests, is imperative to obtain accurate results. Doing so also allows the medical assistant to demonstrate competency to the provider and gain trust and cooperation from the patient.

CHAPTER 12
Phlebotomy

OVERVIEW

Blood testing is a critical component in the proper diagnosis and treatment of patient conditions. Medical assistants are trained and should be competent in *phlebotomy* procedures. Providers rely on the medical assistant to not only perform the phlebotomy procedure, but also follow proper specimen handling and processing guidelines. A fundamental understanding of phlebotomy technique and specimen collection requirements is a cornerstone of a medical assistant's clinical proficiencies. This chapter reviews these techniques and specimen handling standards as they apply to the medical assistant's responsibilities in the ambulatory care environment.

PHLEBOTOMY

Phlebotomy is the process of withdrawing blood from a vein for laboratory testing. This procedure, typically performed by medical assistants in the ambulatory care setting, requires professionalism, the ability to multi-task, and appropriate technique. The provider will rely on the medical assistant to perform this procedure according to laboratory guidelines, adhering to OSHA blood-borne pathogen standards and sharps safety protocols. Performing phlebotomy procedures effectively and processing specimens correctly ensures the provider receives accurate data to aid in diagnosis of the patient's condition.

Objectives

Upon completion of this chapter, you should be able to:

- Verify order details, identify the patient, and determine whether or not the patient followed testing preparation instructions.

- Follow procedures for collecting special testing samples (timed specimens, drug levels, blood cultures).

- Recognize preanalytical factors and how to address them.

- Select appropriate supplies for the tests ordered.

- State tube top colors used for chemistry, hematology, coagulation, and microbiology testing; list additives in each tube; and state the order of draw that should be used when drawing multiple tubes.

- Explain how tubes should be positioned following a blood draw, the number of inversions necessary for each tube, and the importance of fill/level ratios.

- Determine the venipuncture method to be used (evacuated tube method, syringe method, butterfly method) and perform the steps of a venipuncture.

- Perform a capillary puncture and determine the proper order of draw when using microcapillary tubes.

- Perform postprocedure care including bandaging procedures and providing discharge instructions.

- Match and label specimen to patient and completed requisition.

- Handle, process, and store blood samples as required for diagnostic purposes.

- Prepare samples for transportation to a reference (outside) laboratory.

phlebotomy. Withdrawal of blood from a vein

VERIFY ORDER DETAILS

Obtaining the provider's order for laboratory testing is the vital first step to performing any phlebotomy procedure. Never perform a procedure without a provider's order. Verify the order to determine what tests will be run and the identity of the patient before any other part of the procedure begins

Correct interpretation of medical abbreviations is essential to the process of order verification. Lab tests, as well as proper blood collection tubes for the ordered tests, are typically expressed in abbreviations. Review the medical terminology and pharmacology chapters for some of the most common abbreviations used in the laboratory setting.

Review order and lab manual for preparation, collection, handling, and storage instructions

Upon receiving the provider's order, review the order for completion of all required items. Verify accuracy, requested tests, test requirements, and reporting before beginning the procedure.

Some of the required items include the following.

- Ordering provider
- Test and test code (unique to each lab, usually on the *requisition* or in the laboratory reference manual)
- Diagnosis code that correlates with the tests being ordered (ICD-10)
- Special specimen requirements, such as *fasting*
- Patient demographics
- Insurance or other billing information

If there is any question regarding specimen handling requirements or the tube color for each test, consult the facility specific laboratory reference manual. The laboratory reference manual provides all information required for testing (how many and what color tube must be drawn; test code; whether the tube is to be centrifuged, frozen, or if it is light-sensitive).

Procedures for collecting special testing samples

There are some blood tests that require specific timing, specific patient preparation, or particular handling of the blood specimens.

If the provider has ordered a specimen collection at a specific time, the medical assistant is responsible for making sure that the phlebotomy procedure and specimen collection are performed at that time. Timed specimens are crucial for therapeutic drug level monitoring to confirm the patient's medication dosage and compliance.

Blood cultures require specific preparation of the skin, as well as multiple tubes and specific specimen labeling. Failure to adhere to any of these requirements will render a specimen improper for testing or call into question the test results. Consult the laboratory reference manual if performing a blood draw for an unfamiliar test.

requisition. A written or computer generated order for laboratory tests

fasting. Abstinence of food and liquids, except water, for a set number of hours prior to testing

Consider all preanalytical factors

There are several variables to consider when performing a blood collection procedure. Some of these factors are basal state, fasting status, and the condition of the *venipuncture* site. If the veins are sclerotic or the skin is scarred, evaluate an alternative location. Stress can cause elevation in white blood cells, decrease in iron levels, and abnormal hormone levels, among a few possible complications. Other considerations include menstrual cycle, *edema*, current medications, infections, vomiting, and pregnancy. *Hemoconcentration* can also occur if the *tourniquet* is left on the patient longer than the recommended 60 seconds.

Complete lab requisition form and prepare labels for tubes

It is crucial to accurately complete the lab requisition and correctly label specimen containers. Missing or inaccurate information on the laboratory requisition or improper specimen labeling can lead to excessive blood collection, which could be harmful to the patient's health. Accurate lab requisition and labeling helps minimize costly and dangerous errors that result in the wrong diagnosis and treatment.

Verify the following information against the requisition every time with every phlebotomy procedure to minimize errors and ensure proper collection and testing of specimens.

- Provider's order
- Patient's identity
- Labeling of the specimens
- Identification number of the specimens

Identify the patient

Always introduce yourself to the patient and confirm the purpose for the blood collection procedure. In this conversation, verify the patient's identity by confirming the patient's name, date of birth, and any other demographic information needed. Refer to the study guide addendum on the NHA website for details on CLSI guidelines for patient identification specific to specimen collection.

Presenting a calm, professional demeanor can alleviate any fear or anxiety the patient might be feeling regarding the blood draw procedure. This also demonstrates competency and professionalism, which are key attributes of a medical assistant.

venipuncture. The puncture of a vein for the purposes of withdrawing blood

edema. An excessive buildup of fluid in body tissue

hemoconcentration. Increase in the concentration of red blood cells in the circulating blood, which is commonly caused by exceeding tourniquet time of 60 seconds

tourniquet. Flat length of vinyl, rubber, or fabric with Velcro, which restricts blood flow and causes the venous blood to accumulate, enabling better palpation of a vein prior to phlebotomy

Verify the patient followed laboratory preparation instructions

Often there are specific instructions or preparations that need to take place prior to collecting a blood specimen. These are important for accuracy of the testing values. For example, patients should fast for completion of a lipid panel. If the patient just ate a meal prior to having blood drawn, the test values would likely detect fats from the food and the results would indicate elevated lipid levels. Therefore, verify that all specimen guidelines were followed prior to all phlebotomy draws.

Test preparation

- Verify whether test requires fasting. If so, ask the patient when the last time she ate or drank anything other than water and regular medications.
- If testing for drug levels, ask the patient when he last took any medication and the names and dosages of the medications.

Question patient about anxiety and comfort level

Approach each patient with a pleasant, warm demeanor. Some patients have little or no issue with the process of blood collection. Other patients have a great deal of anxiety when having blood drawn. In addition to performing the procedure correctly, it is important to make patients as comfortable as possible and be sensitive to their needs.

Always question patients about previous blood draws and what their reactions have been. Be prepared for a possible adverse reaction to a phlebotomy procedure, including *vasovagal response*.

Throughout the blood collection procedure, check the patient's response. This varies from casual conversation to specifically inquiring how the patient is tolerating the procedure. Be sensitive to verbal and nonverbal communication. If the patient is in obvious distress, stop the procedure and alert the provider.

Explain the procedure

The process of blood collection can be distressing to patients, particularly if they have had a negative experience in the past. It is the responsibility of the medical assistant to put the patient's mind and body at ease. Provide an explanation of the process and purpose of the blood draw to help the patient feel comfortable with the procedure and confident in your abilities.

Give a concise explanation of the procedure, while remaining friendly and professional. Let the patient know that blood will be drawn according to the provider's request. Consult the patient about previous blood draws: good or bad reactions to phlebotomy, sites where blood has been drawn before, and how the patient is feeling about the procedure.

After assembling all of the equipment and identifying and preparing the patient, place the patient in a comfortable, appropriate position for drawing blood.

---

vasovagal response. Fainting because the body overreacts to certain triggers (the sight of blood, extreme emotional distress)

SELECT APPROPRIATE SUPPLIES FOR TESTS ORDERED

Basic supplies and equipment are necessary for collection of all venous blood specimens. Preparing the appropriate equipment prior to the phlebotomy procedure helps ensure the proper collection of blood specimens is completed.

Standard phlebotomy supplies

- Gloves: Ask patients about the possibility of latex allergies as part of the screening questions prior to assembling phlebotomy supplies.

- Tourniquet: Some facilities use latex tourniquets; screening questions about latex allergies with gloves will provide information regarding this issue.

- Isopropyl alcohol wipes: Standard for skin preparation for all draws except blood cultures.

- Nonalcohol prep kits or swabs: Used for blood cultures; can include povidone-iodine or chlorhexidine gluconate swabs.

- Nonsterile gauze: Typically 2 x 2 size; avoid cotton balls.

- Cohesive wrap or paper tape: Applied postprocedure to aid in **hemostasis.**

- Double-pointed needle: Typically 21- to 22-gauge; requires connection to **plastic needle holder** or sleeve.

- Butterfly needle: Also called a **winged infusion**; used for weak or fragile veins prone to collapse, such as in hand draws.

- Blood collection tube: Also called vacuum tube; sterile glass or plastic tube with a vacuum inside and a rubber, color-coded top to indicate chemical additive.

- Plastic or glass capillary tubes with clay sealant tray: Used for capillary blood testing; clay creates a seal at one end of the tube to avoid loss of the specimen.

- Sterile syringe, needle, and syringe transfer device: Used for syringe draws when a butterfly needle is not available.

- Laboratory requisition and labels

- Ice or chemical cold packs: Used for postprocedure care as needed.

---

hemostasis. The stoppage of the flow of blood

plastic needle holder. Adapter that connects to the needle and where the collection tube is inserted during phlebotomy

winged infusion. Butterfly style of needle attached to a length of tubing and affixed to a plastic needle holder; used on small or fragile veins such as those of the hands or pediatric and geriatric patients

Tube colors and additives

Vacuum tubes are identified by stopper color and additives. The tubes are color-coded for easy identification of the chemical additive inside. The tubes must be drawn in the proper order to avoid cross-contamination of the additives. If the tubes are not drawn in the correct order, the additives could inadvertently affect the test. Inaccurate blood-to-additive ratio can also cause inaccurate test results, so fill phlebotomy tubes to the required quantities.

12.1 Order of draw

STOPPER COLOR	ADDITIVE	LAB USE
Yellow	Sodium polyanethol sulfonate (SPS)	SPS for blood culture specimen collections in microbiology
Light Blue	Sodium citrate (*anticoagulant*)	*Coagulation* studies
Red	Plastic: clot activator	For serum determinations in chemistry
	Glass: no additive (plain)	May be used for routine blood donor screening and diagnostic testing of serum for infectious diseases
Gold or tiger top (red-grey)	Serum separator tube (SST)	For serum determinations in chemistry
	Clot activator	May be used for routine blood donor screening and diagnostic testing of serum for infectious disease
	Thixotropic gel (creates barrier)	
Green	Sodium heparin	For plasma determinations in chemistry
	Lithium heparin	
Lavender	EDTA (anticoagulant)	*Whole blood* hematology determinations, routine immunohematology testing, and blood donor screening
Gray	Potassium oxalate and sodium fluoride	Glucose testing (GTT)

There are additional tubes and stopper colors with various chemical additives, but the most commonly ordered blood tests will use the tubes listed. This is considered the order of the draw.

Adhering to the accepted order of the draw, ensures collected specimens produce accurate results and provide reliable data to aid in diagnosis and management of medical conditions.

anticoagulant. A chemical substance that prevents clotting

coagulation. The process by which a clot forms in the blood

whole blood. Total volume of blood including plasma and formed elements; blood that has not been separated by chemical additives or centrifuging

SUPPLIES FOR NONROUTINE TESTS

In addition to routine venipuncture, medical assists may perform various other types of blood collection and testing, such as blood cultures and microcollection. Additional supplies for these types of blood collection can include microcollection tubes for capillary blood requiring a chemical additive, capillary tubes, yellow top tubes, and vacuum culture vials for blood cultures.

DETERMINE VENIPUNCTURE SITE ACCESSIBILITY

It is important to select the safest site for venipuncture (according to patient age and condition) that has the greatest likelihood of successful blood collection. Methods of selection include warming the site to increase blood flow and the use of a tourniquet, palpation, or infrared vein scanner.

Age determinants

Site selection is sometimes determined based on the patient's age. Most often, newborns to infants 12 months of age need only a heel stick and capillary blood specimen unless extensive testing is required.

Patients 12 months to 2 years of age typically require capillary samples obtained through a finger stick. For more extensive testing, traditional venipuncture can be necessary.

For patients 2 years and older, a regular venipuncture is easily accessible and considered routine.

Site restrictions

During site selection, check with the patient regarding possible medical restrictions due to *fistulas*, *ports*, or *mastectomy*. Each of these medical conditions can require specific blood draw procedures to prevent complications and obtain the best specimen for blood testing. Guidance for phlebotomy procedures should come from the provider and the laboratory that will perform the tests. Exercise caution with patients who have these medical conditions and proceed only within your scope of practice and experience level.

fistula. An abnormal connection between two body parts; an arteriovenous fistula may be present at birth or surgically created in patients with renal insufficiency to aid with dialysis

port. A small medical appliance that is installed beneath the skin, used to administer medication or withdraw blood samples

mastectomy. Surgical removal of one or both breasts, typically associated with a diagnosis of cancer

Vein anatomy

The preferred sites for venipuncture procedures performed by a medical assistant are the *median cubital vein*, *cephalic vein*, and *basilic vein*. If these veins within the *antecubital space* are inaccessible, the hand, wrist, and foot are also options. Blood draws from the foot should only be performed under the supervision of a physician due to the risk of *deep vein thrombosis (DVT)*.

Skin integrity and venous sufficiency

Older adult patients have concerns due to physiological changes including muscular atrophy, which changes the integrity of the skin; veins that have lost their elasticity; and venous insufficiency. With loss of venous sufficiency, veins are prone to roll. When veins lose elasticity, they are fragile and easily damaged by venipuncture.

12.2 Anatomy of veins in the arm

- brachial vein
- cephalic vein
- accessory cephalic vein
- median cubital vein
- basilic vein
- radial vein
- ulnar vein

PREPARE SITE FOR VENIPUNCTURE

In preparation of the venipuncture, seat the patient in a comfortable, well-lit area. For patients who have a fainting history, the procedure may be performed with the patient in semi-Fowler's position (back of the patient table lowered to 45°) or laying down.

Positioning the arm

Position the patient with the arm extended to form a straight line from the shoulder to the wrist and the palm of the hand facing upward. It is helpful to have the patient make a fist with the opposite hand and place it behind the elbow of the arm being used for the procedure. This ensures the arm will stay straight and motionless during the procedure.

The seated patient should have both feet flat on the floor and sit up with good posture.

median cubital vein. Located in the center of the antecubital space, most common vein used for phlebotomy procedures

cephalic vein. Located in the lateral antecubital space; one of two preferred veins for phlebotomy procedures

basilic vein. Vein located in the medial antecubital space; superficial to the brachial artery

antecubital space. The inner bend of the elbow; primary site for phlebotomy procedures

deep vein thrombosis (DVT). Formation of a blood clot within a deep vein (most commonly the veins in the legs)

National Healthcareer Association

Arranging supplies

All necessary phlebotomy supplies, including the sharps container for needle disposal, should be within reach. During the procedure, hold the needle in the dominant hand, and avoid switching hands once the skin has bveen penetrated. This will require the remaining supplies be set up on the opposite side of the dominant hand.

Whenever possible, place the sharps container on the dominant side as well. This allows the needle to be disposed of properly without the need for crossing the contaminated needle across the body. Always engage needle safety devices when disposing of a needle in the sharps container.

Cleansing the site

Disinfect the site with 70% alcohol pads with friction using back-and-forth strokes. Allow the skin to air dry, and do not touch the site after cleansing. Do not blow on the area or wave hands over it in an attempt to dry the alcohol faster, as this recontaminates the skin. Refer to the study guide addendum on the NHA website for details on CLSI guidelines for cleansing the venipuncture site.

PERFORM VENIPUNCTURE

Multiple techniques are used to perform venipuncture. The method typically depends on the patient, test ordered, and integrity of the skin. Venipuncture can be performed with either the evacuated tube method using a straight double-ended needle, butterfly needle, or a syringe method (less common in ambulatory care).

Evacuated tube method

The most commonly used technique for phlebotomy procedures is the evacuated tube or vacuum tube method. This collection method uses a straight double-ended needle and color-coded vacuum tubes made from glass or plastic. The tubes come in a variety of sizes depending on the amount of blood needed for testing. The color-coded tops indicate which chemical additive the tube contains and are made of rubber that is punctured by the needle for the collection of blood. The tubes have vacuum pressure to aid in the blood flow into the tube. If the top of the tube is removed or compromised in any way, the vacuum will be lost and the tube should be discarded.

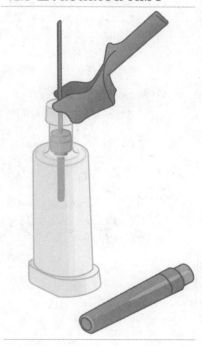

12.3 Evacuated tube

Syringe method

While not commonly performed in the ambulatory care setting, the needle and syringe method of blood collection is still used in some circumstances. Medical assistants should be familiar with the technique and process. This blood collection requires a needle (the same type used for injections; a double-ended needle is not required here) and a sterile syringe from 3 cc to 20 cc, depending on the amount of blood to be collected. This procedure also requires a blood transfer system and appropriate color-coded vacuum tubes.

Butterfly method

Winged infusion or butterfly method is commonly used for smaller or more fragile veins in the dorsal hand, but can also be used in the antecubital area. The butterfly needle has replaced the syringe draw technique in the ambulatory care environment as the method of choice for weak or fragile veins. Butterfly needles are typically smaller gauge (25- to 26-gauge), have small "butterfly wings" on either side of the needle, and have long, thin tubing between the base of the needle and the attachment point on the sleeve. This tubing minimizes the pressure on the vein from the suction in a vacuum tube.

Determining the method to use

Selecting a phlebotomy method is based on the condition of the patient's veins, age, skin conditions, and overall health, as well as the professional experience and judgement of the medical assistant. The method should be the most appropriate for each patient while providing the greatest chance for successful blood collection and limiting patient discomfort during and following the procedure.

Performing the evacuated tube method of venipuncture

Prior to beginning a phlebotomy procedure, verify the provider's order and patient identity. Ask questions regarding fasting state, allergy to latex, use of blood thinning medication, and any other necessary information. This help assess the patient's state of mind and any apprehension about the procedure.

Wash hands and apply nonsterile gloves prior to handling phlebotomy supplies or selecting a vein for the procedure.

Choose the needle gauge size appropriate for the patient to facilitate rapid blood flow and ensure minimization of *hemolysis*; typically a 21- or 22-gauge is appropriate. Needles must be sterile and disposable with a locking safety device as required by OSHA. Some plastic needle holders have a safety mechanism to prevent contaminated needle sticks. If the sleeve has a safety, then an additional safety feature is not required. Always engage safety devices immediately upon completing the procedure and dispose of needles in an appropriate sharps container. Used needles should never be recapped or sterilized for reuse.

Assemble the needle and plastic needle holder prior to tying the tourniquet on the patient or beginning the phlebotomy procedure.

Apply the tourniquet 3 to 4 inches above the venipuncture site. Never leave tourniquets on a patient longer than 1 minute. Extended tourniquet time can lead to increased patient discomfort, accumulation of platelets in restricted veins (affecting laboratory results), and nerve damage.

After applying the tourniquet, if locating the vein takes close to 60 seconds, remove the tourniquet and allow blood flow to return to normal (approximately 2 minutes) before re-applying the tourniquet and beginning the procedure.

---

hemolysis. The rupture of red blood cells, which is commonly caused by performing phlebotomy with too small needle gauge or shaking the blood tubes too hard; blood appears a serum cherry color and sample cannot be tested

Cleanse the skin using the previously discussed technique. Do not touch the skin once it has been cleansed. If reconfirmation of the vein location is needed, disengage the tourniquet and start over. It is not acceptable to touch the alcohol pad with a gloved finger and then palpate the vein; the gloved finger is not properly disinfected, and this practice can lead to increased bacteria at the puncture site.

Anchor the vein by grasping firmly with the thumb 1 inch below the draw site and holding the skin taut. Hold the needle/sleeve unit in the dominant hand and insert the needle with the bevel facing upward at an angle of 15° to 30°. Insert the needle in a smooth, deliberate way; hesitation can increase patient discomfort, cause the patient to move, or result in multiple needle sticks.

While holding the sleeve, direct eyes to the insertion point of the needle. Use the nondominant hand to place the first evacuated tube inside the sleeve with enough pressure to puncture the rubber stopper of the tube with the end of the needle within the sleeve. During tube insertion and exchange, take caution that the needle is not pushed further into the arm or pulled out from the skin. Always confirm when drawing more than one vacuum tube that the tubes are filled in the correct order of the draw.

Once blood flow has been established, release the pressure of the tourniquet (unless it is feared that doing so might cause the vein to collapse), still using the nondominant hand. The vacuum tubes stop filling when a sufficient amount of blood has been collected. Once the last tube has filled, remove the tube while holding the sleeve securely.

Place gauze over the draw site. Remove the needle and immediately apply pressure to the site while activating the needle's safety feature with the dominant hand. (This should only require one hand.) Dispose of the needle sleeve unit in the sharps container. Ask the patient to apply pressure to the gauze covering the site and elevate the arm for 2 minutes. The arm should remain straight, not bent, to allow the vein to repair itself and minimize postphlebotomy bruising to the draw site. While the patient is applying pressure, gently invert the filled vacuum tubes to mix the blood and chemical additives within the tubes. Label the tubes immediately following the procedure and confirm with the patient that label information is correct. Check the gauze covering the draw site prior to the application of bandaging to confirm bleeding has ceased. Then apply clean gauze and paper tape or cohesive wrap.

12.4 Applying a tourniquet

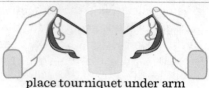

place tourniquet under arm

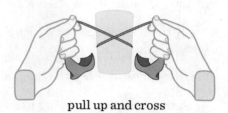

pull up and cross

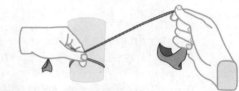

pull one end taut then pinch at base to trap tension

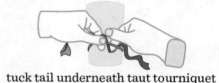

tuck tail underneath taut tourniquet

release

Performing the syringe method

Needle selection is the same for vacuum tube procedures. The size of the syringe depends on the amount of blood required for the ordered tests. Syringe sizes vary, from 3 to 20 mL. Use a locking syringe tip that requires the needle be screwed into the tip of the syringe; this prevents the needle from becoming disconnected from the syringe during the procedure. After assembly of the needle to the syringe, slide the plunger back and forth, taking care not to pull the plunger all the way out from the barrel of the syringe. This helps ensure proper function of the syringe and avoids the plunger sticking when attempting to withdraw blood.

Apply the tourniquet 3 to 4 inches above the venipuncture site. Do not let tourniquet remain on the body longer than 1 minute.

Cleanse the skin using the previously described technique.

Anchor the vein by grasping firmly with the thumb 1 inch below the draw site and holding the skin taut. Hold the needle/sleeve unit in the dominant hand and insert the needle with the bevel facing upward at an angle of 15° to 30°.

Grasp the barrel of the syringe and pull back on the plunger slowly until the required amount of blood has filled the syringe. Applying too much force on the plunger or drawing too quickly can cause the vein to collapse. Syringe draws are typically performed due to a fragile state of the vein, making the vein prone to collapse.

Remove the tourniquet once blood flow is established unless it is feared that doing so might cause the vein to collapse. Place gauze over the venipuncture site. Remove the needle and immediately apply pressure to the site. Follow postprocedure protocol.

12.5 Butterfly needle

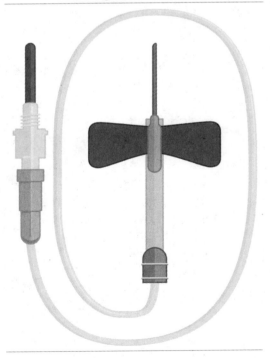

Place the vacuum tubes in a tube rack for transfer of blood from the syringe. Transfer collected blood to the vacuum tube with a safety transfer device, and dispose of the contaminated blood collection device in a sharps container. It is unsafe to puncture the top of a vacuum tube with a needle that has been used for a syringe draw. Use a transfer device to minimize the risk of contaminated needle stick, and follow OSHA needle handling requirements. Invert vacuum tubes to ensure blood and chemical additives have combined completely. Label the tubes and verify their accuracy with the patient.

Performing the butterfly method

The set-up and procedure are the same as for a vacuum tube draw; the only difference is the type of needle.

Butterfly technique takes more time than traditional straight-needle draws due to the smaller needle gauge and length of tubing. Because of this, particular attention must be paid to tourniquet time and the number of tubes that need to be filled. Butterfly needles should also have a locking safety device that is engaged following the phlebotomy procedure prior to disposal in the sharps container.

Tube inversions

Vacuum tubes that have an additive in them should be gently inverted for mixing. While inverting the tubes, completely turn the tube upside down and return it to its upright position. Invert three to 10 times according to manufacturer instructions. Do not shake or forcefully invert tubes due to the risk of hemolysis.

PERFORM CAPILLARY PUNCTURE

Capillary punctures, also called finger sticks, are performed when only a small amount of blood is needed for testing, or when immediate results are required. This method can be useful for infant and adult patients. Capillary blood is a mixture of blood from arterioles, venules, capillaries, and intracellular and interstitial fluids. Due to this mixed composition, not all testing should be performed using capillary blood.

Capillary puncture supplies

- Nonsterile gloves

- Automatic retractable lancets

- Disinfectant pads, such as 70% isopropyl alcohol

- Clean gauze pads

- Bandage wraps

- Micropipette

- Blood collection device appropriate for the test

  ○ Small glass tube (capillary tube)

  ○ Microcollection tube

  ○ Glass microscope slide

  ○ Reagent strip

  ○ Screening card or paper

  ○ Plastic testing cartridge or cassette

- Capillary tube sealer (when capillary tubes are used)

- Biohazard sharps container

12.6 Lancet

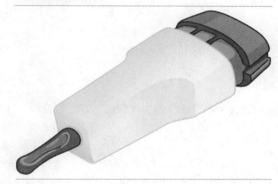

Location of capillary punctures for adults and infants

The preferred puncture site for obtaining a capillary puncture in adults and children is the middle or ring finger of the nondominant hand. Perform the puncture slightly off-center, avoiding the central fleshy part of the fingertip, finger nail, and nail bed. Perform infant capillary puncture on the outer edge of the underside of the heel.

12.7 Location for fingersticks

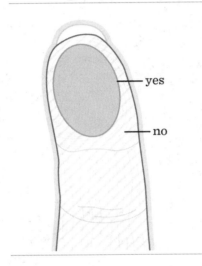

12.8 Location for heelsticks

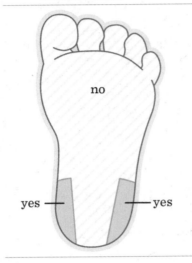

Preparing the site

For the procedure to be successful, the capillaries must have good blood flow. If the patient's hands are cold, the capillaries are somewhat constricted and it can be difficult to collect enough blood. Warm the patient's hands prior to the procedure by having the patient rub them together, run them under warm water, or sit on them for a few minutes. Prep the skin with a 70% isopropyl alcohol pad, and allow the site to air dry completely.

Performing the puncture

Hold the patient's finger between your thumb and forefinger firmly but gently. Hold the lancet device in the dominant hand and at a right angle to the desired puncture site on the patient's finger. Activate the spring or trigger system on the lancet, and discard the used lancet into a sharps container. Always wipe away the first drop of blood to appear after the puncture because of its contamination with tissue fluids. Collect blood. If the blood is slow to flow, a gentle pressure may be applied to the patient's finger; avoid milking the finger.

Once the specimen has been collected, place a clean gauze pad over the puncture site and ask the patient to apply pressure to the area. Properly handle the collection container (for example, inserting the capillary tube into the clay tray to seal the end and avoid losing the specimen). Once the specimen and container are intact, remove the gauze from the patient's finger to assess hemostasis. If blood flow has slowed or stopped, a bandage may be applied. If blood flow is still considerable, apply additional gauze and pressure. For excessive blood flow from the puncture site, elevate the arm over the level of the heart to aid in hemostasis.

Order of draw for microcapillary tubes

The recommended order of draw for capillary blood collection is different from blood specimens drawn by venipuncture. The Clinical and Laboratory Standards Institute recommends the following order of draw for skin puncture.

- Blood gases
- EDTA tubes
- Other additive tubes
- Serum tubes

PERFORM POSTPROCEDURE CARE

The care after any phlebotomy procedure is just as important as the care during the procedure. Patients can have an extreme reaction to a phlebotomy procedure, most commonly fainting or vasovagal syncope. Always assess the patient prior to discharge for any unusual signs or symptoms.

Bandaging needs

Following phlebotomy or capillary puncture, apply a gauze pad over the puncture site with pressure for several minutes or until the bleeding stops. The arm should be extended, slightly bent at the elbow, and elevated above the level of the heart. Once bleeding has stopped, apply a clean gauze pad and bandage to the area.

Discharge instructions

Instruct patients to leave the bandaging in place for at least 15 minutes (longer in some cases, such as donating blood). If the patient has a reoccurrence of bleeding from the site, radiating pain, or dizziness, the clinic should be notified.

HANDLE BLOOD SAMPLES AS REQUIRED FOR DIAGNOSTIC PURPOSES

Proper handling of blood specimens is essential to preserve the viability of the sample. If the sample is mishandled or compromised, the testing might not be able to be performed and the results can be unreliable. In addition to performing blood collection procedures correctly, medical assistants are responsible for familiarizing themselves with proper specimen handling and storage techniques.

Handling instructions

Prior to the handling of any specimen, personal protective equipment (PPE) must be applied to prevent injury and avoid exposure. Change PPE prior to leaving the area in which was used and between each patient.

Each specimen has specific handling instructions (centrifuging of the blood tubes, storage temperature, exposure to light). Consult the laboratory reference manual if there is any question regarding the required handling of a specimen or if the test is unfamiliar. The reference laboratory where the specimen will be sent for testing can also be called for assistance with specimen handling guidelines.

Processing blood specimens for laboratory

The processing of blood samples greatly influences the outcome of the laboratory test values. Remember that once a specimen has been collected from a patient, it will start to break down. Time management in the processing of specimens is crucial to accuracy of testing. A specimen cannot be tested after excessive time has passed.

Centrifugation of serum and plasma

During centrifugation of blood specimens, the blood collection tubes rotate at a high rate of speed. This causes heavier elements within the specimen to be pulled to the bottom of the tube, separating from the lighter specimen elements at the top.

Many centrifuge machines have speed control options because different types of specimens must centrifuge at different speeds (blood vs. urine, for example). The amount of time a specimen needs to be centrifuged varies; confirm prior to starting the machine (laboratory reference manual). Allow serum specimens to clot prior to centrifugation, typically 30 minutes.

Balance tubes in the centrifuge by inserting the tubes across from each other instead of side by side. This ensures balanced weight distribution while the centrifuge is in motion.

Aliquot samples

Aliquot occurs when a single specimen must be divided into multiple tubes for testing on different equipment. Use a single-use pipette for transfer of the serum from one tube to another. When transferring blood in the physician's office laboratory (POL) between containers, wear face and eye protection and use a tube rack for holding the tubes upright during the transfer. Never pour blood specimens from one container to another. Always use a disposable pipette to avoid splashing and spills. Label the tubes appropriately.

Match and label specimen to patient and completed requisition

Labeling of specimen containers is another key step in proper specimen handling. Most laboratory errors occur due to mislabeling of specimens. Continually match the lab specimen to the completed laboratory requisition throughout the collection, handling, and processing. Many lab requisitions come with adhesive numbered labels that should be affixed to all specimen containers associated with that requisition. This is another verification step to help avoid errors.

Completing the requisition form

Upon completion of the phlebotomy procedure, finish the laboratory requisition with the date and time the sample was taken, your initials, and any specific considerations or concerns regarding the sample.

Label the specimen and match it up with the requisition form

Prepare labels at the beginning of the procedure and affix them to the specimen containers immediately following collection. All labels need to match the information on the laboratory requisition. Label information includes the patient's name, unique identification number, date of collection, time of collection, and initials of the person who collected the specimen.

PREPARE SAMPLES FOR TRANSPORTATION TO A REFERENCE LABORATORY

Arrange transportation of the samples as soon as possible after collection. Many reference (outside) labs use a courier service to pick up specimens from clinics. Depending on the frequency of specimen collection, the courier service can have a daily scheduled pick up from a clinic. Other times, the courier service needs to be called for a specimen pick up. It is important to have all specimens labeled, requisitions completed, and everything packaged together in anticipation of the courier's arrival. If the specimens are not ready, the delay in processing could compromise the specimen. Confirm specimen pick up before leaving the clinic each day.

Storage of blood specimens

All specimens should be placed into a clearly marked biohazard bag. Some specimens must be stored and transported at 37º C (98.6º F). Others must be wrapped in foil for light sensitivity, or in a slurry of ice. Store specimens following their specific handling requirements while awaiting retrieval by the lab courier.

Transferring blood specimens to the lab courier

During the transfer of blood specimens to the lab courier, make sure that all specimens have been placed in appropriate biohazard packaging designed for transfer. Specimen bags should be free from punctures or tears to ensure the safety of the courier while handling the specimen bags. All tubes must be labeled along with the appropriate laboratory requisition and contained within the same biohazard bag to process the specimens. Use a separate biohazard bag for each patient's specimens.

RECOGNIZE AND RESPOND TO ABNORMAL TEST RESULTS

An authorized lab supervisor should repeat and verify abnormal or critical lab results. When reporting these results, some require immediate notification of the ordering physician and documentation that the provider was notified. Not all abnormal results are critical. The provider should review all laboratory reports—both normal and abnormal—when they arrive in the clinic prior to being filed or uploaded to a patient's chart.

FOLLOW GUIDELINES IN DISTRIBUTING LABORATORY RESULTS

When the clinic receives laboratory results, forward them to the ordering physician for review. Providers are required to review and acknowledge all results prior to their inclusion in the medical record. Ensure the provider reviews the lab reports in a timely manner and patients are contacted accordingly. The role of the medical assistant often includes notifying patients of their results or scheduling follow-up appointments for patients to review the results with the provider.

SUMMARY

Performing phlebotomy and other blood collection procedures is an important role for the medical assistant, it can also be one of the most rewarding. Medical assistants can work as phlebotomists in reference laboratories, and phlebotomy certification is an opportunity to stack credentials and increase employability.

Providers rely greatly on medical assistants to be knowledgeable in specimen collection and handling processes to ensure the accuracy of the tests they have ordered. By performing these skills correctly, the medical assistant helps provide the best care possible to patients.

CHAPTER 13
EKG and Cardiovascular Testing

OVERVIEW

The electrocardiogram (EKG) is a commonly performed procedure conducted in ambulatory care. EKGs provide a baseline snapshot of cardiac function. The medical assistant must be knowledgeable and skilled with the EKG and other various noninvasive tests used to diagnose cardiovascular conditions. This chapter reviews cardiac circulation and the connection and relationship to the electrical conduction system. In the clinical setting, the medical assistant will be expected to prepare patients for cardiac exams, perform cardiac monitoring, troubleshoot, maintain equipment, and recognize and respond to abnormalities.

Objectives

Upon completion of this chapter, you should be able to:

- Prepare patients for the procedure.
- Perform cardiac monitoring and ensure proper functioning of EKG equipment.
- Recognize abnormal or emergent EKG results.
- Assist the provider with noninvasive cardiovascular profiling.
- Transmit results or report to a patient's EMR or paper chart, and to the provider.

EKGS AND CARDIOVASCULAR TESTING

The medical assistant plays an important role in cardiovascular testing. This includes preparing the patient for the procedure, providing postprocedure assistance, accurately and efficiently performing the testing, noting obvious abnormalities that need immediate intervention, maintaining equipment, and preparing testing materials for provider interpretation. Medical assistants must practice effective communication skills with patients and families to gain the trust and cooperation necessary to get an accurate reading.

Preparing a patient for the procedure

The electrocardiogram is a valuable tool that provides baseline information. This will likely influence the course of treatment or assist in determining an additional plan of action for patients who have cardiac issues. Helping to ensure a pleasant experience can reduce patient anxiety, which will aid in completing the EKG correctly and producing an accurate tracing. In addition, consider preparation of the room and equipment.

Identifying the patient

Use a minimum of two identifiers to confirm a patient's identity. Identifiers such as name and birthdate are commonly used. However, other identifiers—such as an address, telephone number, and the last four digits of a Social Security number—are also acceptable. For privacy and security purposes, patients should not recite their full Social Security number.

Most patients in the ambulatory care setting are conscious and can communicate verbally. Use therapeutic communication techniques; ask "What is your name?" and "What is your birthdate?" rather than asking the patient to confirm the information.

If the patient is unable to communicate, or has dementia or another condition that affects mental functioning, it may be necessary to identify him in another way. In these situations, encourage a family member or caregiver to provide identification for the patient.

Explaining the procedure

Prior to explaining the procedure, introduce yourself and state what will be done. An appropriate introduction would be, "Good morning. My name is Jane Doe, and I am the medical assistant that will be performing your electrocardiogram—or EKG—today." Some patients are aware of the terminology and others are familiar with an abbreviation, so using both can be beneficial in communicating.

Because of the term "electricity," some patients express concern that they will be shocked during the procedure. This is especially true if children need an EKG. Explain that the procedure is harmless. The test records activity of the electrical system within the heart. No electrical current is sent through the body during the procedure.

Instruct patients that the procedure only takes a few minutes. However, they should not move or talk once the medical assistant has the leads connected and is ready to run the tracing.

Always ask the patient if there are any questions prior to starting the procedure.

Disrobing, gowning, and draping instructions

Take great care to protect the patient's privacy and make him feel as comfortable as possible. When disrobing, the patient will be undressed from the waist up and have lower legs or ankles accessible for lead placement. Panty hose or tights should be removed. A drape or gown should be applied with the opening in the front. Female patients often experience more uneasiness with being disrobed than male patients. Therefore, have a light drape or blanket available to place over the patient once the leads are placed. Always ask patients if they would like to have an additional cover. Jewelry (bracelets, necklaces) that can interfere with lead placement or touch the lead wires during the procedure should be removed. All electronic devices, such as cell phones, should be turned off and removed from the patient. These items could lead to *artifacts* on the EKG tracing.

---

artifact. Unwanted external event occurring in an EKG tracing not associated with the heart function

PERFORMING CARDIAC MONITORING (EKG) TESTS

The medical assistant must be familiar with the *electrocardiograph* machine and be able to troubleshoot if not properly functioning. Efficient care of the equipment and proper preparation of the patient can reduce the need to troubleshoot.

EKG equipment and supplies

EKG machines vary in size and shape, but all have basically the same parts.

The multichannel EKG machine is a recorder that monitors all 12 leads at once; it can record three, four, or six leads at a time and print the recording on a single sheet of paper. The three–channel EKG unit is typically found in the ambulatory care setting and, as the name implies, records three leads at once. A single–channel EKG machine records one lead at a time and produces a running strip.

As technology advances, more opportunities are available to record and transmit EKGs. Digital technology allows rapid collection and distribution of data across the health care system. This facilitates effective patient care, whereas ineffective use of fax machines was once necessary to transmit results from one facility or provider to another.

Computer-based monitoring, such as telemetry, is typically conducted in a hospital setting. In these situations, the patient is constantly monitored for any irregularities. Emergency equipment is readily available if interventions are needed.

Other computer-based monitoring systems in the ambulatory care setting provide multiple capabilities including transmission, storage, and retrieval of EKG information.

The electrodes are placed on 10 areas of the body to record heart activity from 12 angles and planes. Each electrode is impregnated with an electrolyte gel that serves as a conductor of the impulses, or a gel is applied and then an electrode and lead wire are attached. Both the electrodes and electrolyte gel are needed to transmit the impulses. Poor-quality or expired electrodes or gel can result in an artifact and interfere with the ability to produce a clean tracing.

13.1 EKG graph matrix

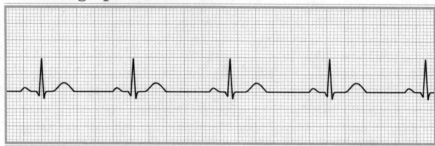

13.2 EKG dot matrix

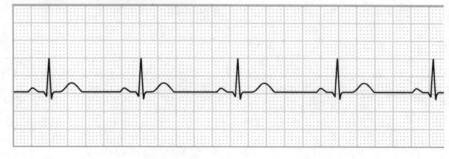

electrocardiograph. The machine that records an electrocardiogram

Electrocardiograph paper can be displayed in graph or dot matrix format, with vertical and horizontal lines or dots at 1 mm intervals. The vertical axis represents gain or *amplitude*. The horizontal axis displays time. Each small vertical square represents 0.1 millivolts (mv). Each small horizontal square represents 0.04 seconds. Large squares are identified by darker lines and include five small boxes horizontally and vertically. The paper should be run at normal speed of 25 mm/second. The normal amplitude is 10 mm or 1 mv. Be familiar with these figures to recognize obvious abnormalities that need to be reported to the provider immediately.

The EKG graph paper is heat- and pressure-sensitive. Waveforms are burned onto the paper via a stylus that heats when the machine is turned on. Take precautions to avoid additional pressure contact via fingernails or other instruments when the EKG is being prepared for the provider.

Performing the EKG

The medical assistant is responsible for connecting the electrodes and lead wires for the EKG. Preparing the patient will likely take longer than the actual test.

If possible, patients should have been instructed to avoid applying any substance to the skin (such as lotions, powders, oils, or ointments) prior to the testing. Help ensure that the skin is clean by using alcohol wipes or soap and water at the attachment sites. Some facilities have electrolyte pads to prep the site.

Excessive chest hair presents challenges with electrode adherence to the skin. If the medical assistant cannot properly place the electrodes with normal skin prep, the next step is to clip the hair. If necessary, small areas might need to be shaved.

Once the patient has been prepped for the procedure, attach the electrodes and leads. The limb electrodes should be placed on fleshy areas of the skin and within the same general vicinity on each limb. For instance, if the left lower leg has been amputated, it can be necessary to place the electrode on the left lower abdomen. Thus, the right lower leg electrode would be placed on the right lower abdomen. The first six recorded leads originate from the arms and legs.

Leads I, II, and III are *bipolar* and record impulses that travel from a negative to positive pole at specific positions in the heart. Lead I records impulses between the left and right arms. Lead II records impulses between the right arm and left leg. Lead III records impulses between the left arm and left leg.

Leads AVL, AVR, and AVF are *unipolar*, but due to poor illustration of the waveforms must be *augmented* and therefore get assistance from two poles to enhance the tracing. In AVL, the left leg and right arm assist with the left arm tracing. In AVR, the left arm and left leg assist with the right arm tracing. In AVF, the right and left arms assist with the left leg tracing.

Once the electrodes are in place, the medical assistant connects the *precordial* lead wires following the contour of the body and taking care to avoid excessive tension or crossing of the wires, which could both lead to artifacts within the tracing.

---

amplitude. Also known as gain is the degree of change; in an EKG tracing, it is represented by the vertical axis

bipolar. Recording of electrical current involving both a positive and negative pole

unipolar. Recording from one location or one pole

augmented. A unipolar recording that requires assisting in magnifying the tracing by drawing from other poles

precordial. Located on the chest in front of the heart

The medical assistant should be familiar with the universal lead wire colors in case markings are not clearly visible.

- *White:* right arm
- *Black:* left arm
- *Red:* left leg
- *Green:* right leg

Precordial leads can be all brown or individually colored.

- *V1:* red
- *V2:* yellow
- *V3:* green
- *V4:* blue
- *V5:* orange
- *V6:* purple

Using anatomical landmarks, place the six chest leads in a systematic order, taking care to avoid placing electrodes over bone (See Figure 13.3). All precordial leads are unipolar and record electrical activity from different parts of the heart.

13.3 Chest lead placement

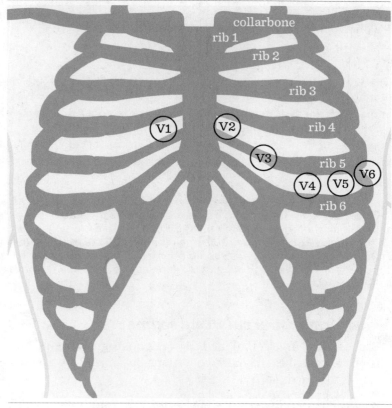

- *V1:* right side of the sternum at the fourth intercostal space
- *V2:* left side of the sternum, directly across from V1 at the fourth intercostal space
- *V4:* left side of the chest, fifth intercostal space, midclavicular line
- *V3:* left side of the chest, midway between V2 and V4 (NOTE: V4 is placed before V3 because of this)
- *V5:* left side of the chest, fifth intercostal space, anterior axillary line
- *V6:* left side of the chest, fifth intercostal space, midaxillary line

Most EKG machines in the ambulatory care setting today perform standardized functions and run automatically once the start button is pushed. It can be necessary to enter specific patient data that includes items such as name, date of birth, sex, medications, and date and time of the procedure. This information will appear on the patient tracing in the electronic record.

CHALLENGE EKG lead placement

The medical assistant is unable to identify the markings on the EKG wires, so she identifies the colors to connect the leads. She attaches them correctly, but the patient shows concern. The medical assistant explains how she remembers colors and where they are attached. "For the arms, I think about the flag and red, white, and black (instead of blue). White matches right, and then black is the opposite arm. For the chest, red is still on the right. And then I use a pneumonic: Your Giant Buffalo is Often Pushy."

QUESTIONS

1. If the medical assistant realizes that the leads were applied incorrectly after looking at the tracing, what should the assistant do?
2. Even if the leads are attached correctly, what other factors associated with the electrode placement or the leads themselves could interfere with the recording?
3. How could the medical assistant have avoided causing concern for the patient?
4. In placing V4 using the midclavicular line, what should the medical assistant do if the patient has large breasts?

Key: 1. *Run a new tracing so that the provider has an accurate tracing. 2. The electrodes could be placed improperly, leading to artifacts. Electrodes should be placed on the fleshy area of the arms and legs, not on bone. Dirty and broken leads can also interfere with the tracing. Leads should always be inspected for damage and cleaned after each use. 3. She should have performed regular maintenance on the machine and checked the equipment before escorting the patient to the room. 4. The leads should not be placed on top of the breast tissue. The medical assistant should gently lift the breast with the back of her hand, preserving the patient's privacy, and place the electrode under the breast on the chest wall.*

Waveforms, intervals, and segments

Each waveform, interval, and segment has significant meaning on the EKG. The medical assistant is not expected to diagnose conditions but must have an awareness of obvious normal vs. abnormal tracings.

P wave: Represents atrial **depolarization** or contraction.

QRS wave: Represents ventricular depolarization or contraction (atrial **repolarization** is not visible but occurs during this phase).

T wave: Represents ventricular repolarization or relaxation.

U wave: Not always visible but represents a repolarization of the **bundle of His** and **Purkinje fibers**.

P-R interval: Starts at the beginning of the P wave and ends at the beginning of the Q wave. It represents the time it takes from the beginning of atrial depolarization to the beginning of ventricular depolarization.

P wave. The first wave in the cardiac cycle representing atria depolarization

depolarization. Systole; contraction

QRS wave. Also known as QRS complex; the second wave in the cardiac cycle representing ventricular depolarization

repolarization. Asystole; relaxation

T wave. The third wave in the cardiac cycle representing ventricular repolarization

bundle of His. A collection of fibers that conduct the electrical impulses from the AV node to the ventricular septum

Purkinje fibers. The fingerlike projections that spread through the ventricular muscle and initiate ventricular contraction

P-R interval. The length of time from the beginning of atrial depolarization to the beginning of ventricular depolarization

QT interval: Starts at the beginning of the Q wave and ends at the end of the T wave. It represents the time it takes from the beginning of ventricular depolarization to the end of ventricular repolarization.

ST segment: Starts at the end of S wave and ends at the beginning of the T wave. It represents the time from the end of ventricular depolarization to the beginning of ventricular repolarization.

The medical assistant should monitor the tracing as it is being recorded to ensure that leads were connected properly and that artifacts are not appearing. Items that should be visible include a universal standardization mark, a baseline that is tracking through the middle of the tracing, no abnormal spikes in the baseline, and visible P, QRS, and T waves. Unless there is cardiac pathology, waveforms should also be positively deflected.

13.4 Waveforms, intervals, and segments

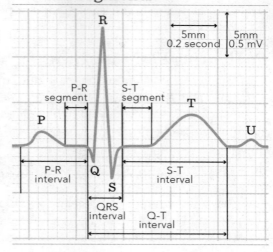

The procedure should be relatively quick and noninvasive, but constant monitoring is required. Take any complaints of chest pain seriously and notify the provider.

Patients who are in a recumbent position can experience syncope upon rising. This can be minimized by having the patient sit for a short while before standing.

Patients can experience dyspnea when lying flat if they have COPD or other lung disorders. Avoid or minimize this by elevating the head of the bed to a semi-Fowler's position and efficiently complete the EKG.

Once *electrocardiography* is completed, detach all leads from the electrodes, and remove and discard electrolyte pads. Inspect the skin for irritation at the connection sites. Thank the patient for cooperating and provide privacy for redressing.

QT interval. The length of time from the beginning of the ventricular depolarization to ventricular repolarization

electrocardiography. The process of recording an electrocardiogram

ENSURING PROPER FUNCTIONING OF EQUIPMENT

The electrocardiograph must be serviced according to manufacturer recommendations. However, the medical assistant is responsible for day-to-day care and maintenance to ensure proper functioning.

Calibrating EKG equipment

The universal *standardization* mark of 10 mm high and 5 mm wide should be visible on an EKG tracing. This represents 1 mv of amplitude. If the QRS complex is too large and goes off the paper, the standardization can need to be reduced to 0.5, which will result in a standardization mark of 5 mm high and 5 mm wide.

If P waves are absent, the heart rate can be elevated. It can be necessary to change the standardized speed from 25 mm/second to 50 mm/second.

Although most newer equipment does this automatically, if adjustments to the amplitude or speed need to be made, they should be documented on the tracing and communicated to the provider so that appropriate adjustments are made in the interpretation.

Checking EKG strips for artifacts

External interferences can occur and lead to artifacts within the EKG tracing.

Somatic tremor is characterized by irregular spikes throughout the tracing and is related to muscle movement. If the patient is chilled, shivering can occur. Medical conditions such as Parkinson's Disease can also result in somatic tremor.

13.5 Somatic tremor

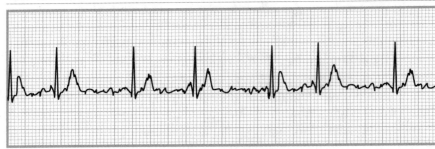

AC interference, or 60-cycle interference, is characterized by regular spikes in the EKG tracing. It is related to poor grounding or external electricity interfering with the tracing. Things such as lights, computers, and crossed lead wires can result in AC interference.

13.6 AC interference

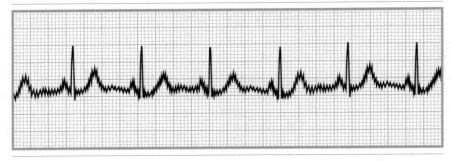

standardization. The universally acceptable speed of the tracing and gain (height) used for accurate interpretation of the tracing

somatic tremor. Muscle movement causing irregular spike in an EKG tracing

alternating current (AC) interference. 60-cycle interference; an artifact in the EKG tracing caused by electrical interference

A *wandering baseline* results from poor electrode connection. It can be associated with lotions, oils, or powders on the skin. The baseline will wander away from the center of the paper, causing difficulty in tracing interpretation.

An *interrupted baseline* is obvious when there is a break in the tracing. It is usually related to a disconnected or broken lead wire.

13.7 Wandering baseline

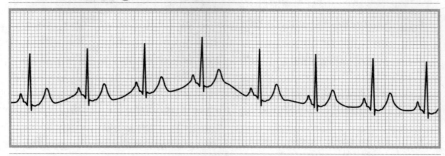

Eliminating artifacts

Somatic tremor can be reduced by decreasing patient anxiety, and providing warmth and comfort as needed. If patients have conditions that lead to uncontrolled muscle movement, have them lay their hands palms down under their buttocks to reduce somatic interference. Ensure proper grounding of the machine to aid in reducing AC interference. Do this by using a three-prong plug, avoiding crossed wires, moving the bed away from the wall, and turning off unnecessary electronic devices. Clean the skin prior to attaching the electrodes and instruct the patient to avoid using creams and lotions to assist in reducing a wandering baseline.

EKG machines are typically equipped with filters to remove external interference. Check to make sure that the filter is turned on.

The medical assistant must be able to detect artifacts and then determine the cause to reduce or eliminate them. In addition to the methods described previously, regular cleaning, maintenance, and inspection of the lead wires will alert the medical assistant to potential lead wire concerns.

wandering baseline. Inconsistency in the baseline location on the EKG tracing likely caused by poor lead contact or skin applications

interrupted baseline. A break in the tracing usually caused by a disconnected or broken lead

RECOGNIZING ABNORMAL OR EMERGENT EKG RESULTS

The medical assistant is not expected to interpret the EKG tracing but should be able to recognize obvious abnormal rhythms or waves that might need to be communicated immediately to the provider.

Abnormal rhythms

Arrhythmias originating from the *sinoatrial (SA) node* are easily detected.

Sinus bradycardia is a normal EKG tracing of a heart rate less than 60/min. Sinus tachycardia reflects a heart rate greater than 100/min. A slight irregularity in the rhythm is sinus dysrhythmia and is associated with normal breathing patterns. A break in the normal EKG may be sinus arrest. In this condition, the SA node failed to fire; it is not significant unless the arrest lasts longer than 6 seconds.

13.8 Sinus bradycardia

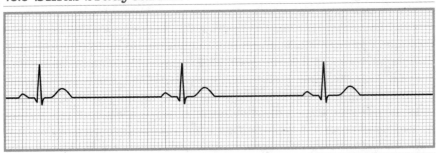

13.9 Sinus tachycardia

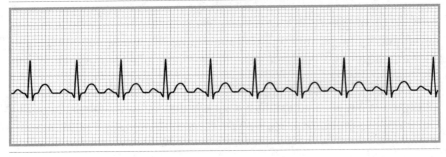

13.10 Sinus arrest

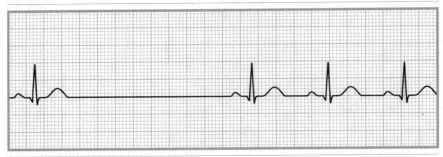

arrhythmia. Also known as dysrhythmia; a change from a normal EKG rhythm

sinoatrial (SA) node. The natural pacemaker of the heart located in the upper right atrium

13.11 Atrial flutter

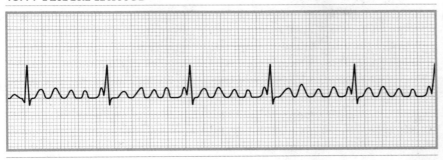

13.12 Atrial fibrillation

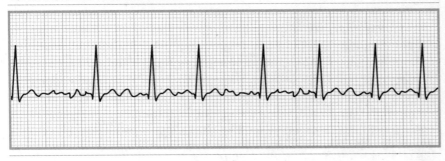

13.13 Ventricular fibrillation

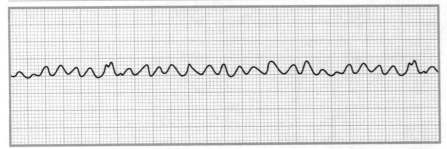

13.14 Asystole

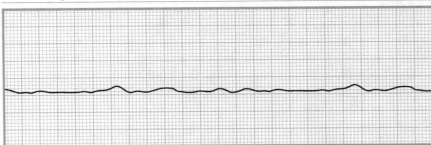

More severe atrial arrhythmias include atrial flutter and atrial fibrillation. In atrial flutter, the atria are contracting at a rapid rate much faster than the ventricles are contracting. In atrial fibrillation, there is no organized contraction of the atria. They are in a quivering state where blood clot formation due to stagnation of the blood in the ventricles is possible.

Ventricular arrhythmias that need immediate intervention include ventricular fibrillation, in which the ventricles are not contracting but quivering, and there are no discernible waves noted throughout the tracing. If the heart stops, the patient has no rhythm noted and the EKG will demonstrate asystole.

Abnormal waves

The medical assistant should be familiar with the normal configuration of the P, QRS, and T waves.

The normal P wave should be *positively deflected*. In the event it is *negatively deflected*, a junctional dysrhythmia is likely present. This means that the typical impulse pathway from the SA to *atrioventricular (AV) node* is not occurring. The initial impulse is originating in the AV junction, AV node, or from some ectopic source.

If the QRS appears wide and bizarre, the medical assistant should suspect that a ventricular arrhythmia is occurring. One of the most common abnormal waves associated with the ventricles is premature ventricular contractions (PVCs). Although occasional PVCs can be insignificant, these are abnormal waves. The provider should be notified.

13.15 P wave negative deflection

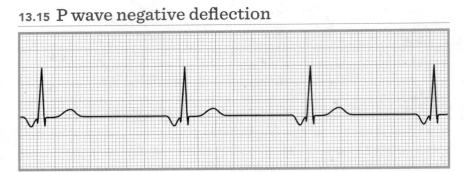

13.16 Premature ventricular contraction

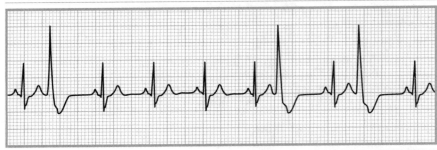

TRANSMITTING RESULTS

If a single-channel EKG machine is used, it can be necessary to mount the tracing prior to delivering it to the provider for interpretation. If the EKG is a multi-channel machine, it is likely that the tracing is complete and ready for provider interpretation. Some machines even provide an interpretation. For both formats, the EKG becomes part of the patient medical record. It might need to be scanned by the health information management department to add to the electronic record after discharge.

Patients in the home environment might need to transmit their results through the telephone. In this case, an EKG with phone transmission capabilities is used like a fax machine. If the tracing is not saved digitally, then the print-out would need to be added to the medical record and forwarded to the provider for interpretation. Patients who have ambulatory monitors deliver the equipment back to the office. The recording is interpreted using a Holter scanner or computer.

Regardless of the method used to compile the results, the EKG becomes part of the legal health record.

positive deflection. An upward curvature of waves in an EKG tracing

negative deflection. A downward curvature of waves in an EKG tracing

atrioventricular (AV) node. The secondary pacemaker located at the junction of the atria and ventricles

ASSISTING PROVIDERS WITH NONINVASIVE CARDIOVASCULAR PROFILING

Besides an EKG, other noninvasive procedures can be done to evaluate heart function. This includes stress testing and Holter, or *ambulatory monitoring*. Echocardiograms can be done in a specialist's office to assess the cardiac structures and their movement, such as the atrioventricular and semilunar valves.

Stress testing

Stress testing is typically completed in hospital environments where thorough monitoring and emergency equipment is available. One of the greatest risks associated with this testing is cardiac arrest. However, stress testing can be conducted in a cardiology specialty setting. Patients are typically attached to heart monitoring equipment, and they exercise on a treadmill or stationary bike to see how the heart handles the stress. They might receive thallium, which is a dye that provides additional information on blood flow.

The medical assistant can assist the provider by attaching leads and monitoring vital signs throughout the procedure. The medical assistant can be responsible for patient education, including pre- and postprocedure instructions.

Holter monitoring/event monitoring

Ambulatory monitoring is fairly common in cardiology practice and sometimes in family practice. The medical assistant is responsible for attaching electrodes to the trunk and providing patient education. Prior to placement of electrodes for ambulatory monitoring, the medical assistant should review the manufacturer's guidelines.

Patients are instructed to assume their normal activities and keep a diary of those activities. They should also press the event monitor if they experience any cardiac symptoms (such as palpitations) or neurological symptoms (such as syncope). Patients should not move the electrodes. They should avoid showers until the electrodes are removed. Exposure to electrical forces such as metal detectors should also be avoided.

SUMMARY

The most common cardiac test done in ambulatory care is the EKG. The medical assistant is a valuable part of the health care team in ensuring that the test is completed accurately. The medical assistant is also responsible for properly preparing the patient, maintaining equipment, and troubleshooting when necessary. A thorough knowledge of the anatomy and physiology of the heart and the electrical conduction system aids the medical assistant in identifying obvious abnormalities in a recording, which could affect patient outcomes.

ambulatory monitoring. Often referred to as Holter monitoring; an EKG conducted over a period of time while the patient resumes normal activities

CHAPTER 14

Patient Care Coordination and Education

OVERVIEW

The medical assistant plays an important role in patient *care coordination* and education. The medical assistant coordinates care between medical specialists and different agencies to provide the best outcome for patients. Education to promote active participation of patients and their family or caregivers is a key component to effective medical interventions and treatments. The medical assistant is part of a team caring for patients by providing quality care, promoting health, providing education, and assisting with medical *compliance*.

PATIENT CARE COORDINATION AND EDUCATION

Lack of care coordination has contributed to the increase in health care costs. Repeated diagnostic testing, multiple prescriptions, adverse medication interactions, unnecessary emergency department visits, and hospital readmissions are some of the reasons for the increased health care costs. The value of care coordination has increased as a result of the Affordable Care Act (ACA). Activities such as value–based payments instead of fee–for–service payments, reduced payments to hospitals that have high readmission rates, financial incentives for reduced hospital readmissions, and meeting federal performance standards are necessary for health care organizations to remain viable. Even if this act is repealed and replaced, it is likely that similar payment models will continue to keep patients healthier and minimize health care costs.

Objectives

Upon completion of this chapter, you should be able to:

- Participate in team-based patient care.
- Discuss models that practice team-based care and population health.
- Collaborate with health care providers and community-based organizations.
- Participate in transition of care for patients.
- Review patient records prior to visit to ensure health care is comprehensively addressed.
- Assist providers in coordinating care with community agencies for clinical and nonclinical services.
- Facilitate patient compliance (continuity of care, follow-up, medication compliance) to optimize health outcomes.

14.1 Annual global mortality by chronic illnesses

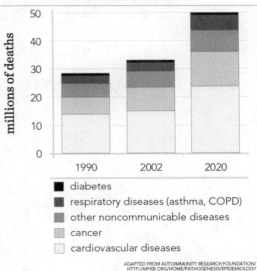

ADAPTED FROM AUTOIMMUNITY RESEARCH FOUNDATION/
HTTP://MPKB.ORG/HOME/PATHOGENESIS/EPIDEMIOLOGY

---

care coordination. The deliberate organization of patient care activities between two or more participants involved in a patient's care to facilitate the appropriate delivery of health care services

compliance. Meeting the standards and regulations of the medical practice's established policies and procedures

With the increase in chronic conditions, the shift from treating illness to promoting health has become imperative. As of 2012, 117 million Americans had one or more chronic conditions. This is expected to increase by more than 1 percent each year through 2030. Patient care coordination and education is the responsibility of the entire health care team.

14.2 Projected prevalence of chronic illnesses in the U.S.

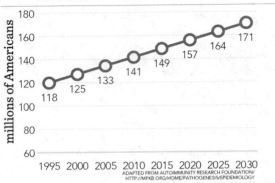

ADAPTED FROM AUTOIMMUNITY RESEARCH FOUNDATION/
HTTP://MPKB.ORG/HOME/PATHOGENESIS/EPIDEMIOLOGY

TEAM-BASED PATIENT CARE

Team-based health care creates a partnership between providers and patients to ensure patients are educated and actively involved in their care. Every team member is accountable for providing quality care. This approach requires communication among all members of the team. Two common health care delivery models that practice team-based patient care include the *patient-centered medical home (PCMH)* and *accountable care organization (ACO)*. In both models, the patient is the focus with all members of the team working to provide the best outcome for the patient using a *holistic health care* approach.

Roles and responsibilities

The implementation of payment models such as "pay for performance" requires a specific mindset for those delivering health care. The patient's health is everyone's responsibility.

In organizations that practice team-based care, team members work collaboratively to provide seamless care. This allows patients to obtain the best care possible without interruptions. Everyone works at the top of their license or credential in these settings by aligning staff responsibilities to their credentials.

For team-based care to be effective, many clinicians are needed to address all needs of the patient. Primary care providers include the physician, nurse practitioner, or physician assistant. Other health care providers include mental health specialists; physical, occupational, and speech therapists; pharmacists; nutritionists; and dentists.

Patients who have chronic conditions are usually assigned a nurse case manager to follow them throughout their disease. Support staff (medical assistants, administrative staff members) also play a key role in team-based care settings.

14.3 Team-based patient care

family/support	patient	providers
home care	medical history	primary care
informal caregivers	goal setting	specialty care
education and support	self-management	inpatient care
medications and pharmacy	compliance	long-term care
community resources	preferences	mental health services

patient-centered medical home (PCMH). A model philosophy intended to improve the effectiveness of primary care

accountable care organization (ACO). An association of providers and third-party payers that assumes a defined range of responsibilities for a specific population and is held accountable, financially as well as through specific quality indicators, for its members' health

holistic health care. Comprehensive or total patient care that considers the physical, emotional, social, economic and spiritual needs of the person.

Specific roles of team members

The *primary care provider (PCP)* is the first provider the patient seeks care from. One of the PCP's main goals is to coordinate preventative health care services (regular check-ups, screening, tests, immunizations, health coaching). PCPs can be family practitioners, internal medicine or doctors of osteopathy (DO), or pediatricians. Pediatricians offer preventative care services and treat common pediatric conditions such as viral infections or minor injuries.

A *specialist* is a provider that diagnoses and treats conditions that require a specific area of expertise and knowledge. Primary care providers may refer patients to a specialist to diagnose or treat a specific short-term condition. For chronic diseases, patients can work with specialists for an ongoing period of time.

Physician assistants (PAs) have similar training to physicians and are licensed to practice medicine as long as they are supervised by a medical doctor (MD). PAs can conduct physical exams, provide preventative care, prescribe diagnostic tests, assist with surgical procedures, diagnose illnesses, and prescribe medicine.

Advanced practice nurses have more education and experience than RNs and can usually perform the same tasks as a physician assistant. Clinical nurse specialists, nurse anesthetists, nurse practitioners (NP), and nurse midwifes are common advanced practice nurses.

With a nationwide shortage of physicians going into primary care, PAs and NPs are a solution that is more cost-efficient than physicians.

Registered nurses (RNs) are licensed by individual states and have an associate or bachelor's degree in nursing. RNs usually oversee the case management of patients who have complex chronic conditions. They also coach patients about their overall health.

Practical nurses (PNs) are sometimes referred to as vocational nurses and are also licensed by individual states. PNs usually train for approximately 1 year at a community college or vocational school, receiving a diploma or associate degree. These health care professionals often triage phone calls, administer medications, and assist with other clinical duties in the clinical setting.

Pharmacists prepare and dispense medications prescribed by authorized providers. They must be knowledgeable of individual and various combinations of medicines to be able to educate patients on their use and answer questions about side effects. Using a pharmacist to implement medication therapy management is relatively new to ambulatory care.

Dentists diagnose and treat issues relating to the teeth and mouth. Dentists also educate patients on ways to prevent problems with oral health. Many community health centers include oral health services to patients.

Occupational therapists assist and educate patients on how to perform everyday tasks after a physical, mental, or developmental disability has occurred.

Physical therapists assess a patient's pain, strength, and mobility and then develop a treatment plan to improve any areas of concern.

Speech therapists or speech-language pathologists work with patients who have problems with speech and swallowing due to an injury, cancer, or stroke. They focus on helping a person work toward improving, regaining, and maintaining the ability to communicate, chew, and swallow.

Some clinics offer rehabilitation services. Having therapy services within the clinic is an added convenience for many patients and improves the communication process between providers and therapists.

Psychiatrists are MDs who diagnose, prescribe medications, and treat mental, behavioral, and emotional disorders.

Psychologists are not MDs but have a doctor of psychology (PsyD) or a doctor of philosophy degree (PhD). They work with patients who are experiencing mental health challenges, especially during times of stress or emotional turmoil.

Social workers assist patients and families in times of transition or crisis. They assist patients in a clinical or hospital setting with physical, emotional, and financial issues related to an illness or injury. Social workers often coordinate additional services (transportation, housing, access to meals, financial resources, long term, hospice services).

Providers on the mental health team that work in the PCMH or ACO usually contract with the facility to work a specific number of hours per week. Clinics with a large census can include a full-time social worker as part of their permanent staff.

A **registered dietitian nutritionist (RDN)** is an expert in diet and nutrition. RDNs educate patients on the connection between chronic disease and poor nutrition, assist with menu planning, and help low-income patients obtain healthier foods at lower prices.

Some patients rely on religion or spirituality to cope with an illness or injury. Priests, ministers, and rabbis are some clergy members who often to provide patients with this spiritual support.

Support staff

Administrative and clinical staff professionals are also key players in providing the best possible experience for health care consumers. Scheduling appointments, answering phones, greeting patients, maintaining medical records, assisting providers during exams/procedures, performing measurements, processing billing, completing insurance forms, performing laboratory or other diagnostic services, and managing financial records are some of the responsibilities of the administrative and clinical support staff in a medical office. Here are a few examples of these jobs.

- Clinic coordinator
- Medical administrative assistant
- Clinical medical assistant
- Medical records specialist
- Medical billing specialist
- Financial counselor
- Scheduler

Patients and family members

The role of the patient and family members is more active in patient-family centered health care than the traditional delivery of health care. The wants and needs of the patient and family are the focus areas in this type of delivery. All parties have a say in how the patient receives treatment, what those treatments will be, the desired outcome, and education and counseling to achieve these goals. The key to achieving full participation of patients and their families is good communication. When this is successful, patients report improved symptoms and overall better outcomes. When patients feel like they are in partnership with their provider, they have increased satisfaction with their care. Fewer hospitalizations, less testing, and fewer treatments are also achieved with successful patient-family centered health care. As a result, health care costs are also decreased.

Institute for Health Care Improvement Triple Aim

The Institute for Health Care Improvement (IHI) has a rubric for health care transformation. The three goals are:

- Improving the experience of care.

- Improving the health of populations.

- Reducing costs of health care.

Methods for meeting these goals are the implementation of either a PCMH or ACO. These models both use the team-based or patient-family centered care model. For the IHI Triple Aim to be met, all three goals must be accomplished.

Health care models that practice team-based care

The enactment of the Affordable Care Act emphasized the need for team-based medicine. The three main goals of ACA were to:

- Expand health insurance coverage.

- Shift the focus of health care delivery system from treatment to prevention.

- Reduce costs and improve the efficiency of health care.

PATIENT-CENTERED MEDICAL HOME

The PCMH is a care delivery model whereby patient treatment is most often coordinated through the primary care provider to ensure they receive the necessary care when and where they need it. The goal of a PCMH is to have a centralized setting that facilitates partnerships between the patient, the provider, and the patient's family (when appropriate).

There are five core functions and attributes of the PCMH.

Comprehensive care is an approach that cares for all of the patient's needs—that is, the whole patient and not just medical and physical concerns. This involves the providers as well as the entire health care team.

Patient-centered care positions patients and their families as core members of the team. The focus is on individual needs and preferences of the patient throughout various stages of life.

Coordinated care means that all specialty care, hospitals, home health care, and community services are overseen by the provider-directed medical practice. The PCMH works at creating and maintaining open communication between the patient and other members of the team. This is aided by information technology (EMR, EHR).

Accessible services include providing tools (open-scheduling, extended hours, communication with providers) through patient information web portals.

Quality and safety commitments include delivering quality health care. This is met by delivering evidence-based medicine that is assessed by collecting safety data and measuring and responding to patient experiences and satisfaction.

PCMHs save money by reducing emergency department visits, hospital admissions, and readmissions, and provide an overall improvement in patient health.

ACCOUNTABLE CARE ORGANIZATIONS

ACOs are made of providers associated with a defined patient population who are accountable for the quality and cost of care delivered to those patients. ACOs are at the delivery system level in response to payment reforms instigated by the Affordable Care Act. As with PCMHs, the focus is on care coordination but with many practices within one organizing entity. This includes multiple providers, hospitals, and specialty clinics. ACOs can also include ambulatory care, inpatient care, or emergency care services. Because the focus is on more than the patients in one practice, there is a relationship to the community in which the organization is located and emphasis on public health issues to prevent illness. To promote wellness, the ACO might have outreach programs (smoking cessation, weight loss clinics, nutritional programs, online education) that are available to anyone.

TRANSITION OF CARE FOR PATIENTS

Successful transitional care occurs when there is appropriate coordination and continued quality in health care as a patient moves from one care setting to another. Transitions are areas that fall short when it comes to providing quality care. Lack of communication between providers regarding patient histories, medication therapies, and overall patient needs are the main reasons for increased risk for rehospitalization, adverse clinical events, increased spending, and poor care quality. To overcome these shortfalls, an effective transitional care model can be implemented. This model focuses on comprehensive inpatient hospital planning and home follow-up for chronically ill patients. The key components are the individualized, interprofessional protocols that prevent or reduce readmissions. The nurse in the transitional care model communicates frequently with the provider's office and accompanies the patient to follow-up visits. The nurse also educates the patient regarding managing their own care and encourages the patient and family caregivers to take an active role in maintaining health. This model does not provide ongoing care but is designed to help the patient and family caregivers develop the knowledge and resources to prevent future health declines. The key is excellent communication between the primary care provider and the patient. The medical assistant often acts as the bridge between the patient and the provider.

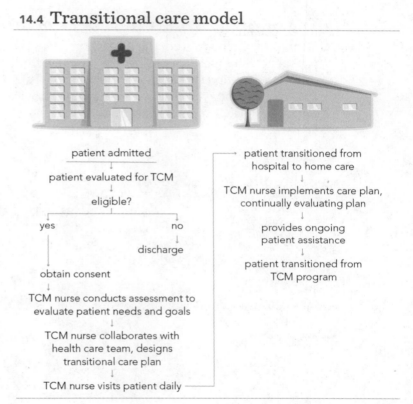

14.4 Transitional care model

patient admitted
↓
patient evaluated for TCM
↓
eligible?
- yes
- no
↓ (no)
discharge

(yes) ↓
obtain consent
↓
TCM nurse conducts assessment to evaluate patient needs and goals
↓
TCM nurse collaborates with health care team, designs transitional care plan
↓
TCM nurse visits patient daily

patient transitioned from hospital to home care
↓
TCM nurse implements care plan, continually evaluating plan
↓
provides ongoing patient assistance
↓
patient transitioned from TCM program

Collaborating with providers and community-based organizations

Upon admission to a critical care facility, the planning for patient discharge begins. The nurse assesses the patient to determine what services are needed to transition to home or to a skilled nursing facility. If the patient is transferred to a nursing facility, the hospital nurse or social worker will inform the provider of the facility and determine who will be providing care. If the patient is being discharged to home, the nurse or social worker will provide information as to what community based organizations will be involved (hospice, home care nursing). The medical assistant often ensures the patient information is documented and communicated to the provider in a timely manner, so discharge is not delayed.

Setting up appointments following inpatient stays

At the time of discharge, the patient will be given instructions on when to follow up with the primary care provider. Sometimes, the hospital nurse or social worker will call to make the arrangements. It is important when scheduling the follow-up appointments to do so in a timely manner. The patient can have an illness that is resolving but not completely gone, or might have a surgical incision that needs to be evaluated for continued healing and to prevent infection. The patient might also be taking a medication that requires bloodwork monitoring.

Making sure reports are available prior to the visit

Confirm that all reports from the hospital stay are available to the provider before a scheduled appointment. If a report is missing, the provider will lose valuable time waiting for the reports to be sent from the facility. On the day of the scheduled appointment, a request for all reports including the discharge summary needs to be sent to the provider. If electronic health records are used, the patient's chart needs to be checked to ensure all documentation is available and in the system.

14.5 Example discharge form

Patient Discharge Form

Health Care Providers
1234 Main Street
Shermer, IL 12345
1.800.555.1234

Name: _____
Address: _____
Email address: _____

Date admitted: _____
Phone number: _____
Attending physician: _____

Reason for admittance: _____

Diagnosis at admittance: _____

Treatment summary: _____

Discharge reason:
☐ Needs met
☐ Patient deceased
☐ Hospital admission
☐ Moved away
☐ Refused services
☐ Discharge to outpatient therapy
☐ Transferred: hospice services
☐ Transferred: other home health services
☐ Transferred: nursing home

Discharge state:
☐ Independent
☐ Assistance required: minimal
☐ Assistance required: moderate
☐ Assistance required: maximal
☐ Assistance required: total

Date discharged: _____
Physician approved: ☐ Yes ☐ No
Diagnosis at discharge: _____

Further treatment plan: _____

Follow up with provider? ☐ Yes ☐ No
Follow-up date: _____

Notes: _____

Medication information: _____

Signature: _____
Date: _____

REVIEW PATIENT RECORD

The patient's record is reviewed by several members of the team prior to the patient's visit. The nurse case manager often oversees patients who have chronic or terminal conditions. Notes are entered into the chart instructing support staff of items that need to be addressed during the appointment. The medical assistant usually preplans visits of patients who have noncomplicated cases.

Each workday starts with a team meeting to go over the patient list for the day. This provides each team member with an opportunity to share any new findings or concerns about a particular patient, so the right resources are available during the visit. For example, the pharmacist can be asked to talk to a patient about diabetes medications, the dietician can be asked to educate a patient about better food choices, and the social worker can be asked to help the patient get a hospital bed.

Preventive medicine and wellness

To comply with the Triple Aim initiative, improvement of overall population health should be a high priority. Prevention of illness must be a main goal for all health care workers. It is imperative for the shift from illness care to wellness care to occur. Teach patients the importance of a healthy lifestyle and the need for preventive wellness checks, including recommended immunizations.

Determinants of health

Determinants of health include several social factors, health services, individual behaviors, and genetic factors. The interaction of personal, social, economic, and environmental factors influences a person's health in some way. However, behavior determinants can often be altered by modifying factors (diet, exercise, smoking cessation, avoiding illicit drugs). Other determinants (biology, genetics) cannot be modified. Determinants such as age, sex, or inherited conditions are examples of biological or genetic determinants that cannot be modified. Sickle cell anemia, hemophilia, cystic fibrosis, heart disease, and cancer are examples of common conditions that have strong biologic or genetic connections.

The environment in which a person lives also influences overall health. The social determinants are the accessibility of resources to meet daily needs, such as:

- Education and employment opportunities

- Grocery stores with adequate fresh foods

- Minimal exposure to crime and violence.

- Adequate transportation.

- Exposure to mass media and emerging technologies.

14.6 Example environmental and physical health determinants

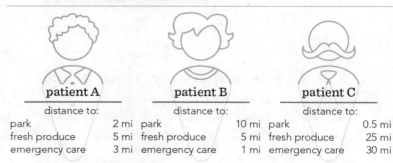

patient A		patient B		patient C	
distance to:		distance to:		distance to:	
park	2 mi	park	10 mi	park	0.5 mi
fresh produce	5 mi	fresh produce	5 mi	fresh produce	25 mi
emergency care	3 mi	emergency care	1 mi	emergency care	30 mi

Where a person lives can be an influence on health. Not all patients have equal access to health determinants like parks, fresh produce, and emergency care.

Physical determinants are the influence of the natural environment on health including weather or climate change, housing and neighborhoods, work sites, and recreational settings (parks, green space). Exposure to toxic substances and physical hazards also fall into this category.

Availability of health services or the ability to afford health care are also determinants of health. Individuals who are unable to see a provider often have unmet health needs, delay in receiving care, and no preventative care. This is why policymaking is a determinant of health. Examples of how policies have influenced health include raising taxes on tobacco products, resulting in fewer users, and the enforcement of seat belt laws, resulting in fewer fatal motor vehicle accidents. The Affordable Care Act made health insurance available to more individuals who might otherwise go uninsured.

Tracking and reporting technologies

The Medicare Access and CHIP Reauthorization Act (MACRA) was signed into law on April 16, 2015. MACRA replaces the former Medicare reimbursement schedule with a new pay-for-performance program that focuses on quality, value, and accountability. Two new payment tracks are available through MACRA, the Merit-Based Incentive Payment System (MIPS) and Advanced Alternative Payment Models (APM). These tracks determine what Medicare will reimburse providers. The new payment models include payment bonuses, penalties, or adjustments based on performance scoring. The four performance categories are:

- Quality.

- Cost/resource use.

- Clinical practice improvement activities.

- Advancing care information.

MACRA implementation is slated to start in 2019, using data from 2017 to determine payments. Small samplings of areas that will be tracked and scored in the new payment structures include:

- Using claims data to calculate population based measures (HgbA1c scores in diabetic population, blood pressure ranges in hypertensive populations).

- The promotion of EHR use (getting all providers to use EHR technology).

- Achieving health equity (seeing Medicaid patients in a timely manner).

- Expanded practice access (providing 24/7 access to MIPS providers).

Checking preventive care section of chart

The medical assistant often has elevated responsibilities in team-based care settings and may be responsible for pre-visit planning. Pre-visit planning can begin days before the appointment and includes going through the patient's chart to establish the following.

- Due dates of preventive testing (Pap smears, colonoscopies, mammograms)

- Due dates of immunizations (Check the CDC website [www.cdc.gov] for immunization schedules.)

- Due dates of patient care management items (HgbA1c, diabetic foot check, cholesterol testing)

- Expired or soon-to-be-expired prescriptions

Review the preventive care section of the patient's electronic medical record to determine if any preventive/diagnostic testing, immunizations, or exams are due, such as diabetic foot checks. Also review the medication section of the chart to see if the patient needs new prescriptions. Electronic orders for diagnostic testing or prescriptions are then created in the order's section of the patient's EHR. The provider will review the orders and either sign off on the orders or make revisions. Having the orders signed prior to the appointment allows the medical assistant to start carrying out the orders at the beginning of the patient's visit.

Responsibilities during the visit

Part of the medical assisting routine consists of gathering specific information from the patient. This will facilitate a smooth patient visit with the provider and eliminate additional work that could delay the patient and provider.

When escorting the patient to the exam room, perform height and weight measurement. Once in the room, measure blood pressure, radial pulse, respirations, and temperature.

Begin acquiring information from the patient. Ask about the reason for the visit, any questions or concerns the patient wants addressed during the visit, and if they are experiencing any health status changes. Perform medication reconciliation, determining if the patient requires any refills that were not obvious during the pre-check and confirming any allergies. Then screen for any health conditions per facility protocols (fall risks, mental health status, various developmental screening tests), update the health history, educate the patient regarding preventive services based on standing orders, and discuss any needed or recommended immunizations.

During the provider interview with the patient, the medical assistant can transcribe for the provider. This involves listening to the interview and examination as it is occurring and documenting all information into the medical record using a template. After the visit is concluded, the provider proofreads the gathered information, revises or confirms it is accurate, and signs off on the note. The medical assistant can also assist the provider with the examination.

Medical assistants often meet with patients and their relatives to discuss the diagnosis, symptom management, treatment options, prescribed medications, dietary restrictions, and other key matters related to conditions and recovery. While medical assistants are not authorized to give recommendations or advice, they are often the liaison between the provider and the patient and help to reinforce instructions and ensure comprehension.

Health coaching

Assist the provider by communicating vital information. Help educate the patient in regards to compliance, treatment options, and adopting a healthy lifestyle. Developing a rapport with the patient is paramount to the patient feeling involved and responsible for their own health, which is a key component of team-based health care. Effective communication allows the medical assistant to convey information necessary for effective health coaching. Establishing trust helps reinforce the instructions given by the provider. Patient compliance is supported by giving accurate information and the patient being comfortable with the information being conveyed.

Learning styles

There are three ways people can attain new information.

Auditory learning is achieved by hearing the information. This can be accomplished with providing information verbally while the patient listens.

Kinesthetic learning involves movement or performing the task. Someone who learns this way needs to see the action and then perform it themselves. A demonstration of the skill needed with a return demonstration or an anatomical model the patient can touch works best.

Visual learning involves reading information and seeing diagrams or graphics. The patient can have overlaps in these learning styles, so it is important to ask what they consider to be their best methods of learning.

14.7 Engaging learning styles

teaching about blood sugar testing

kinesthetic
demonstrate procedure

auditory
describe procedure

visual
pamphlet about procedure

Education delivery methods and instructional techniques

There are many ways to provide education to patients. Knowing a patient's learning style will give the best way to present material. Provide visual material for those who learn by seeing; this can include DVDs or approved online videos. For kinesthetic learning, provide demonstration materials, so the patient can practice the skill. Active involvement allows the patient to have ownership of the skill he is learning. Demonstration with a return demonstration and repetition of the skill will help information retention and allows the patient to perfect the skill with positive feedback.

No matter the learning style of the patient, ask for feedback. This is crucial to evaluating the effectiveness of the teaching session. Restating, repeating, and rephrasing the material is a method for evaluating the patient's understanding of the material. Providing positive reinforcement gives the patient the motivation to learn information that can seem scary or makes the patient apprehensive. Therapeutic communication allows the patient to be comfortable and engaged in the learning process. Have the patient restate or demonstrate the provided information before ending the education session. Provide any written material and make sure the patient takes it with them when exiting the office. If this step is forgotten, mail the information to the patient.

Provide a quiet location for the teaching session, as distractions are detrimental to learning. Speak at an adequate pace, not too fast or slow, and make eye contact with the patient. Provide written material in lay language, at the patient's reading level, and in the patient's primary language. Provide large-print material for patients who have low vision.

Barriers to learning

Barriers to learning can be developmental or physical. This needs to be considered when providing the information to patients.

If the patient is a child, make sure to speak at the appropriate grade or developmental language level. Do not stand over the child, because this can be intimidating. Have the child repeat information or demonstrate the skill, then educate the parent on the information or skill to perform.

For individuals who have visual impairments, provide large-print or Braille resource. Demonstration may also be used with the patient handling the needed materials. For patients who have hearing loss, it is important to speak face-to-face. Having the patient repeat information confirms comprehension. Provide written material so the patient can see information as it is being discussed. DVDs or other visual material can also be used. For patients who have language barriers, the material needs to be made available in the patient's primary language. Speak to the patient and not the translator. Look for nonverbal cues that the patient understands the material as it is presented.

COORDINATING CARE WITH COMMUNITY AGENCIES

There are many services within the community that can benefit patients. Be aware of what services are offered and offer contact information for those services. Brochures from the organizations are usually free and available to hand out. Keep a list of community resources in an easily accessed location so that information can be provided to patients without any delays. Depending on the specialty of the practice, lists can be organized according to patients' condition, age, or socioeconomic status. The Centers for Disease Control and Prevention website has resources that provide services within specified geographic locations. Local hospital websites also provide information regarding outreach programs offered in the community. Document all information provided to the patient documented in the health record; this aids in promoting *continuity of care*.

FACILITATE PATIENT COMPLIANCE TO OPTIMIZE HEALTH OUTCOMES

Checking in with the patient or patient's family

The best method to promote compliance is through communication. This can be achieved through telephone calls or e-mailing through a secured server, depending on the patient's preference. This is part of maintaining HIPAA compliance. Also check to see if any family members are authorized to receive the patient's health information. It is the patient's right to restrict who receives any information. Follow-up communication is critical to promoting compliance and for clarity of goals. Any questions the patient has are easily answered, and any worries or fears regarding medication side effects can be alleviated. The patient feels cared for, and the provider is aware that the treatment plan is being followed.

---

continuity of care. Continuation of care smoothly from one provider to another, so that the patient receives the most benefit and no interruption to care

SUMMARY

The rising cost of health care has brought about changes in the overall delivery of care. Prevention is the key to decreasing the burden of providing care to a population suffering from increasing chronic conditions. Patients need to be aware they are members of the health care team. The medical assistant is in one of the best positions to help them with this role. The medical assistant has both the administrative and clinical knowledge to provide the best care for the patient and assist the provider more effectively.

CHAPTER 15
Administrative Assisting

OVERVIEW

The administrative duties of medical assistants are extensive and crucial to quality health care. Examples include scheduling, basic bookkeeping, completing insurance documentation, and maintaining compliance with government regulations. The unique combination of providing patient care and performing administrative duties makes medical assistants vital and versatile members of the health care team.

SCHEDULING AND MONITORING PATIENT APPOINTMENTS

Several methods can be used when scheduling patient appointments. While the most common practice is use of electronic software, some offices still use an *appointment book*. Either method is acceptable, but the use of practice management software to develop a *matrix* or an electronic *template* can make appointment scheduling easier. Consider the type of appointment scheduling to be used, as well as the protocols for scheduling specific types of appointments. Written policies regarding routine, acute illness, *no-show*, and rescheduled appointments are needed for consistency.

Objectives

Upon completion of this chapter, you should be able to:

- Schedule and monitor patient appointments using electronic and paper-based systems.
- Manage electronic and paper medical records.
- Identify and check patients in and out.
- Verify insurance coverage and financial eligibility.
- Verify diagnostic and procedural codes.
- Prepare documentation and billing requests using current coding guidelines.
- Ensure that documentation complies with government and insurance requirements.
- Facilitate/generate referrals to other providers and allied health professionals.
- Obtain and verify prior authorizations and precertifications.
- Bill patients, insurers, and third-party payers for services performed.
- Perform charge reconciliation.
- Resolve billing issues with insurers and third-party payers, including appeals and denials.
- Provide customer service and facilitate service recovery.
- Enter information into databases or spreadsheets.
- Maintain inventory of clinical and administrative supplies.
- Participate in safety evaluations and report safety concerns.

appointment book. A book used to schedule, cancel, and reschedule appointments; can be color-coded or arranged so a week is shown at a glance

matrix. A table used for scheduling

template. An outline used to make new pages with a similar design, pattern, or style

no-show. Appointment that an individual fails to keep without giving notice

Electronic vs. paper-based systems

Medical records consist of an electronic medical record system or a paper-based medical record system. The preferred method for tracking and documenting patient data has become the electronic health record. Paper charts are tangible records comprised of documented proof of patient care. However, paper charts have some significant disadvantages. They can only be used by one person at a time, can easily be misplaced due to filing errors, and cannot be easily shared with other providers. The electronic medical record can accomplish a significant number of tasks using one system. Many tasks can be performed within the electronic medical record. Electronic medical records help decrease medical errors, as well as time spent correcting diagnoses and procedure coding for medical billing. This decreases the time needed for insurance reimbursements. In addition, the electronic medical record provides a secure way to communicate with the patient regarding medication refills, upcoming appointments, and the status of *referrals*.

15.1 Electronic medical record

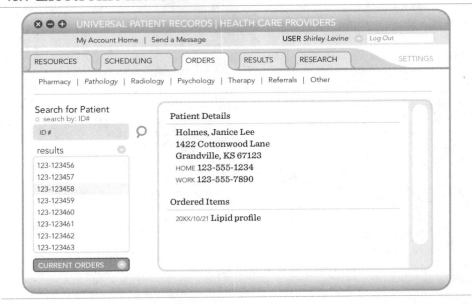

15.2 Scheduling matrix

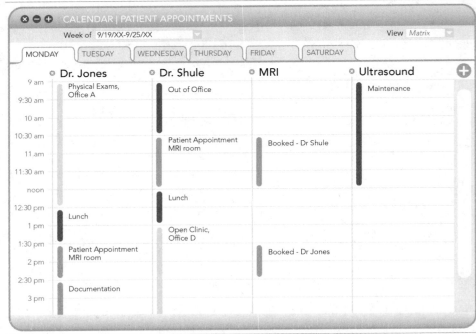

Scheduling software

Medical assistants use practice management software to search for appointments with criteria such as specific providers, available times, types of appointments, and additional search functions based on a set matrix.

---

referral. Directing a patient to a specialist

Establishing a matrix

The use of a template allows the medical assistant to establish a matrix for setting appointments and blocking off specific time periods for holiday, meetings, and lunch breaks. The template for each matrix can be used repeatedly for each provider over any length of time. Appointments may be grouped by provider, appointment types (new patients, OB patients, allergy patients) and available resources (surgery room, laboratory). Additionally, the matrix can be adjusted based on future needs as they arise.

Types of scheduling

Several types of scheduling methods can be used based on the facility's, provider's, and patient's needs. *Wave scheduling*, *modified wave scheduling*, and *double-booking* are some common types of scheduling. Wave scheduling allows three patients to be scheduled at the same time, to be seen in the order in which they arrive. In this method, one patient arriving late does not disrupt the provider's schedule. Modified wave scheduling allocates two patients to arrive at a specified time and the third to arrive approximately 30 minutes later. This timely sequence is continuous throughout the day. Double-booking is when two patients are scheduled at the same time to see the same provider. This is often used to work in a patient with an acute illness when no other time is available. It creates delays in the provider's schedule that continues throughout the rest of the day.

Internal appointments or established patients

The first piece of necessary information for scheduling an internal appointment with an established patient is the patient's name and date of birth. Next, determine the reason for the visit, as well as the amount of time the patient and provider will need for the visit. Lastly, determine if there is any day of the week or time the patient prefers. All elements should be considered, including availability, provider's preferences, and patient's habits.

15.3 Wave scheduling

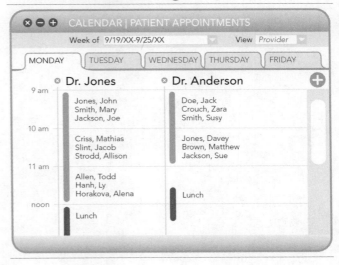

15.4 Modified wave scheduling

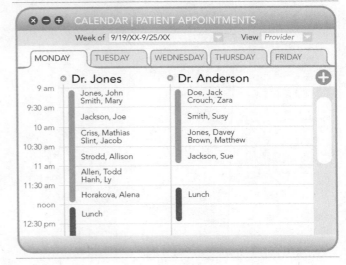

wave scheduling. Scheduling three patients at the same time to be seen in the order in which they arrive

modified wave scheduling. Allocating two patients to arrive at a specified time and the third to arrive approximately 30 minutes later, repeated throughout the day

double-booking. Scheduling two patients at the same time with the same provider, often to fit in a patient who has an acute illness

External appointments or new patients

Information needed for scheduling an external appointment for a new patient begins with obtaining demographic information. This includes full name, address, date of birth, contact phone numbers, insurance information for billing purposes, Social Security number, and emergency contact information. Have new patients complete a registration packet prior to the visit, if possible. These packets usually comprise new patient forms for documenting demographic information, *Notice of Privacy Practices*, and patient medical history form, which includes current medications.

15.5 Notice of Privacy Practices

Health Care Providers
1234 Main Street
Shermer, IL 12345
1.800.555.1234

Notice of Privacy Practices

This notice describes how your medical information may be used and disclosed (provided to others) and how you can get access to this information. Please review this notice carefully.

Our Responsibilities

Health Care Providers takes the privacy of your health information seriously. We are required by law to keep your health information private and provide you with this Notice of Privacy Practices. We will act according to the terms of this Notice. We reserve the right to change this Notice of Privacy Practices and to make any new practices effective for all Protected Health Information that we keep. Any changes made to the Notice of Privacy Practices will be posted in the Patient Registration area and given to you at your next appointment. Health Care Providers is required to notify you if your protected health information is breached (seen by anyone who is not authorized to see it).

How We May Use and Share Your Medical Information

For Treatment
We may use your medical information to give you medical care. We may share your medical information with doctors, nurses, technicians. For example, departments may share your medical information to plan your care. This may include prescriptions, lab work, and x-rays. We may share your medical information with people not at our facility. This may include referring physicians and home health care nurses who are treating you.

For Payment
We may use and share your medical information with your insurance plan or others who help pay for your care. We do this to find out if your plan will pay for the treatment.

For Health Care Operations
We may use and share your medical information for our operations. These uses and disclosures help us run our programs and make sure our patients receive quality care. For example, we may use medical information to review our treatment and services. We may use medical information to measure the performance of our staff and how they care for you. We may share medical information with doctors, nurses, technicians, students, and other health care workers for teaching purposes or preparatory research.

Appointment Reminders
We may contact you to remind you about your appointment for medical care.

Treatment Alternatives
We may use and share medical information to tell you about different types of treatment available to you. We may use and share medical information to tell you about other benefits and services related to your health.

Your Health Information Rights

Health Care Providers is required to
• maintain the privacy of your medical record
• abide by the terms of this notice
• notify you if we are unable to agree to a requested restriction
• accommodate reasonable requests you may have to communicate health information by alternative means or at alternative locations or phone numbers

We reserve the right to change our practices and to make new provisions effective for all protected health information we maintain. We will post a copy of our current notice in a visible location at all times. We will not use or disclose your protected health information without your authorization, except as described in this notice.

15.6 Patient medical history form

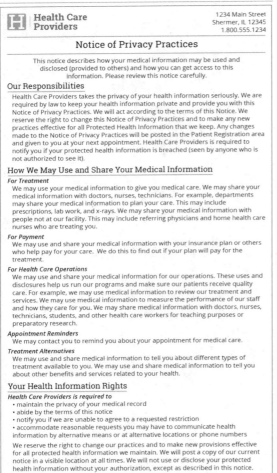

Health Care Providers
1234 Main Street
Shermer, IL 12345
1.800.555.1234

Health History Questionnaire

Name:
DOB:
Occupation:

Today's Date:
Chart Number:

Part I - Present Health History

Reason for today's visit:

List any conditions for w

List any medications yo

List any allergies (foods

Habits and Genera

Do you smoke?
Do you drink?
Do you exercise?
Do you have sleep trou
Has your appetite chan
Do you drink coffee or

Do you:
Feel nervous?
Feel depressed?
Feel indecisive?
Lose your temper?
Worry a lot?
Tire easily?
Use drugs?
Do you wish to talk a

Have you recently
Marital status?
Employment?
Place of residence?
Financial status?

Health Care Providers
1234 Main Street
Shermer, IL 12345
1.800.555.1234

Health History Questionnaire

Name:
DOB:
Occupation:

Today's Date:
Chart Number:

Part II - Past Health History

Family Health History

Check any condition if there is a history amongst immediate family

☐ Asthma   ☐ Diabetes   ☐ Cancer
☐ Blood disease   ☐ Glaucoma   ☐ Epilepsy
☐ Rheumatoid arthritis ☐ Tuberculosis   ☐ Gout
☐ High blood pressure ☐ Heart disease   ☐ Mental problems
☐ Seizures   ☐ Suicide

Hospitalizations and Surgeries

Please list all times you have been hospitalized and any surgical procedures you have undergone

Illness and Health Indicators

Check any condition you have previously experienced (or still experience)

☐ Eye or eyelid infection ☐ Glaucoma   ☐ Other eye problems
☐ Ear trouble   ☐ Decreased hearing ☐ Deafness
☐ Thyroid trouble   ☐ Strep throat   ☐ Bronchitis
☐ Emphysema   ☐ Pneumonia   ☐ Allergies / Hay fever
☐ Asthma   ☐ Tuberculosis   ☐ High blood pressure
☐ Heart attack   ☐ High cholesterol   ☐ Arteriosclerosis
☐ Heart murmur   ☐ Ulcer   ☐ Colitis
☐ Other bowel problem   ☐ Hepatitis   ☐ Liver disease

Notice of Privacy Practices. A notification by providers required by the HIPAA Privacy Rule that provides an understandable explanation of patients' rights with respect to their personal health information and the privacy practices of their providers

Duration of appointment

Always adhere to the office policies and protocols when scheduling patient appointments. When determining the duration of a patient appointment, consider the provider's preferences, the patient's needs, whether the patient is established or new, and room availability. With effective scheduling, the patient should not wait more than 15 minutes in the waiting area for the appointment.

Urgency of appointment

All calls that come in to the office should be evaluated and prioritized based on a *screening* process. Obtain the caller's full name, phone number, and address at the beginning of a call when the patients symptoms point toward a life threatening condition. A list of questions should be prepared by the provider or practice manager for the medical assistant to reference when determining whether the call is routine, urgent, or life-threatening. If the situation is deemed critical and emergency services are needed, keep the caller on the phone until emergency medical services arrive to ensure the safety of the caller.

Handling cancellations and no-shows

The medical practice should have a policy for individuals who fail to keep appointments or routinely cancel appointments. Patients cancel and miss appointments for a variety of reasons that can be beyond their control. Each incident should be recorded as part of the medical record to keep a detailed legal record of how many times a patient has cancelled or missed scheduled appointments. Some practices have policies that allow for charging a fee for the missed visit. Providers may discharge the patient from the practice if continued cancellations or missed appointments take place, as this demonstrates noncompliance. It is imperative that all appointments missed are documented to protect the provider from legal action. The medical assistant should be familiar with the established office policies for these situations.

Recalls (electronic and manual)

An *automated call routing* system offers patients the option of cancelling, confirming, or rescheduling an appointment. This automated system keeps track of which patients have confirmed, which patients will not be coming for their regular scheduled appointment, and which patients request a call back to reschedule. It is also good practice to contact patients who have opted to cancel to ensure continuity of care and good customer service.

---

screening. Examining and separating into groups

automated call routing. A software system that answers phones automatically and routes calls to staff after the caller responds to prompts; also used to call patients to remind them of upcoming appointments

MANAGING ELECTRONIC AND PAPER MEDICAL RECORDS

Management of electronic or paper medical records requires an accurate and efficient system that includes filing protocols. These protocols involve processes for developing and categorizing the medical record. The medical assistant takes part in maintaining and operating system software, security measures, documentation guidelines, and provider order entries. The medical assistant is also responsible for sending medical release forms to obtain previous medical records, abiding by legal requirements related to chart maintenance, and retention and appropriate destruction of charts.

Verifying accuracy of a patient's medical record ensures all clinical findings are documented, which provides continuity of care for the patient and legal protection for providers. Statistical data is gathered from the documentation, and supports insurance claims for reimbursements. Quality control ensures there is an adequate degree of value put into processes, management, and guidelines.

Filing systems and processes

Each office has its own filing system for paper records, but there are five basic steps for filing.

- *Conditioning* involves grouping related papers together, removing all paper clips and staples, attaching smaller papers to regular sheets, and fixing damaged records.

- *Releasing* is marking the form to be filed with a mark of designated preference (ready to be filed, the provider's initials, using a stamp).

- *Indexing and coding* is determining where to place the original record in the file and whether it needs to be cross-referenced in another section. A chart number is typically used for this.

- *Sorting* involves ordering papers in a filing structure and placing the documents in specific groups.

- *Storing and filing* is securing documents permanently in the file to ensure the medical record documents do not become misplaced.

There are three basic filing methods.

- *Alphabetic filing* is a traditional system for patient records in providers' offices and the most widely used. Files are arranged by last name, first name, and middle initial.

- *Numeric filing* is typically combined with color coding and used for larger health centers or hospitals. This method allows for unlimited expansion without the need to shift files to create room. It saves time for retrieving and filing charts, and provides additional patient confidentiality.

- *Subject filing* is used for general correspondence using the alphabetic or alphanumeric filing method. With this method, all correspondence dealing with a particular subject is placed under a specific tab with subject headings.

Maintenance, storage, and disposal of medical records

There are legal requirements related to the maintenance, storage, and destruction of medical records. Charts should never leave the office. Transcription should be processed in a timely manner, and chart documents that have yet to be filed in a patient record must be locked away at closing. In addition, prescription pads should be kept in a locked, tamper-proof safe.

Typically, the first step when deciding whether to purge, transfer, or retain a medical record is to determine whether it is active, inactive, or closed. Laws relating to the retention of medical records vary by state, and several government platforms have their own policies and procedures for retaining records. In most cases, when there are no specific guidelines for retaining medical records, facilities preserve records for a minimum of 10 years. Any patient covered by Medicare or Medicaid must have their records retained for a minimum of 10 years.

Upon determination of a patient's chart status and based on retention guidelines, the medical record should be shredded by a professional and confidential document destruction service. The *Health Insurance Portability and Accountability Act (HIPAA)* does not require a specific method for the disposal of medical records, but the medical facility should keep a detailed record of when, how, and by whom the medical records were destroyed.

15.7 Medical release form

Health Care Providers
1234 Main Street
Shermer, IL 12345
1.800.555.1234

HIPAA Privacy Authorization for Release of Medical Information

Authorization

I, _____ _____ _____
Print patient's name   Date of birth   Social security number
hereby authorize Health Care Providers to release information records, including HIV Antibody Testing, Psychiatric/Psychological, Alcohol and/or Drug Abuse, to:

To:
Address:
For the purpose of:
Appointment on:
Other:
Please specify reason for disclosure:

I understand that if I consent to the release of any of my medical records, the results of any HIV Antibody Testing, Psychiatric/Psychologocal, Alcohol and/or Drug Abuse information will be released.

I understand this consent may be cancelled upon written notice to the hospital, except that action by the hospital has been taken in reliance on this authorization, and that this authorization shall remain in force for a 90-day period in order to affect the purpose for which it is given. Alcohol and drug abuse information, if present, has been disclosed from records whose confidentiality is protected by Federal Law.

Federal Regulations (42CFR, part II) prohibit making any further disclosure of records without the specific written authorization of the undersigned, or as otherwise permitted by such regulations.

The confidentiality of HIV antibody test results is protected by law, which prohibits any further disclosure by a person to whom this information has been disclosed, without specific written consent of the undersigned or as otherwise permitted by law.

Date of Authorization   From   To

Patient's Signature

Parent, Legal Guardian, or   Relationship to Patient
Authorized Representative Signature

Witness

Health Insurance Portability and Accountability Act (HIPAA). A law implemented in 1996 to improve the portability and continuity of health insurance coverage; contain costs, fraud, and abuse in the health care industry; set a higher standard for electronic health information communications; and promote the privacy of health information

Categories of the medical record

Categories within a patient's medical record are comprised of laboratory reports, radiology reports, nurses' notes, medications, flow sheets, and provider progress notes. In addition, administrative forms such as demographic information, HIPAA privacy notices, photo identification, and insurance cards are all filed in chronological or *reverse chronological order*.

Creating and preparing medical records

When creating and preparing medical records, each section should be grouped according to type, progress notes, laboratory, and radiology. This is a source-oriented medical record (SOMR). There are two methods commonly used to document information on the progress sheet: SOAP and CHEDDAR.

SOAP arranges the progress notes according to:

- Subjective impressions

- Objective findings or clinical indication

- Assessment or medical diagnosis

- Plan for treatment

With CHEDDAR the progress note is arranged by:

- Chief complaint

- History

- Examination

- Details

- Drugs and dosages

- Assessment

- Return visit information

15.8 New patient demographic form

Health Care Providers
1234 Main Street
Shermer, IL 12345
1.800.555.1234

New Patient Demographics Form

Name: SSN:
Address: DOB:
Email address: Sex: ☐ Male ☐ Female

Home phone: Cell:
Marital status: ☐ Married ☐ Single ☐ Other
Spouse / Next of kin: Number:
Emergency contact: Number:
Employer name: Number:

Primary insurance:
    Group No: ID No:
Secondary insurance:
    Group No: ID No:

Preferred provider:
Preferred pharmacy:
Address:
Referring physician:
Phone:
How did you hear about us?
    ☐ Previous patient
    ☐ Referral: doctor
    ☐ Referral: friend or family
    ☐ Referral: other
    ☐ Website
    ☐ Billboard
    ☐ Yellow pages
    ☐ Newspaper advertisement
    ☐ Other

15.9 SOAP progress note

Progress Notes

Name:	Shipley, Donna	**Date of Service:**	1 Oct 20XX
ID #:	BBB111111	**DOB:**	21 Sep 19XX
Provider:	Richardson, E.	**Sex:**	Female

Description: Postoperative Care

Procedures	**CPT Code**
Incision and removal - complicated	10121-22
Lab draw	36415
General health panel	80050

Subjective
Patient came into office today pain on left forearm that has been there for 5 days. Patient also here today to receive lab work for physical exam already scheduled.

Objective
Examining the left forearm shows that the cyst is tender and measures at 6cm in size. Left arm has a severe case of edema with redness. There is obviously some infection present in the cyst that needs to be drained right away.

---

reverse chronological order. Arranged so that the most recent item is on top and older items are filed further back

Record management systems and software

Medical record management and software interface systems include filing and storage of archived files. Tickler files are customarily used when following up on something by a specific date. Archived charts are to be stored for the required amount of time and purged to make space for upcoming records to be archived. Having a variety of processes in place that keep current records easily accessible and older records stored properly assists in efficient work flow.

The use of electronic medical records management software can assist medical offices in compliance with federal guidelines. However, it can also be useful by providing tools such as scheduling, which tracks appointments and sends out reminders and confirmations; an electronic medical billing system; or electronic eligibility verifications and referral management program. Medical offices may choose programs or software from multiple companies to meet their needs. To meet current federal criteria to qualify for CMS incentives, the provider must use the system for e-prescribing, communicating with patients, and computerized provider order entry (CPOE), which includes laboratory and radiology orders.

Security measures

It is imperative that any personal information given to the provider and medical assistants be secured by passwords, encryption, and firewalls. All staff members in the medical office should have individual passwords to protect computers, networks, and data from unlawful usage. Encryption is when the data is translated into code that requires the use of a password to unlock. Additionally, viruses are often uploaded to computers and programs via emails and unsecured networks that quickly use all available memory and steal or destroy valuable data. Antivirus programs should be used to protect the network and computer system from patient data being infiltrated or stolen. Firewalls help to protect systems from viruses by blocking unauthorized programs from accessing the network.

Documentation guidelines

Accurate medical records ensure continuity of care among all health care providers. Medical record documentation must be accurate, thorough, and judicious to comply with office, local, state, and federal policies. The medical record functions as evidence in courts of law for legal actions regarding specific medical management and medical practice methods that support patient care. In addition, maintained and accurate medical records aid researchers in gathering statistical information.

Computerized physician order entry

CPOE is an electronic medical record system function that allows providers to digitally order laboratory and radiology testing, treatments, referrals, and prescriptions. In 2009 when the federal government implemented the HITECH Act and the Meaningful Use program, CPOE use rapidly increased in inpatient and outpatient facilities. The majority of hospitals and outpatient practices now use some form of CPOE. The CPOE system structure was created to improve the safety of medication orders, but modern technology allows electronic ordering of tests, procedures, and consultations as well.

Sending records to patients and other providers

All requests for medical records need to be provided in writing, and the release filed into the patient's chart. The patient's attorney, mediator, or arbitrator must obtain approval from the patient prior to obtaining access to the patient's medical records. However, the patient's attorney may present a legal power of attorney document that authorizes them to view the medical records on behalf of the patient if necessary.

IDENTIFYING AND CHECKING PATIENTS IN/OUT

Greeting patients as they enter the medical office is the first step in the check-in process. Welcoming patients by name is a courteous and cordial way to acknowledge them before checking them in. Establish eye contact and smile while introductions are being made. After the greeting is conducted, obtain identifiable information along with other required registration processes.

Reception room environment

The reception room should be appealing, welcoming, and clean. Throughout the day all magazines, office brochures, and educational patient material should be picked up and stacked neatly. The Notice of Privacy Practices should be available to patients at all times for their review. At the end of each working day, sanitize the office chairs, reception counters, and door knobs.

Identifying and greeting patients

A patient's first impression often leaves a lasting perception of an office and the staff. Greet patients politely as they enter the building and as they complete their visit. The tone of voice used, body language, facial expression, and other nonverbal communication methods can make a significant impression on the patient.

Collecting demographic information

Collect demographic information using a registration form during the check-in process. Most registration forms request the following information to be obtained.

- Patient's full name
- Date of birth
- Guarantor name and their relationship to the patient
- Address
- Telephone number
- Marital status
- Spousal information (if any)
- Place of employment
- Social Security number
- Driver's license number
- Emergency contact information

Q: Why are the demographic and registration forms important for the patient to fill out?

A: The patient demographic and registration forms are important because they provide all the necessary information to identify the patient, contain emergency contact information, and Privacy Notice and HIPAA information.

Q: What are the two primary forms of identification the patient needs to provide during the check-in process?

A: The patient's driver's license or state-issued identification and insurance cards are the two primary forms of identification to provide when checking in.

Q: Does the patient sign the consent to treat form before or after seeing the provider?

A: The patient needs to sign a consent to treat form before the provider sees them, unless it is an emergent situation. This is necessary for any treatment or procedures, including examinations.

Collecting payments

It is important to review the patient insurance information for each visit to ensure the correct fee is collected. Insurance policies and allowed amounts can vary greatly. Some patients are responsible for the full allowed amount, which applies to their deductible before the coinsurance amount applies to patient responsibility. Other insurance policies have a specific contracted copayment due at the time of service.

Required information for patient to review and sign

Provide all patients with a consent to treat form to review and sign before the provider can move forward with any treatment. A written informed consent is required when an invasive procedure or treatment will be performed. Any situation that requires an in-depth understanding of a treatment or procedure needs an informed consent signed in advance. Implied consent is given when the patient has a minimally invasive procedure, such as a venipuncture or an electrocardiogram.

Using basic office equipment

It is vital that a medical assistant know how to operate all basic office equipment (copier, scanner, fax machine, computer, multi-line telephone system). This equipment is used multiple times a day to ensure all duties are completed.

15.10 Consent to treat form

Health Care Providers	**Consent to Treat**
1234 Main Street	Name: _____ Today's Date: _____
Shermer, IL 12345	DOB: _____ Chart Number: _____
1.800.555.1234	Occupation: _____

Consent to Treat

I authorize the health care providers of Health Care Providers to administer treatment as deemed necessary for care of the patient named above. This pertains to today's visit and any future visits involving treatment by Health Care Providers. I certify that I am the patient or the parent or legal guardian of the patient. I also certify that no guarantee or assurance has been made as to the results that may be obtained from the treatment.

Assignment of Benefit

All professional services rendered are charged to the patient. As a service to the patient, necessary forms will be completed to help expedite insurance carrier payments. The patient/parent/responsible party is responsible for any unpaid balances. Co-payments will be made at the time of service. I request that payment of authorized Medicare, Medicaid, or other insurance compnay benefits be made to the Health Care Providers for any services issued to me by Health Care Providers. All regulations pertaining to Medicare and Medicaid assignment of benefits apply.

I fully understand and accept the information provided by this consent.

_____ _____ _____
Signature   Printed name   Date

Handling visitors other than patients

It is a common office policy to have all visitors (pharmaceutical representatives, vendors) sign in and receive a visitor badge prior to entering the back portion of the medical office. These types of visitors are usually only welcomed when the schedule permits, proper identification is provided, and the requested provider is willing to spend time with the representative.

Explaining general office procedures

General office procedures include opening the office for the day by ensuring all necessary equipment (computers, laboratory equipment, lights) are turned on. Prepare for the day ahead by printing daily schedules, answering messages from the night before, and ensuring all exam rooms are stocked.

VERIFYING INSURANCE COVERAGE AND FINANCIAL ELIGIBILITY

Health insurance coverage is verified by contacting the patient's insurance carrier for benefits. The medical assistant documents any exclusions or noncovered services, if referral or authorizations are required for specific services, and obtains the necessary payment amounts due from the patient at the time of service. The patient's financial eligibility is also determined to make appropriate payment plans or offer a self-pay discounted rate for services rendered.

Insurance terminology

A medical assistant must be proficient and knowledgeable regarding insurance terminology to determine a patient's coverage, benefits, and financial responsibility.

Copay is a specified sum of money based on the patient's insurance policy benefits due at the time of service.

Coinsurance is an amount a policyholder is financially responsible for according to their insurance policies provisions. For example, the policyholder must meet a specified deductible amount before the medical insurance company will contribute their portion. Typically, an 80/20 ratio allows for 80% of the allowable charges be paid by the insurance company with the remaining 20% to be paid by the policyholder.

Deductibles are specific amounts of money a patient must pay out of pocket before the insurance carrier begins paying for services. Deductible amounts are usually on a calendar year accrual basis.

An *explanation of benefits (EOB)* is provided to the patient by the insurance company as a statement detailing what services were paid, denied, or reduced in payment. An EOB also includes information pertaining to amounts applied to the deductible, coinsurance, or allowed amounts.

explanation of benefits (EOB). A statement from an insurance carrier describing what services were paid, denied, or reduced in payment

Remittance advice (RA) is an explanation of benefits sent to the provider from the insurance carrier. Similar to the EOB, the RA contains multiple patients and providers. Also included is the electronic fund transfer information or a check for payment. Remittance advice statements are used to post payments to patient accounts.

Advance beneficiary notice (ABN) is a form a Medicare patient will sign when the provider thinks Medicare might not pay for a specific service or item. The patient has the option to choose to have Medicare billed, so an official payment decision is made and a Medicare Summary Notice sent to the patient with an explanation for noncoverage, or to not have the charges submitted to Medicare, and receive the services from the provider with the understanding that the patient is responsible for payment at the time of service without the ability of appealing to Medicare or deciding not to receive the services. This form needs to be signed by the patient before services are provided, with a copy to be kept on file and a copy to be given to the patient.

Types of insurance plans

There are several types of insurance policies available, classified as federal or private.

Federal policies include Tricare, which covers military personnel and their dependents. Medicaid is funded by the federal government and managed by the state; it covers those who meet specific eligibility criteria set by the state. Medicare is a federal program that covers individuals age 65 and older or who need coverage due to specific medical issues. Workers' compensation is a state legislative law that protects employees against the cost of medical care resulting from a work-related injury.

Private policies include group policies offered through an individual's employer who will usually pay a portion of the premium and deduct the remainder of the premium from the employees' paycheck. Individual policies are insurance plans that an individual funds themselves. Patients might pay the entire premium themselves if they are self-employed.

Verifying insurance coverage

When verifying a patient's health insurance, the following information is needed.

- Patient's full name
- Date of birth
- Policy number
- Social Security number (depending on insurance company requirements)

When obtaining eligibility and benefit information, ask for the effective dates, deductible, copayment, or coinsurance amounts. In addition, verify if there are any coverage or plan exclusions or limitations, and if any authorizations or referrals are required. The medical assistant will also need to confirm where the claims are to be sent and who they spoke with to obtain the information.

Financial eligibility, sliding scales, and indigent programs

Some medical practices occasionally provide medical care for individuals who are unable to pay for services. In most cases, indigent programs are available through social services or community hospitals. Medical assistants should be familiar with local agencies and organizations that can aid patients in times of need. If a provider decides to provide services on a payment schedule, the patient is often asked to sign a Federal Truth in Lending Statement to arrange for payments that extend longer than 4 months.

VERIFYING DIAGNOSTIC AND PROCEDURAL CODES

Diagnostic and procedural coding translates written descriptions of diseases, ailments, injuries, or any health encounter into numeric or alphanumeric codes. The correct use of diagnostic and procedural coding is ensured by accurate and efficient medical record maintenance and claims processing. Each code identifies a specific encounter, ailment, or injury. Each diagnostic and procedural code allows for submission of services for reimbursement from insurance companies and to provide statistical data for research studies.

Medical coding systems

For an illness to be properly coded, a recognized and established structure for coding must be used.

ICD-10-CM

ICD-10-CM coding was implemented on October 1, 2015, after unexpected delays by Congress. ICD-10-CM coding contains approximately 55,000 more codes than ICD-9-CM and allows more specific reporting of diseases and newly recognized conditions. There are three to seven characters used. The first character is alphabetical. The second and third characters are numeric, with fourth, fifth, sixth, and seventh being either alphabetic or numeric. A potential placeholder provides for future expansion of the codes. This allows for more specificity and laterality.

ICD-10-PCS

ICD-10-Procedure Coding System (ICD-10-PCS) is a system comprised of medical classifications for procedural codes typically used within hospitals that record various health treatments and testing. These codes are a replacement for ICD-9-CM, Volume 3.

CPT codes and modifiers

Current Procedural Terminology (CPT) codes and modifiers are used to document procedures and technical services based on services by providers in outpatient settings. All information in the medical record must be accurate for the correct code to be documented. In addition, using the appropriate codes assists in communicating data on procedures and services, correct filing of insurance claims, and provides basic information for statistical analysis of health care services.

HCPCS

Healthcare Common Procedure Coding System (HCPCS) is a group of codes and descriptions that represent procedures, supplies, products, and services not covered by or included in the CPT coding system. Similar to CPT codes, HCPCS codes are updated every year. They are designed to enhance uniform reporting and collection of statistical data on medical supplies, products, services, and procedures. These codes are typically used for Medicare and Medicaid insurance plans.

Current Procedural Terminology (CPT) codes. Five-digit numeric codes used to describe an evaluation/management service rendered by providers

Healthcare Common Procedural Coding System (HCPCS). Codes created by the Centers for Medicare and Medicaid Services to report supplies, materials, and other procedures and services not defined in the CPT manual

PREPARING DOCUMENTATION AND BILLING REQUESTS

Medical assistants are responsible for preparing documentation and billing requests according to current coding guidelines. Forms used to obtain information necessary to send out claims include the patient encounter form, treatment or progress notes, history and physical exam notes, and discharge summaries. Depending on whether the patient had surgery or laboratory services, an operative report or pathology report may also be needed to prepare documentation and billing submissions.

CMS billing requirements

Information required for completion of the CMS-1500 Form requires several fields to be correctly completed for the claim to be accepted by insurance carriers. All new patients are asked to fill out a registration form detailing all demographic and insurance information. Then verify the insurance information for eligibility and specific requirements. During this process, determine whether the patient requires an authorization or referral from the insurance carrier. Next, review patient medical records for accurate documentation for the visit. The medical assistant receives an encounter form or superbill from the provider for the visit to determine the correct procedural coding and diagnoses are used. The medical documentation is then reviewed to substantiate the correct charges and confirm accurate diagnoses are used for each procedure. Finally, the claim is sent to the insurance company for reimbursement for services rendered.

The CMS-1500 form is divided into sections and blocks that need to be accurately completed. *Chapter 1: Health Care Systems and Settings*, has additional information regarding the sections and blocks on this form.

15.11 Patient encounter form

Health Care Providers

1234 Main Street
Shermer, IL 12345
1.800.555.1234

Patient Encounter Form

Patient Information
Patient ID #
Patient name
Address
City/State
Contact #
DOB/Age

Payment Method
Primary
Primary ID #
Primary group #
Secondary
Secondary ID #
Secondary group #

Visit Information
Date
Physician
Referral
Reason for visit

Office Visits

New Patient

99201	Minimal office visit	
99202	20 min	
99203	30 min	
99204	45 min	
99205	60 min	

Established Patient

99211	Minimal office visit
99212	20 min
99213	30 min
99214	45 min
99215	60 min

Preventive Medicine Visits

New Patient

99381	Less than 1 year
99382	1 to 4 years
99383	5 to 11 years
99384	12 to 17 years
99385	18 to 39 years
99386	40 to 64 years
99387	65+ years

Established Patient

99391	Less than 1 year
99392	1 to 4 years
99393	5 to 11 years
99394	12 to 17 years
99395	18 to 39 years
99396	40 to 64 years
99397	65+ years

Vitals
BP
Pulse
Temp
Height
Weight

Procedures

81002	Urine, dip
82948	Glucose, blood stick
85018	Hemoglobin
99173	Visual acuity
92551	Hearing screening
36415	Venipuncture
36416	Finger stick
86580	PPD
46600	Anoscopy

Immunizations

90471	IZ Admin # 1
90472	IZ Admin # 2
90472	IZ Admin # 3
90472	IZ Admin # 4
90472	IZ Admin # 5
90713	IPV
90718	Td
90700	DTaP
90721	DTaP/HIB
90648	HIB
90633	Hepatitis A
90744	Hepatitis B
90707	MMR
90716	Varicella
90669	Prevnar 13
90658	Influenza

Other Visit Information
Lab orders

Notes

Diagnosis - ICD-10-CM

Abd pain, unspec	R10.9
Anemia, unspec	D64.9
Bronchitis, unspec	J20.9
Burn	T30.0
Conjuctivitis	H10.13
Contact dermatitis	L25.9
Contusion	T14.9
Cough	R05
Dental caries	K02.9
Disorders of teeth	K08.9
Enuresis	F98.0
Foreign body, eye	T15.9
Foreign body, soft tis.	M79.5
Headache, unspc	R51
Hearing problem	R68.8
Hygiene	Z72.9
General exam, normal	Z00.00
General exam, abnormal	Z00.01
Immunization	Z23
Impacted cerumen	H61.23
Impetigo	L01.0
Injury to eye	S05.9
Injury, superficial	T07.0
Lice, head	B85.0
Medication dispensed	Z76.0
Nausea & vomiting	R11.2
Otitis media, acute	H66.009
OM w/ rupture of TM	H66.019
Pharyngitis	J02.9
PPD screen	Z11.1
School exam	Z02.89
Splinter, finger	S60.45
Tonsillitis, acute	J03.90
URI, acute, NOS	J06.9
UTI, unspec	N39.0
Vision problem	H54.7

Follow up with provider? ☐ Yes ☐ No
Follow-up date:
Further treatment plan:

Signature:
Date:

Generating insurance claims for payment

Medical assistants can generate two types of claims to submit for payment for services rendered. A paper (hard copy) claim is manually filled out and mailed to the insurance carrier. Ensure that each entry is clear and concise, formatted correctly, all uppercase letters, no punctuation included, nothing is photocopied, nothing is handwritten, and no staples are attached. Any errors could result in the claim being sent back as unable to be processed. Most medical practices have phased out the use of paper claims and are submitting insurance claims electronically. Most medical records software is designed to generate claims processing submissions electronically. It requires all the same information as the paper-based claim, but can be processed through a direct billing system or a clearinghouse vendor to scrub (correct errors or complete missing information) claims and remit for payment.

15.12 Patient discharge form

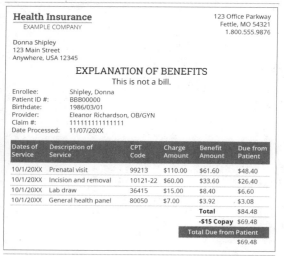

Interpreting the explanation of benefits

An explanation of benefits (EOB) is sent to the patient after the claim has been processed by their insurance carrier to detail the payment made to the provider for each service, the allowable amount covered by the insurance, the amount the patient owes, and the amount to be adjusted off of the account. If the claim is denied or reduced, information is provided as to why. The EOB uses language easily understood by the insurance beneficiary.

15.13 Explanation of benefits

Health Insurance
EXAMPLE COMPANY

123 Office Parkway
Fettle, MO 54321
1.800.555.9876

Donna Shipley
123 Main Street
Anywhere, USA 12345

EXPLANATION OF BENEFITS
This is not a bill.

Enrollee: Shipley, Donna
Patient ID #: BBB00000
Birthdate: 1986/03/01
Provider: Eleanor Richardson, OB/GYN
Claim #: 11111111111111
Date Processed: 11/07/20XX

Dates of Service	Description of Service	CPT Code	Charge Amount	Benefit Amount	Due from Patient
10/1/20XX	Prenatal visit	99213	$110.00	$61.60	$48.40
10/1/20XX	Incision and removal	10121-22	$60.00	$33.60	$26.40
10/1/20XX	Lab draw	36415	$15.00	$8.40	$6.60
10/1/20XX	General health panel	80050	$7.00	$3.92	$3.08
				Total	$84.48
				-$15 Copay	$69.48
				Total Due from Patient	$69.48

COMPLIANCE WITH GOVERNMENT AND INSURANCE REQUIREMENTS

Medical assistants should be familiar with requirements for individual, third-party, and government insurance plans. In addition, it is part of the daily routine to handle tasks associated with an insurance carrier's handbook, contracts, and forms necessary for plan benefits and any preauthorization or referral requirements. This equips the medical assistant with the knowledge and skills to ensure documentation complies with government and insurance requirements.

Chart reviews

Chart reviews consist of collection and clinical review of medical records to ensure that payment is made only for services that meet all plan coverage and medical necessity requirements. Chart review activities are directed toward areas where data analysis indicates vulnerabilities in recent billing patterns. The goal of the chart review program by insurance companies is to reduce payment errors by identifying and addressing documentation issues or billing errors concerning coverage and diagnosis coding inaccuracies.

Evaluation and management services

The medical assistant must understand important differences and variations to properly code evaluation and management (E/M) services. There are three factors in determining the level of service with E/M coding: history, examination, and medical decision making. The provider should document whether the patient has a problem-focused, detailed, or comprehensive history. The provider will also document their examination of the patient regarding specific body areas and organ systems, as well as the level of examination provided. Other factors are place of service and patient status. Once the appropriate level of E/M service code has been determined, it must be documented with full detail in the patient's medical record and noted on the encounter form for billing procedures.

Auditing methods, processes, and sign-offs

Auditing methods, processes, and sign-offs used to examine medical records or claims for accuracy and completeness can be performed manually or electronically. Medical records are sorted and sent in sets to each insurance carrier to ensure all fields are completed and reporting data is accurate, as well as to generate informative statistical data reports. The provider will also review and sign-off on progress notes after they have been dictated.

REFERRALS TO OTHER PROVIDERS AND PROFESSIONALS

A referral is a document or form required by insurance companies that is used when a provider wants to send a patient to a specialist. Depending on the records system that is used, referrals can be sent manually or electronically. All referrals sent and received should be documented as part of the patient's permanent medical record.

Referrals should only be submitted after the approval of the provider and authorization from the insurance company has been obtained.

The type of referral will determine how long it will take to process before it is authorized. Regular referrals usually take 3 to 10 business days for evaluation and approval. Urgent referrals generally take 24 hours for authorization. However, a stat referral for an emergent situation can be approved via telephone immediately once it has been faxed to the insurance companies' utilization review department. In some cases, the provider might have to provide additional information to justify a stat referral request via peer-to-peer review with the utilization review department.

The medical assistant should include in a referral the patient's demographic and insurance information, provider's identification information including National Provider Identification (NPI), diagnosis, and planned procedure or treatment.

PREAUTHORIZATIONS AND PRECERTIFICATIONS

Using the information on the reverse side of the patient's insurance card or on the insurance website, medical assistants can determine what type of services need preauthorizations or precertification. Preauthorization is a process required by some insurance carriers in which the provider obtains permission to perform specific procedures or services or refers a patient to a specialist. Most managed care and HMO insurances require preauthorization prior to patients receiving any procedures or treatments outside of the primary care office. Patients need to be made aware of covered and noncovered benefits, as well as financial information (required copayments, deductibles) when seeing specialists, as the financial obligations are typically higher. These services are typically for nonemergent surgeries, expensive medical tests, and medication therapies. The medical assistant needs to include the following when obtaining or verifying prior authorization.

- Authorization code
- Date the authorization is effective
- Date the authorization expires
- Authorized diagnosis and procedural codes
- Contact information for the specialist office
- How many visits are authorized
- What the authorization has been issued for

Procedures that need to be precertified

If a patient is hospitalized, most insurance companies usually require precertification within 24 hours of the admission. A precertification is a process required by some insurance carriers in which the provider must prove medical necessity before performing a procedure. Precertifications are also sometimes required for specific types of laboratory tests, diagnostic testing, and procedures that are considered unusual or expensive (MRI, chemotherapy medications).

Participating providers

Patients can contact a provider's office to inquire if the office or provider are participating with their insurance plan. If a provider is nonparticipating and the patient is seen, the claim will be denied or reimbursement will be reduced because the provider is not in-network with that insurance company. Participating providers with any insurance company agree to adjust the difference between the amount charged and the approved contracted amount the insurance company will reimburse. If the provider's office is participating, they agree to bill the patient for only the deductible, copay, coinsurance, or amounts due based on allowed fees set forth in the contract between the provider and insurance company. In return, the insurance company agrees to pay the provider's office directly for covered services rendered to the insured.

BILLING PATIENTS, INSURERS, AND THIRD-PARTY PAYERS

Medical offices process insurance claims for patients as a courtesy because most patients do not understand the process that is involved. Medical assistants are responsible for working to obtain maximum benefits and reimbursement from the patient's insurance and third-party payers for services rendered. Make sure all procedures and services that were performed by the provider are listed correctly and appropriately on the claim so that the correct reimbursement will be received.

Financial terminology

Medical assistants should be familiar with the following financial terminology, definitions, and how to use these terms. *Account balance* is the total balance on an account; it can be a *debit* (negative) or *credit* (positive). *Accounts receivable* is the amount owed to the provider for the services rendered. *Accounts payable* is debt incurred but not yet paid; this can be for supplies or utilities. Debits represent a record on an account as an addition to expenditure or asset accounts or a subtracted amount from income. *Credits* are an entry on an account represented as an addition to profits. *Assets* are property of an individual or organization that is subject to payments for debts owed. *Liabilities* are items that are outstanding (debts).

Billing methods

Two types of billing methods are manual and computerized systems. A computerized billing system uses software to generate a report for accounts according to the last time a payment was made. Medical assistants can use this report to determine which accounts are 30, 60, or 90 days old. The manual billing system is also used this way, but with a different process. Accounting forms, ledgers, or receipts are often used on a peg board system. Manual billing still provides the medical assistant with all record entries, collections, and receivables. However, it is cumbersome and time-consuming, and requires significantly more time to process than computerized billing systems.

Once a report is generated, the medical assistant will use the data to determine which patient accounts need to be sent their monthly billing statement and which need to be sent to collections. Once a month billing is generated, it is usually sent before the 25th of each month to reach the patient by the last day of the month. This form of billing encourages the patient to send payment at the beginning of the month. Some offices prefer cycle billing, which divides accounts into small alphabetic or color-coded groups, regardless of changes on the account. This method ensures statements will be sent by specific dates so the payments on the accounts remain distributed throughout the month. When billing is spread out over the course of the month, more time and care are given to each statement. This reduces the likelihood of accounting errors.

account balance. The amount owed on an account

debit. An amount owed

accounts receivable. Money owed to the provider

accounts payable. Debts incurred, not yet paid

credit. The monetary balance in an individual's favor

assets. The entire saleable property of a person, association, corporation, or estate applicable or subject to the payment of debts

liabilities. Amounts owed; debts

Payment methods

Most medical offices accept credit cards, debit cards, checks, and cash. Credit and debit cards are widely accepted for convenience, but there is a small fee charged for each transaction. In the case of a hardship or a large bill, credit arrangements may be made. The medical assistant must provide a detailed explanation of fees, services, and charges, as well as convey a tactful and courteous explanation of the payment plan. Discussion of the payment processes and all other information must be documented and signed by an authorized member of the office and the patient. This documentation must be attached to the patient's financial record with a copy given to the patient. If a check is returned to the medical office for nonsufficient funds (NSF), the medical office has the right to charge additional fees to the patient's account. This information needs to be displayed prominently throughout the office and be shared with each patient prior to their first encounter.

Posting charges and payments

Charges and payments to patients' accounts are either entered into the computer system or manually entered onto a ledger and a day sheet using the pegboard method. As soon as the patient submits the payment, the medical assistant can mark the charges as paid. It is important to include the check number or type of credit card used, and where the payment originated (patient, insurance). This allows for easy tracking in case of any discrepancies.

Making adjustments

When the provider participates with insurance, medical assistants have to make adjustments to patient accounts for insurance disallowances. Other circumstances may be for professional discounts, account write-offs, or payments sent to the practice after the account has been placed in collection status. If the patient or guarantor files for bankruptcy, all charges must be adjusted off the account.

Online banking for deposits and electronic transfers

Online banking allows for electronic fund transfers (EFTs) for payroll disbursements, money owed to business institutions, and payments from insurance companies and other governmental organizations. When insurance payments are made through EFTs, the amount is deposited 1 to 2 weeks faster than a conventional check. EFTs are processed through an automated clearinghouse that follows federal rules and regulations.

Medical assistants are responsible for promptly making daily deposits to ensure accuracy in daily reconciliation of the cash drawer, day sheets, and patient accounts. When checks are received, it is important that deposits are made daily. This allows for funds to pay accounts payable and reduce any issues with stop payments or stolen checks, and it is also a courtesy to the payer.

CHARGE RECONCILIATION

The medical assistant is responsible for completing charge reconciliation. The first step in this process is to add deposits, deduct outstanding checks, and deduct bank service charges, NSF checks and fees, and check-printing charges. Next, add the interest earned along with any notes receivables (EFTs) collected by the bank. If the bank statement and office accounts do not balance, initiate a full investigation. When the error is discovered, add or deduct errors in the company's cash account. Compare the adjusted balances and record all adjustments to reconcile the balance. This is an audit to confirm accounts are accurate and the bank is managing funds correctly.

Obtaining accounts receivable total

Balance and obtain an accounts receivable total once a month after posting all charges and payments have been completed. To obtain the total, pull a list of all accounts with a balance and then add all balances for a total figure. This figure should equal the accounts receivable balance from the daily control cumulative total. If a pegboard system is used, the total for daily, weekly, monthly and yearly amounts will be listed on the side of the day sheet. All ledgers should be tallied and compared to the totals on the day sheet on a monthly basis.

Aging reports, collections due, adjustments, and write-offs

Before a medical practice submits any accounts to collections, all avenues for collection should be exhausted. To determine if an account is delinquent, run an aging report. Aging reports are grouped by day of last payment or by the date of service if no payments have been made. The date categories are 0 to 30 days, 30 to 60 days, 60 to 90 days, and 90 to 120 days. Depending on office policies, the medical assistant makes a friendly reminder call, letters are mailed encouraging the patient to make a payment or set up a payment plan, and if all else fails, a certified letter is mailed requesting payment before the account is sent to collections. When the final notice is sent, the account must be sent to collections and all further patient contact regarding the account must be discontinued. Always treat the patient with respect and follow office policies and procedures when making payment arrangements.

RESOLVING BILLING ISSUES WITH INSURERS AND THIRD-PARTY PAYERS

There are two primary reasons claims are denied or rejected: technical errors and insurance policy coverage issues. Medical assistants can reduce claim issues with insurers and third-party payers by ensuring insurance is verified prior to the patient being seen and that guidelines are followed when reviewing claims prior to submission. This helps reduce the amount of claim denial.

Billing inquiries

All billing inquiries should be handled in a prompt and courteous manner. If the patient is calling about an error, place the patient on hold while the account is being pulled up for review, thank the patient for holding, explain the charges carefully, and make sure all questions and concerns have been answered. If the medical assistant is unable to resolve the issue, obtain the patient's contact information so the appropriate staff can contact them once the issue has been investigated and the solution has been determined.

Steps to appeal a denial

When filing an appeal for a denial received from an insurer, first determine why the claim was denied. Then obtain and complete the insurance company's appeal document. The appeal document must be filed as quickly as possible so that it doesn't exceed the time needed for filing. Include a letter from the provider to provide support for medical necessity, progress notes from the treating provider, and relevant results from any testing performed.

CUSTOMER SERVICE AND SERVICE RECOVERY

Always strive to provide excellent customer service with every patient encounter. One of the most important traits a medical assistant can have is a good attitude. This can influence the atmosphere and the perception patients have of an office. Patients expect to receive superior customer service. In addition, due to the nature and sensitivity of health and medical history, always ensure confidentiality.

Telephone etiquette

Medical assistants must be professional and courteous while communicating via the telephone at all times. Actively listen to the caller, enunciate clearly, and speak in a friendly voice. Hold the handset or headset mouthpiece approximately 1 inch away from the lips and directly in front of the mouth to promote clarity. Lastly, always maintain confidentiality. The use of a speaker phone is prohibited because other individuals might overhear private medical information, which is a violation of HIPAA.

Facilitating service recovery

Medical assistants work with patients to provide care and excellent customer service. Good communication is just as important as good care. Always listen to patients to properly understand their needs and be able to respond accurately. When the medical assistant conveys their message to the patient, it is important to display sensitivity and use language that the patient can understand. The patient in turn interprets that message according to how they comprehend the words used and in what context the message is being communicated. It is important when dealing with a difficult patient for the medical assistant to remain professional. This is displayed by a calm demeanor and tactful, courteous manner.

ENTERING INFORMATION INTO DATABASES OR SPREADSHEETS

Medical assistants often use spreadsheets for reports or entering information into the electronic medical record database. After new information has been entered, periodically save the spreadsheet. In addition to tracking patient data, spreadsheets can be used for inventory lists and personnel functions.

Computer literacy

The medical assistant should be familiar with basic computer terms. For example, a network is a group of two or more computer systems that are connected together. Be careful when accessing outside sources from a workplace computer.

Any website visited needs to comply with the organization's network security protocols and policies. The use of unauthorized websites and suspicious downloads can increase the chances of violations of patients' protected health care information (PHI). All patients are entitled to the utmost confidentiality regarding the personal nature of their medical records.

Word processing and typing

It is necessary to be familiar with programs such as Microsoft Word, Excel, PowerPoint, and Outlook, which are used in many medical offices. Medical assistants use word processing software, such as Microsoft Word, to create and modify documents. Features like Mail Merge are useful for developing a set of emails, letters, faxes, or printing labels and envelopes for correspondence and mass mailings.

Data entry and data fields

A data field is a location where data is stored within a computer program. The term generally denotes an area in a database or a section in a form that needs to be completed, on paper or electronically. Data entry is the act of typing or writing the information into the field.

Common databases used in health care

The most commonly used database in health care is the *electronic medical record (EMR)* and the *electronic health record (EHR)*. Electronic health records can be created, managed, and consulted by authorized clinicians and staff from more than one health care organization. Electronic medical records can be created, gather, managed, and consulted by authorized clinicians and staff within a single health care organization. In both the EHR and EMR, information is arranged into different areas within the system. Examples are demographics, insurance, clinical information, and accounts. Each database holds information that can be grouped by using certain criteria. This allows for reporting on specific conditions or demographic information across a large population.

EHR vs. EMR

Electronic medical records (EMRs) are digital charts to be used within a facility.

Electronic health records (EHRs) include the EMR and other information to be used between facilities.

electronic medical record (EMR). An electronic record of health-related information about an individual that can be created, managed, and accessed by authorized individuals within a single health care organization

electronic health record (EHR). An electronic record of patients' health-related information that conforms to nationally recognized interoperability standards, and can be created, managed, and accessed by authorized individuals from multiple health care organizations

Responsible behavior in social media

Social media and networking creates an innovative way for medical facilities to attract new patients. Medical assistants might have access to interact with others in virtual communities and social networks. Adhere to HIPAA rules and regulations when interacting on social media websites. Patient information is sensitive and should always be protected to the fullest extent. Never share information regarding patients or unofficial pictures taken at the office on professional social media sites. When using personal social media, avoid befriending a patient, as this could be considered a violation of personal-professional boundaries and create licensing or legal issues. Any health information that could be linked to an individual patient (names, pictures, physical descriptions) should never be shared on social media sites. Even if the patient offers written permission to provide a testimonial or quote on a site, use careful restrictions that allow minimal information to protect privacy. Maintain discretion both on and off the job. Many employers search for applicants on the Internet and review social media posts prior to hiring.

INVENTORY OF CLINICAL AND ADMINISTRATIVE SUPPLIES

Medical assistants can be responsible for maintaining inventory and ordering supplies for the office. This is to ensure administrative and clinical staff have all the supplies they need to properly function on a daily basis. Supplies should be ordered, checked against the shipping or packing list when they arrive, and stocked in a secure location in the office that is easy to access by personnel. Communication in the office is essential when stock is running low. Without the appropriate supplies stocked, the provider and medical assistants might not be able to complete all their duties or perform needed tests and procedures. This can create an inconvenience for patients if they need to return to the office at a later date.

Administrative and clinical supplies

A few administrative supplies are essential to everyday work functions.

- Pens
- Pencils
- Reams of paper

- Toner cartridges
- Paper clips
- Registration forms

- Patient information sheets
- Clipboards

The supplies needed are dependent on the office specialty and amount of in-office procedures performed. If the office is computerized, the needed supplies may be decreased. Inventory of supplies is very important to maintain the workflow of the office.

SAFETY EVALUATIONS AND CONCERNS

Safety and security are important aspects of a medical assistant's duties. Be alert for any suspicious individuals visiting the practice. Understand the protocol for handling any threats to security and the required steps involved. In the case of fire or a natural disaster, the medical assistant needs to know the location of smoke alarms, fire extinguishers, fire exits, and exit routes, and the protocol for evacuating the office. Make sure all patients have been evacuated and are accounted for prior to exiting.

Equipment inspection logs, required schedules, and compliance requirements

A compliance requirement from the Clinical Laboratory Improvement Amendments (CLIA) requires that controls and settings be performed on all equipment. These requirements are intended to ensure that patient testing is accurate and the results are reliable. Maintenance must be completed by an authorized user of the equipment. For example, if a medical assistant is authorized to use the equipment, the medical assistant must also be responsible for the maintenance issues of that equipment. Failure to perform regular maintenance can result in malfunction or inaccurate results.

Safety notebooks

Occupational Safety and Health Administration (OSHA) is a division of the federal government overseen by the Department of Labor agency. The responsibility of OSHA is to reduce workplace injuries, illnesses, and fatalities. OSHA requires all facilities with more than 10 employees to have a written emergency plan of action. This plan must include reports of emergencies, an emergency evacuation plan, exit routes, protocols for employees who operate equipment, a method to account for all employees after evacuation, name of the individual responsible for the plan, and a list of personal protective equipment to be used to prevent exposure to bloodborne pathogens.

An exposure control plan can be part of the standard safety plan written for the facility, but it must encompass all the components required by OSHA. It is required that this plan be in writing, be reviewed annually, and for written documentation to exist that the plan was reviewed and updated or revised. A hard copy must be given to employees upon their request within 15 working days, and the plan must be available at all times in the workplace.

Safety Data Sheets (SDSs) detail vital information about any product or chemical used in the medical facility. The SDS clarifies the correct use of the product and the proper action if a spill occurs.

SUMMARY

Medical assistants play a significant role in medical facilities. They have administrative and clinical skills, making them versatile and flexible members of the health care team. Whether dealing with billing issues, ordering supplies, or assisting the provider with a procedure, the medical assistant is often present in all stages of health care delivery. The medical assistant must be prepared to handle all aspects of the medical office from greeting the patient on arrival to the patient exiting the office. Medical assistants need to be organized, provide quality patient care, and be ready to adapt to patient needs. All of this must be done in a friendly, efficient, and professional manner.

CHAPTER 16

Communication and Customer Service

OVERVIEW

The medical assistant must understand the importance of effective *communication* in the health care environment and be able to apply that knowledge when interacting with patients, caregivers, or anyone on the health care team. This chapter focuses on a variety of communication strategies, including therapeutic communication techniques. The medical assistant often acts as the representative of the provider, the profession, the practice, and themselves. Therefore, there is a great responsibility to provide professional and compassionate communication at all times.

COMMUNICATION AND CUSTOMER SERVICE

Effective communication and great *customer service* go together in any work setting. Customer service is ensuring customer satisfaction during a workplace transaction. A positive experience for a patient in a health care setting often begins with the medical assistant, but every member of the health care team plays an important role in delivering effective communication to ensure customer satisfaction. Open communication and quality customer service are important for maintaining positive relationships between the patient and the health care team. Allowing patients to communicate how they feel, listening to their viewpoints, and taking measures to assist in solving problems can increase customer satisfaction and provide a better experience for the patient.

Objectives

Upon completion of this chapter, you should be able to:

- Clarify and relay communications between patients and providers.
- Facilitate and promote teamwork and team engagement.
- Modify verbal and nonverbal communication for diverse audiences.
- Modify verbal and nonverbal communications with patients and caregivers based on special considerations.
- Communicate on the telephone with patients, caregivers, providers, and third-party payers.
- Prepare written and electronic communications.
- Handle challenging customer service occurrences.
- Recognize and respond to common defense mechanisms
- Engage in crucial conversations with patients, caregivers/health care surrogates, staff, and providers.

communication. The process of exchanging information via verbal or nonverbal methods
customer service. Providing quality attention and assistance to a consumer of a product or a service

CLARIFY AND RELAY COMMUNICATION BETWEEN PATIENTS AND PROVIDERS

Clear and accurate communication between patients and providers helps achieve patient compliance. The medical assistant often clarifies and relays communication between patients and providers. Ensuring the patient understands the provider's orders pertaining to prescriptions, medical care at home, and diet is a key role of the medical assistant.

16.1 Medical assistant's role in communication

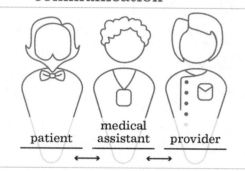

patient   medical assistant   provider

The medical assistant acts as a bridge to ensure communication between patients and providers.

16.2 Communication cycle

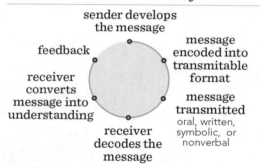

sender develops the message

feedback

message encoded into transmitable format

receiver converts message into understanding

message transmitted
oral, written, symbolic, or nonverbal

receiver decodes the message

Professionalism

Displaying professionalism is the first step in providing a positive experience for a patient. Some components of professionalism are what the medical assistant is wearing and how they communicate with the patient. First impressions are lasting impressions. The way a medical assistant appears and acts is a reflection of the provider and practice. Practice good personal hygiene, wear professional attire, and display a positive attitude at all times. Keep hair, fingernails, piercings, and visible tattoos simple, and follow office-specific policies.

Not only is professionalism important for making the patient feel at ease and comfortable, it also carries legal responsibilities. Conducting oneself in a professional manner also means keeping patient information confidential. HIPAA gives patients rights regarding the disclosure and transmission of their health information, establishing rules and limits on who can look at and receive their health information. Only access and communicate patient information when it is necessary to provide care or services and when authorized to do so. To prevent HIPAA violations, protect patient privacy in communications and disclosures.

Communication cycle

The communication cycle consists of sequential steps involved in transferring a message and receiving *feedback*. This process starts with an idea or message by a sender and ends with a response from a receiver. The sender develops the subject matter he wishes to communicate. Once this idea is put into a translatable format, the sender decides on the route of delivery. This step can be done via an oral, written, symbolic, or nonverbal communication method.

Once the message is transmitted to the receiver, she begins to decode the sent message. This means the receiver converts the message into thoughts and tries to understand it. Effective communication occurs only when both the sender and receiver assign similar meanings to the conveyed message.

The final step of the communication process is feedback. This is the part of the cycle when the receiver provides a response to the sender's message. This step determines whether the receiver has correctly understood the intended message.

feedback. Information given in response to an action to reinforce or improve the behavior

Verbal vs. nonverbal communication

Communication can be conducted as verbal or nonverbal. *Verbal communication* is the sharing of information between individuals by speech that employs recognized spoken words. Nonverbal communication consists of the behaviors and elements of speech aside from the words used. These can include gestures, facial expressions, body posture, stance, eye movements, and appearance. Both verbal and nonverbal communication elements are important when providing quality customer service and patient care.

Communication styles

To be an effective communicator, it is important to recognize that people communicate in different ways. There are several communication styles, as well as tools to determine which communication style an individual uses. Labeling a communication style can assist in determining how one manages information. Learning how to relate to and understand various styles will help you be more effective in communicating with diverse populations.

Analytical communicator: Prefers to work with real numbers, facts, and data, and places very little emphasis on feelings or emotions.

Intuitive communicator: Prefers to look at the big picture. While this can be an efficient style, it sometimes can result in more questions than answers if too broad of an approach is used.

Functional communicator: Prefers an organized approach to work with timelines and detailed plans. Uses a step-by-step method to solve problems and communicate information. This can be an effective style of communication if the patient does not become overwhelmed with too many details.

Personal communicator: Uses emotional language and connections. Cares about what people think and feel in response to the information given. Often good listeners and have the ability to resolve conflict fairly easily.

Communication with providers and other members of the health care team

Effective communication among health care professionals and other members of the health care team is important for efficient and effective patient care. Communication amongst team members can be challenging at times, because health care is complex and unpredictable. These traits can further complicate the situation and lead to ineffective communication. Recognizing differences and displaying mutual respect can alleviate some of these challenges.

16.3 Communicating with health care professionals

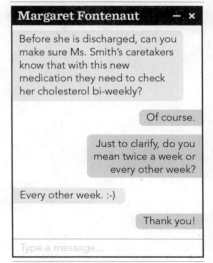

Margaret Fontenaut   — ×

Before she is discharged, can you make sure Ms. Smith's caretakers know that with this new medication they need to check her cholesterol bi-weekly?

Of course.

Just to clarify, do you mean twice a week or every other week?

Every other week. :-)

Thank you!

Type a message...

---

verbal communication. The use of spoken words to convey information

Communication with patients

Effective, positive relationships with patients and their families is built on an trust and honesty. With health care becoming more technologically complex, patients and families need to take an active role in health care decisions. The following list provides a few methods that can increase trust and communication.

- *Display professionalism:* Details such as physical appearance, eye contact, and displaying an understanding and knowledge of the situation enhances confidence of patient with the provided care.

- *Use skilled interviewing techniques:* Ask patients a variety of open- and *closed-ended questions* that encourage them to explain more about their health and daily behaviors. "Can you tell me more about yourself?" or "Can you explain what you were doing when you started to feel that pain?" can help to open communication by allowing the patient to explain their point of view.

- *Provide empathy:* Avoid jumping to conclusions or passing judgment by being empathetic and providing encouragement.

- *Practice collaboration:* Patients are more likely to positively respond to recommendations and questions in collaborative settings. When the patient is part of the health care team, communication is more effective and overall care improves.

- *Embrace technology:* Technology provides health care professionals many ways to communicate with patients. However, take care not to overwhelm the patient. Instead of flooding patients with messages from multiple platforms, select no more than three communication channels, and use them well. If a patient is only comfortable with one method, it is best to just provide communication via the preferred method.

Therapeutic communication

Therapeutic communication aims to enhance the patient's comfort, safety, trust, or health and well-being. It is a process in which the medical assistant consciously influences a patient or helps the patient gain a better understanding through verbal or nonverbal communication. Therapeutic communication involves specific strategies that encourage the patient to express feelings and ideas that convey understanding and respect.

closed-ended questions. Questions that have a limited number of possible responses

Interviewing and questioning techniques

There are reasons to ask questions. The information medical assists gather helps determine the types of questions the provider will ask.

Open-ended questions can provide qualitative and quantitative information and are often used at the beginning of the interview to determine the reason for the visit. Examples are "What brings you into the office today?" or "What types of concerns do you have to share with the provider today?" Allow patients to use their own words to describe what they hope to discuss or determine with the visit.

Closed-ended questions provide a set of answers from which the respondent must choose. They have yes or no answers or multiple choices. These questions can provide clear and concise information and are used to identify specific information such as, "Does it hurt when you take a breath?" or "What day did the pain begin?"

Leading questions are phrased in a manner that tends to suggest the desired answer. Avoid these types of questions because they risk the possibility of coercing the patient into a desired response.

Active listening

Listening is the most fundamental component of communication. Active listening is mindfully hearing and attempting to comprehend the meaning of spoken words. It can involve making sounds that indicate attentiveness, as well as giving feedback in the form of a paraphrased rendition of what has been said. Signs of active listening include a smile, eye contact, erect posture, and attention to what is being said.

Boundaries of the medical assistant

Boundaries are necessary to keep the patient as the priority and focus of each encounter. Discussing personal life with a patient is inappropriate and alters the role of the medical assistant from a caregiver to a person in need of care. When these limits are altered, what is allowed in the relationship becomes vague and possibly unethical. Avoid sharing personal stories or experiences with patients, even if they seem relevant to the situation. This behavior can be misunderstood as advice or treatment recommendations, which are outside of the medical assistant's scope of practice.

The giving or receiving of gifts between a patient and health care professional is also discouraged. This can blur the lines of the professional relationship and can have a negative effect on communication. The health and well-being of the patient depends upon a collaborative effort between the medical assistant and the patient.

leading questions. Questions that tend to lead the respondent into the desired answer

FACILITATE AND PROMOTE TEAMWORK AND TEAM ENGAGEMENT

Teamwork is an essential component in an effective health care environment. Diversity, communication, leadership, and team building exercises promote teamwork. Communication among team members should be clear and open. High-quality teamwork breeds high-quality patient care and satisfaction. Medical assistants can assist in strengthening the team and thus strengthen patient communication, relationships, and collaborations.

Effective ways to engage with other team members

Communication is more than just exchanging information. It's about understanding the emotion and intentions behind the information. Engaging with team members effectively is important for delivering efficient and effective health care. There are many ways to engage with other members of the team. Communicating, interacting, and developing professional relationships takes time. It is important to demonstrate a professional image and treat all co-workers and health care staff with respect. Each member of the health care team addresses the patient with a specific process in mind, but team communication prioritizes the ultimate goal of quality patient care.

Effective ways to engage with the patient and patient's family

Patients and their family are also part of the health care team. Engaging with them is just as important as engaging with other members of the team. Focusing on the diagnosis and treatment of the patient is key for the provider, but other facets of patient care cannot be ignored. Assist the provider by engaging the patient and acting as the liaison between the provider and the patient. Learning to work with patients and families as partners in their own care is neither easy nor intuitive. It involves significant changes, both cultural and logistical. Effective ways to engage with patients and their family include the following.

- *Include the patient in the process.* Asking patients about their expectations provides a channel for an honest dialogue that moves beyond the caregiver giving instructions to an inclusive approach that includes the patient's preferences. The best way to know those preferences is to simply ask.

- *Practice active listening.* A partnership involves more than just giving information. Providers and other members of the health care team must be willing to seek and value input from patients and family members. Learning to listen to and trust patients and family members can require a significant adjustment for all those involved.

- *Communicate effectively.* Effective communication is a two-way street. It is not only how one conveys a message; it is also how one listens to gain the full meaning of what is being said. This is especially important when obtaining patient histories.

The importance of superior customer service

Consistently offering superior customer service makes patients feel they are valued and that the health care staff cares about developing a long-term caregiver-patient relationship. Focusing on superior customer service benefits a health care organization in a number of ways. Established patients who are satisfied with their care often share their experiences with others. This repeat business and informal recruiting of new patients allows for business growth. A positive environment with quality customer service has overall positive staff morale. The staff, culture, and patient population all benefit from superior customer service.

Patient satisfaction surveys

Patient satisfaction surveys produce data about patients' perspectives of care. Survey results are used to create new incentives for health care facilities, improve the quality of care, enhance accountability by increasing transparency, or alter office policies and procedures to address patient needs. The questions often relate to responsiveness of staff, cleanliness of the environment, presence of effective communication, and overall satisfaction with services provided.

Coaching and feedback

Positive reinforcement is the process whereby desirable behavior is encouraged by presenting a reward at the time of such behavior. It can produce new behaviors and open communication. Being positively motivated aids the growth, success, and overall well-being of a person. Consistency with this reinforcement is of the utmost importance. Something that is considered "good" behavior today should not be labeled otherwise tomorrow. Inconsistencies can be counterproductive, leading to confusion and indecisiveness about acceptable behavior in the future. In positive reinforcement, the end result is to increase the behavior. Use positive reinforcements with patients and fellow staff members.

MODIFY COMMUNICATION FOR DIVERSE AUDIENCES

Everyone has experiences and values that shape the way they see the world. Be conscious of different viewpoints and your own personal biases, and take care to examine your words and actions to avoid miscommunication. To ensure effective communication, avoid figurative language, remember that nonverbal communication is critical, and keep the conversation straightforward and brief. It takes practice and patience to accomplish all this while remaining compassionate and caring.

16.4 Avoiding figurative language

While figurative language is common in everyday speech, it can be confusing for some patients. Speak directly to avoid misunderstandings.

DON'T SAY:	SAY:
"He passed away."	"He died"
"I'm all ears."	"I'm listening."
"You're fit as a fiddle."	"You're in good health."

Medical terminology and jargon

Every health condition comes with its own language and medical terminology, which can be difficult for patients to understand, especially those with low health literacy levels. Patients do not know how to communicate their concerns in this language; this can lead to adverse consequences for their health.

Take time to be sure the patient understands the medical terminology and offer explanations as needed using appropriate terms.

positive reinforcement. Rewarding of a desirable behavior

MODIFY COMMUNICATION BASED ON SPECIFIC CONSIDERATIONS

Patients who have impaired vision, hearing, or speech use a variety of ways to communicate. Patients who are blind can give and receive information audibly, and patients who are deaf can give and receive information through writing or sign language. A *telecommunication* relay service, video relay service, or a translator can be used to communicate with patients who need accommodations.

Patient characteristics affecting communication

Barriers to communication include differences in language, culture, cognitive level, developmental stage, sensory issues, and physical disabilities. When patients and health professionals have different language proficiency, there is a barrier to effective communication. Unfortunately, this language barrier is often not immediately evident. Patient and providers can underestimate the language barrier. Cultural differences are also a barrier; culture affects understanding of a word or sentence and even perception of the world. Low health literacy is a barrier due to the inability to understand the provider's medical jargon or complex instructions. Patients have the right to be fully informed about their care. Effective communication is a prerequisite to safe health care.

TELEPHONE COMMUNICATION

Phone communication with physicians, pharmacists, medical staff, third-party payers, patients, and family members of patients can result in miscommunication that leads to billing and collection errors or even treatment and prescription errors. Telephone communication can be error-prone due to technical issues and an absence of visual cues. Despite the potential drawbacks, phone communication with patients can benefit patient health and a medical facility's profitability. Patients who have chronic and high-risk conditions have significantly fewer hospital admissions when effective phone communication is used.

Basic telephone etiquette

Always adhere to basic telephone etiquette tips to maintain professionalism. When answering or making a call in the medical office, identify yourself in a calm and confident tone at the beginning of the call. If possible, conduct calls in a quiet environment without distractions. When leaving a message, think through what needs to be communicated, speak slowly, and use clear and concise language. It is also helpful to repeat necessary information while leaving a message so the listener can avoid replaying the message.

Calls from providers

Every health care organization has a specific way to handle incoming calls from providers. Many offices expect calls from providers to be transferred to the primary care physician without question. Regardless, the most important thing to remember is to be businesslike and task-oriented, determining the reason for the calls efficiently and effectively as possible. Focus on reducing the hold time and offer a call back if necessary.

---

telecommunication. Using of technology to exchange information

Calls from third-party payers

Calls from third-party payers are important for the reimbursement process. Each health care organization may have different ways of handling these calls. Many have a department that these callers can speak with to provide consistency. Third-party payers can need to speak with a member of the team regarding medical codes, documentation, claim submissions, and denials. Making sure these callers talk with the right department is vital for office revenue.

Calls from patients and caregivers

Medical assistants handle calls from patients and caregivers on a daily basis. Good telephone skills can maximize patient health and safety, particularly for patients who have chronic and other serious conditions. When discussing health matters over the phone, verify that the person speaking is either the patient or has been given proper authority to discuss patient information via the phone. When giving instructions, ask the person to repeat back the information to ensure understanding. Once the phone call is complete, document the call and what was discussed in the patient's health record as a part of their permanent file.

PREPARE WRITTEN AND ELECTRONIC COMMUNICATIONS

Written communication involves any interaction that uses the written word. Written communication used internally for health care organizations includes memos, reports, bulletins, job descriptions, employee manuals, and email. One advantage of electronic business correspondence is that messages do not have to be delivered on the spur of the moment; instead, they can be edited and revised several times before they are sent to ensure the message is clearly communicated. It also provides a permanent record of messages that have been sent and can be saved for future reference.

There are potential pitfalls associated with written communications. Unlike oral communication in which impressions and reactions are exchanged instantaneously, the sender of written communication does not generally receive immediate feedback. Written messages often take more time to compose due to their information-packed nature and the difficulty that many people have in composing such correspondence.

Internal communications

Sharing information within an organization for business purposes is considered *internal communication*. Internal communication includes face-to-face conversations, telephone calls, interoffice mail, paging, faxing, closed-circuit television, and email.

---

internal communication. Sharing information within a business or organization

External communications

External communication is the transmission of information between a business and another person or entity outside of the company's environment. It is important for all formats, grammar, and spelling to be accurate. External communication includes face-to-face communication, print media (newspapers, magazines, fliers, newsletters), broadcast media (radio, television), and electronic communication (websites, social media, email). All external communication is a representation of the medical practice and must be professional and appropriate.

16.5 Example business letter

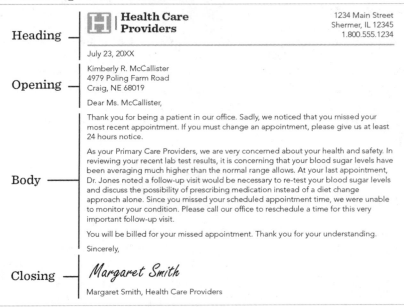

Heading

Health Care Providers

1234 Main Street
Shermer, IL 12345
1.800.555.1234

July 23, 20XX

Opening

Kimberly R. McCallister
4979 Poling Farm Road
Craig, NE 68019

Dear Ms. McCallister,

Body

Thank you for being a patient in our office. Sadly, we noticed that you missed your most recent appointment. If you must change an appointment, please give us at least 24 hours notice.

As your Primary Care Providers, we are very concerned about your health and safety. In reviewing your recent lab test results, it is concerning that your blood sugar levels have been averaging much higher than the normal range allows. At your last appointment, Dr. Jones noted a follow-up visit would be necessary to re-test your blood sugar levels and discuss the possibility of prescribing medication instead of a diet change approach alone. Since you missed your scheduled appointment time, we were unable to monitor your condition. Please call our office to reschedule a time for this very important follow-up visit.

You will be billed for your missed appointment. Thank you for your understanding.

Sincerely,

Closing

Margaret Smith

Margaret Smith, Health Care Providers

16.6 Example cover sheet

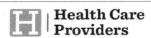

Health Care Providers

1234 Main Street
Shermer, IL 12345
1.800.555.1234

Confidentiality Notice

Confidential Health Information Enclosed

Protected Health Information (PHI) is personal and sensitive information related to a person's health care. It is being faxed to you after appropriate authorization from the patient or under circumstances that do not require patient authorization. You, the recipient, are obligated to maintain it in a safe, secure and confidential manner. Re-disclosure without additional patient consent or as permitted by law is prohibited. Unauthorized re-disclosure or failure to maintain confidentiality could subject you to penalties described in federal and state law.

IMPORTANT WARNING: This message is intended for the use of the person or entity to which it is addressed and may contain information that is privileged and confidential, the disclosure of which is governed by applicable law.

If you are not the intended recipient, or the employee or agent responsible to deliver it to the intended recipient, you are hereby notified that any disclosure, copying or distribution of this information is Strictly Prohibited. If you have received this message by error, please notify the sender immediately to arrange for return or destruction of these documents.

Business letter formats

Business letters are written with the intention of getting the reader to respond. They should be written with a clear purpose, error-free, friendly, and pertinent. All business correspondence should be on company letterhead and written in a standard format. Business letters have the following elements.

- Heading: The letterhead and dateline (month fully spelled out, day, and year)

- Opening: The recipient's address and salutation

- Body: The content and information to be communicated

- Closing: The complimentary closing and signature

Preparing faxes

Fax machines are still used in the health care industry. Fax machines allow documents to be securely transmitted with end-to-end encryption. Always use a cover sheet that discloses that confidential information is attached.

external communication. Sharing information between a business or organization and an outside entity

E-mail communication

E-mail is inexpensive, efficient, and can be used internally and externally to convey information. It can be easily archived for reference or printed if hard copies are needed. With all of the advantages, remember that e-mails provide a permanent, traceable record of communication. Be sure to use proper punctuation and grammar, appropriate subject lines, and clear and concise verbiage.

Communicating with patients through the patient portal

Medical assistants can communicate with patients through a patient portal. Patient portals typically offer around-the-clock access to personal health information. Some portals allow patients to request prescription refills, make scheduling requests, communicate with providers, and make payments. Patients can view recent testing and lab reports once the provider has signed off on them. Strict security measures require each patient to have a unique login. One of the main reasons for offering a patient portal is to increase communication between the health care team and the patient. Satisfaction and overall quality of care increase when patients are more engaged in their health care; the use of a patient portal can facilitate this engagement.

16.7 Example patient portal

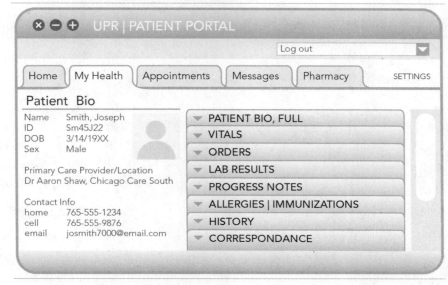

HANDLE CHALLENGING CUSTOMER SERVICE OCCURRENCES

It is inevitable that problems will occur, and patients will rightly voice their concerns when warranted. Conflict can often lead to valuable solutions to complex problems. The following techniques can assist a health care professional in navigating interactions with challenging health care consumers. Allowing patients to communicate how they feel, listening to their viewpoints, and providing an appropriate solution alleviates some stress in the clinical setting.

Cause-and-effect analysis

Business should be focused on understanding conflicts and issues, as well as analyzing the associated causes and outcomes. Complaints often expressed by patients include long wait times on the telephone or in the office, inconvenient office hours, and feeling rushed when seeing the provider. Once these issues are identified, the organization can take appropriate actions toward correcting the problem. For example, the schedule can be altered to allow more time for each patient encounter with a provider, or an automated phone system can be incorporated to expedite and filter calls for faster service. Regardless, patients should be viewed as customers. Customer satisfaction is an important component in maintaining an efficient patient-centered practice.

Techniques to work with angry patients

The medical assistant will likely interact with rude or angry patients. Regardless of the reason for the patient's anger, remain professional and assist the patient as well as possible to ensure the patient receives a satisfying experience.

When encountering a patient who is upset, remain calm. By using active listening skills, the medical assistant can gain a sense of why the patient is upset and hopefully be able to provide a solution. Even if a solution is not readily available, use therapeutic communication techniques to let patients know they are being heard and their concerns are being addressed. Displaying empathy and apologizing for a mishandled situation can reassure patients that they are a priority. If a solution can be offered, do so as soon as possible or explain when the solution will be provided. If an immediate solution cannot be anticipated, continue communicating with the patient regarding the status of the conflict.

When to refer problems to a superior

No matter how professional and courteous the medical assistant is, on occasion, patients get upset. An important part of handling these types of incidents is to recognize when the situation warrants an additional level of expertise. If the patient is upset and it appears as though there is no solution that can be offered, consult with a supervisor or refer the patient to a staff member who can provide solutions. This is also needed if the patient requests a referral or demonstrates aggressive behavior.

Documentation of an event

Incident reports are used to document incidents or events involving patients, visitors, and staff that can affect the quality of patient safety or care, or that can become a potential liability for the institution. Incident reports should be housed in the office in a designated secure area but not be put in the patient record. Detailed and accurate documentation is vital for these unusual occurrences. The following are reminders for medical assistants to use when completing an incident or unusual occurrence report.

- Only staff involved in the incident should complete the form.

- Make sure all of the text is legible when using handwriting or electronic documentation. Do not leave any sections blank.

- Only include factual information on the report, such as objective symptoms. If a quote or subjective information is shared, be sure to identify the source. Provide sufficient detail and include additional documentation if needed.

- If medical care is warranted, be sure to document this in the report.

- Notify the supervisor based on office policies and procedures, and present the completed report to the appropriate personnel.

RECOGNIZING DEFENSE MECHANISMS

Patients who have illnesses or who have experienced traumatic events often use defense mechanisms, which are designed as a means of coping, protecting the ego, and surviving. Some defense mechanisms are healthy, and others can result in unsafe situations for both the patient and health care professionals. Be alert to displays of defense mechanisms, and seek additional assistance or adjust communication based on the action being displayed.

Denial

Denial is one of the most commonly used defense mechanisms in which an individual refuses to accept what is being communicated. For example, a patient is told he has a disease, refuses to believe the diagnosis, and demands a second opinion. It can be considered healthy in early stages, but eventually the patient will learn to recognize the news as reality and then begin to cope and deal with it appropriately. The medical assistant or health care professional will not be successful in having effective communication until the patient has begun to accept the information presented. Allowing the patient time to digest the information and then providing further communication is the best approach for this defense mechanism. A support system of family and friends is important to assist the patient through denial.

Regression

Regression involves a patient reverting to a previous action or time in her life when she felt more secure. This defense mechanism is often seen in children who have recently had a traumatic experience or change in situation. For example, a child who has a newborn sibling can perceive a change in family status and feel insecure. This child might revert to sucking a thumb, wetting the bed, or using "baby language." This is an unconscious defense mechanism that medical assistants should be aware of to assist in educating caregivers. Patience and support are important during this regressive defense mechanism.

Projection and displacement

These defense mechanisms are used to protect the ego by placing blame on something or someone and displaying verbal or physical actions (which is a form of displacement) aimed at releasing the anger. For example, a patient is asked to get a chest x-ray to evaluate a cough, but doesn't do it. Later, the patient receives a diagnosis of lung cancer and is angry with the health care professional for not insisting the x-ray be completed and for not following up. The patient is projecting the guilt he is feeling for not following through with the test onto the health care professional. He then experiences displacement if he goes home and yells at a loved one to release frustration and anger. The medical assistant must be aware of these mechanisms, take measures to ensure personal safety, and not become defensive when reinforcing reality with the patient.

Repression

This is an unhealthy mechanism used to protect the individual from remembering devastating events. Do not inform the patient of the reality; this should be addressed carefully with a psychologist or psychiatrist. Examples of repressed traumas include child sexual abuse or experiences of military personnel in a war zone. Do not confuse repression with posttraumatic stress syndrome. In posttraumatic stress syndrome, the patient is often aware of what the stressors are and has psychological complications related to that reality. In repression, the patient has repressed the memory and it is not obvious or known to them.

Sublimation

This defense mechanism is displayed when an individual uses a socially acceptable and constructive substitute for an unacceptable action related to an impulse. For instance, a patient is angry about a breast cancer diagnosis, but knows it is not morally and legally right to blame the provider because the patient was late in getting the mammogram done. As a means of coping and protecting the ego, the patient becomes a spokesperson for early breast cancer detection. Use good active listening skills to detect this type of defense mechanism.

ENGAGE IN CRUCIAL CONVERSATIONS

Conducting crucial conversations with patients, caregivers, staff, and providers is often a stressful process. Adequate preparation and experience make these difficult discussions go smoother, but they can still be challenging. The following steps can help with these important and inevitable conversations.

- *Consider safety first.* The patient needs to feel comfortable and secure to trust the health care team and engage openly in conversation.

- *Demonstrate empathy, not sympathy.* In any conversation, consider what others might be experiencing, but displays of sympathy are nonproductive.

- *Stick with the facts.* It is easy to divert away from the primary conversation and begin to develop personal opinions. In both of these situations, stick to the facts and remain objective to ensure comprehension of the material being presented.

- *Watch words and actions.* Using sarcasm and humor, or displaying negative *body language*, is not appropriate during crucial conversations. Approach conversations with purpose and appropriate dialogue to maximize the level of communication.

- *Use active listening.* This skill demonstrates concern and interest in what is being communicated.

16.8 Using appropriate body language

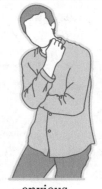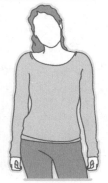

anxious
indirectly faced
hunched stance
covering neck (protective)
crossed arms (defensive)

calm
directly faced
open stance
relaxed arms

body language. A method of communication that uses body movements, expressions, or positional changes to express a person's feelings

SUMMARY

Effective communication and great customer service are vital in providing quality health care. Every member of the facility plays an important part in communication to ensure customer satisfaction. The medical assistant is often responsible for clarifying and relaying communication between patients and providers. To accomplish this task, the medical assistant must be effective at interpreting verbal and nonverbal communication, handling difficult customer service occurrences, and communicating on the telephone with patients, caregivers, providers, and third-party payers. Medical assistants facilitate and promote teamwork and team engagement. Great customer service is important to maintaining ongoing patient relationships and requires active participation from the entire medical team to be successful.

CHAPTER 17
Medical Law and Ethics

OVERVIEW

The health care industry is highly regulated in response to an ever-changing society. Medical law is composed of legal terms, federal law, state law, regulatory requirements, patient privacy, and health care standards. It is necessary to have a thorough understanding of these requirements and regulations as well as recognize when violations occur and how to report such incidents.

MEDICAL LAW AND ETHICS

To understand medical law and ethics, medical assistants must first know the legal terms associated with the profession. Many of these terms are used when discussing patient privacy, state or federal regulations, and various patient-care practices. In addition, medical assistants should also research the Medical Practice Act of the state where they practice to become familiar with tasks that can legally be delegated to medical assistants and which providers have delegation authority. These tasks will provide the framework for the medical assistant's scope of practice. Institutional policies will complete that framing process. An overzealous medical assistant, who becomes familiar with routine practices of the provider, might be tempted to perform diagnostic testing or direct the patient to take an over-the-counter medication during a telephone encounter without a direct prescription from the provider. These actions are beyond the medical assistant's scope of practice and can jeopardize the well-being of the patient.

Being familiar with health care regulations, recognizing ethical violations and responding appropriately to those violations are all essential responsibilities of a medical assistant.

Objectives

Upon completion of this chapter, you should be able to:

- Comply with legal and regulatory requirements.
- Protect patient privacy and confidentiality, including medical records.
- Adhere to legal requirements regarding reportable violations or incidents.
- Adhere to professional codes of ethics.
- Identify personal or religious beliefs and values and provide unbiased care.
- Obtain, review, and comply with medical directives.
- Obtain and document health care proxies and agents.
- Provide, collect, and store Medical Order for Life-Sustaining Treatment (MOLST) forms.

LEGAL AND REGULATORY REQUIREMENTS

To comply with legal and regulatory requirements, the medical assistant must understand the legal system. The following section provides some basic terminology used in the legal system.

Legal fundamentals

Criminal law addresses the rules and statutes that define wrongdoings against the community as a whole. Crimes can be classified as *misdemeanors* or *felonies*. A misdemeanor is considered less serious than a felony and carries a lesser penalty, usually a fine or imprisonment for less than a year. Examples of misdemeanors include reckless driving and discharging a firearm in city limits. A felony is more serious than a misdemeanor and constitutes a stiffer penalty, usually imprisonment greater than 1 year and, in extreme cases such as murder, can result in a death sentence. An *assault* is an instance in which someone threatens to cause harm to an individual. *Battery* is intentional touching or the use of force in a harmful manner, without the individual's consent. A *plaintiff* is the individual that files a lawsuit to initiate a legal action. A *defendant* is the person that is being sued or accused of a crime in a court of law. A *subpoena* is a written order that commands someone to appear in court to give evidence. Oftentimes, attorneys will depose a defendant or a witness before a case is brought to trial. A *deposition* is a formal statement in which the individual who is being deposed promises to tell the truth. These statements are often used during a court proceeding, especially when the defendant or witness changes their view of what occurred from the time of the deposition to the day of the hearing.

criminal law. Laws that deal with crimes and their punishments

misdemeanor. An offense that is considered less serious than a felony and carries a lesser penalty, usually a fine or imprisonment for less than 1 year

felony. A crime declared by statute to be more serious than a misdemeanor and deserving of a more severe penalty. Conviction usually requires imprisonment in a penitentiary for longer than 1 year

assault. The crime of trying or threatening to hurt someone physically

battery. Intentional touching or using force in a harmful manner, without the person's consent

plaintiff. A person who files a lawsuit initiating a legal action

defendant. A person who is being sued or accused of a crime in a court of law

subpoena. A written order that commands someone to appear in court to give evidence

deposition. A formal statement that someone who has promised to tell the truth makes so that the statement can be used in court

Civil law is applied most often in medical malpractice cases. Civil law governs the private rights of individuals, corporations, and government bodies and includes cases involving *contracts*, family matters, and property issues. A contract is a legally binding agreement between two or more individuals or entities to do something. For example, a contractor agrees to provide services in exchange for a fee. In order for a contract to be valid, it must contain the following four elements.

- **Mutual assent:** An agreement by all parties to contract; must prove there was an offer and acceptance

- **Consideration:** A benefit of some type for entering into the contract, such as financial reimbursement

- **Capacity:** Parties must be legally able to contract (legal age and of sound mind)

- **Legality:** Subject matter must be legal

When a party fails to hold up their part of a contract, they may be sued for *breach* of contract. This is why medical consent forms often include risks associated with the procedure and unsatisfactory disclosures statements, which state that the provider does not guarantee satisfactory results. This is common for cosmetic procedures.

In civil law cases, there are usually no fines or imprisonment. However, plaintiffs may receive a monetary award for injuries sustained as a result of a particular incident. In a medical *negligence* case, the plaintiff may receive compensation for medical expenses, lost wages, and for the pain and suffering associated with the negligence.

Administrative law is the body of law in the form of decisions, rules, regulations, and orders created by administrative agencies under the direction of the executive branch of the government used to carry out the duties of such agencies. In general, administrative agencies are responsible for protecting the civil rights, privacy, and safety of its citizens. The Health Insurance Portability and Accountability Act (HIPAA) came out of administrative law. The HIPAA Privacy Rule is designed to protect the patient's personal and medical information. Administrative judges at the state or federal level usually oversee these cases.

The legal system is a guide that is used in health care to ensure patients' and providers' rights are protected. When the legal system is violated, *litigation* can occur. Litigation is a lawsuit that will include a defendant and a plaintiff. Patients, providers, and health care workers need to understand their legal rights.

---

civil law. Laws that deal with the rights of people rather than with crimes

contract. A legal agreement between two or more parties (e.g., people, companies)

breach. Infraction or violation of a law, obligation, tie, or standard

negligence. The failure to do something that a reasonably prudent individual would do under similar circumstances

administrative law. The body of law in the form of decisions, rules, regulations, and orders created by administrative agencies under the direction of the executive branch of the government, used to carry out the duties of such agencies

litigation. A lawsuit or legal action that determines the legal rights and remedies of the person or party

Federal laws that affect medical practices

Medical assistants should be familiar with laws that affect the medical community. Here are some of the most common laws that affect medical practices.

Affordable Care Act (ACA): The ACA was put in place to reform the health care system by providing more Americans with affordable, quality health insurance to ultimately curb the growth in health care spending in the United States. Future modifications or replacement of this act will likely include prevention, wellness, and collaborative care strategies.

Occupational Safety and Health Administration (OSHA): OSHA states that employers are accountable for providing a safe and healthful workplace for employees by setting and enforcing standards and by providing training, outreach, education, and assistance.

Health Insurance Portability and Accountability Act of 1996 (HIPAA): HIPAA gives patients rights over their health information and sets rules and limits on who can look at and receive patients' private information. HIPAA applies to protected health information, whether electronic, written, or oral.

Controlled Substances Act (CSA): CSA is a federal policy that regulates the manufacture and distribution of controlled substances. Controlled substances can include narcotics, depressants, and stimulants. The CSA classifies medications into five schedules, or classifications, based on the likelihood for abuse, status in international treaties, and any medical benefits the substance might provide.

Title VII of Civil Rights: Title VII of Civil Rights Act prohibits an employer with 15 or more employees from discriminating on the basis of race, national origin, gender, or religion.

Equal Pay Act: The Equal Pay Act mandates the same pay for all people who do substantially equal work regardless of sex.

Americans with Disabilities Act (ADA): ADA forbids discrimination against any applicant or employee who could perform a job regardless of a disability. ADA also requires an employer to provide accommodations that are necessary to help the employee perform a job successfully, unless these accommodations are unduly burdensome.

Family Medical Leave Act (FMLA): FMLA is a federal law that requires certain employers to give time off to employees for familial or medical reasons.

The Joint Commission (TJC): Accreditation with TJC helps organizations position for the future of integrated care, strengthen patient safety and the quality of care, improve risk management and risk reduction, and provide a framework for organizational structure and management.

State laws that affect medical practices

State medical practice acts and laws that affect what responsibilities may be delegated to a medical assistant are different for each state. In addition, other providers (nurse practitioners, chiropractors) have their own state medical practice acts. Be aware of the tasks that can legally be delegated to a medical assistant based on laws of the state in which the practice is located.

Some states have a clearly defined scope of practice for medical assistants. However, the majority of states do not specifically mention medical assistants but instead use the broad term "unlicensed agents" or something similar. Some states require a medical assistant to be certified or registered to administer medications. General procedures that fall in the recognized scope of practice for a medical assistant can include the following.

- Schedule patients for procedures and treatments within the medical office or outside specialty clinic.
- Greet patients and assist them with registration processes.
- Prepare patients for provider exams by positioning and educating them regarding the procedure.
- Prepare examination rooms and necessary equipment and supplies.
- Obtain and document vital signs.
- Obtain and document patient history using medical terminology.
- Provide therapeutic communication to the patient, and accurately convey clinical information from the provider to the patient.
- Perform basic wound care (dressing changes, retrieving wound cultures).
- Remove superficial sutures or staples.
- Operate approved diagnostic equipment without test interpretation.
- Provide patient education and instructions for procedures.
- Administer medications orally, topically, sublingually, vaginally, rectally, and by injection (as permitted by supervising provider).
- Be certified to perform CPR and provide first aid in an emergency.
- Perform venipuncture and capillary blood collection.
- Perform simple laboratory and screening tests, such as urinalysis.
- Conduct filing, bookkeeping, and inventory.
- Process insurance claims and perform basic transcription for medical records dictation.
- If approved by the provider, call in prescriptions or refills to the pharmacy.

Standard of care

Health care professionals have a standard of care they are expected to follow while performing professional duties. Standard of care is the degree of care or competence that one is expected to exercise in a particular circumstance or role. Negligence is the failure to do something that a reasonably prudent individual would do under similar circumstances. Negligence cases use standard of care to decide whether a provider met the standard of care necessary to adequately perform their role. As part of the standard of care, health care workers must not stray from their scope of practice. Medical assistants that perform tasks outside their scope of practice breach the standard of care. An *expert witness*, which is usually someone who has similar training and credentials as the party being sued, is often used during negligence cases to establish what the standard of care is for a particular situation and whether that standard was met.

Tort law

A *tort* is an action that wrongly causes harm to an individual but is not a crime and is dealt with in a civil court. There are two major classifications of torts: intentional and negligence.

An *intentional tort* is a deliberate act that violates the rights of another. Examples of intentional torts include assault, battery, defamation of character, invasion of privacy, and administering an injection without the consent of the patient. The plaintiff in an intentional tort case does not need to prove the defendant intended to cause harm, just that the willful act of the defendant caused harm to the plaintiff. *Defamation of character* is hurting someone's reputation. *Slander* is verbal defamation, while *libel* is written defamation. Invasion of privacy is intrusion into the personal life of another individual without just cause. Prying into a patient's medical record or sharing information about a patient to another party without their consent are examples of invasion of privacy.

Negligence is a common tort in malpractice cases. *Res ipsa loquitur* and *respondeat superior* are two Latin terms that can be used to describe certain aspects of negligence. *Res ipsa loquitur* literally means "it speaks for itself." In other words, the negligence is obvious. In these cases, the burden of proof falls on defendants to prove they were not negligent. An example of a *res ipsa loquitur* case would be finding an instrument inside the patient following a surgical procedure or a patient sustaining burns while lying on a heating blanket. *Respondeat superior* is a doctrine that states that employers are responsible for the actions of their employees when the actions are performed within the constraints of their position. This doctrine came from the *common law* "master–servant rule."

expert witness. A witness in a court of law who is an expert on a particular subject

tort. An action that wrongly causes harm to someone but that is not a crime and that is dealt with in a civil court

intentional torts. An intentional wrongful act by a person or entity who means to cause harm, or who knows, or is reasonably certain, that harm will result from the act

slander. To make a false spoken statement that causes people to have a bad opinion of someone

libel. A false accusation that is made with malicious intent to hurt the reputation of a person who is living or the memory of a person who is dead, resulting in public embarrassment, contempt, ridicule, or hatred

res ipsa loquitur. A doctrine or rule of evidence in tort law that allows an inference or presumption that a defendant was negligent in an accident injuring the plaintiff on the basis of circumstantial evidence if the accident was of a kind that does not usually happen in without negligence

respondeat superior. A doctrine in tort law that makes an employer liable for the wrong of an employee

common law. The laws that developed from English court decisions and customs and that form the basis of laws in the U.S.

Negligent torts are unintentional. To prove negligence, the plaintiff must prove the following, often referred to as the "Four D's of Negligence."

- A *duty* existed.

- There was *dereliction* of duty.

- The misconduct of the defendant was the *direct cause* of the injury.

- *Damages* (usually substantial) occurred as a result of the misconduct.

Violation of state medical practice acts can result in the provider or health care worker being accused of the following.

- *Malfeasance* is performance of an unlawful, wrongful act; for example, performing a procedure on the wrong patient.

- *Misfeasance* is performance of a lawful action in an illegal or improper manner; for example, performing the procedure on the correct patient, but doing so incorrectly.

- Negligence is the failure to do something that a reasonable person of ordinary prudence would do in a certain situation, or the doing of something that such a person would not do.

- *Nonfeasance* is failure to perform a task, duty, or undertaking that one has agreed to perform or has a legal duty to perform; for example, waiting to treat a patient until it is too late.

Types of consent

In the clinical setting, there are two types of consent: implied and informed. *Informed consent* is a clear and voluntary indication of preference or choice, usually oral or written, and freely given in circumstances where the available options and their consequences have been made clear. An example is signing consent forms prior to a procedure. *Implied consent* is a voluntary agreement with an action proposed by another. An example is patients rolling up their sleeves to give blood. Consent is an act of reason. The person giving consent must be of sufficient mental capacity and be in possession of all essential information to give valid consent. Consent must be free of force or fraud. *Fraudulent* actions relate to actions that purposely intend to deceive someone.

---

malfeasance. Performance of an unlawful, wrongful act

misfeasance. The performance of a lawful action in an illegal or improper manner

nonfeasance. Failure to perform a task, duty, or undertaking that one has agreed to perform or has a legal duty to perform

informed consent. A clear and voluntary indication of preference or choice, usually oral or written, and freely given in circumstances where the available options and their consequences have been made clear

implied consent. Voluntary agreement with an action proposed by another

fraudulent. Relating to actions that purposely intend to deceive

PATIENT PRIVACY AND CONFIDENTIALITY

Patient privacy should be a priority for health care staff at all times. This includes the use of a fax machine, copy machine, or email.

- Never leave confidential patient information on a fax machine.

- Always use a cover page.

- Verify the correct fax number.

- Shred medical documents when necessary.

- Be sure the fax machine, copier, and computer are not visible to patients.

The medical record contains sensitive information about the patient history, current health status, and planned treatment. Never release this information to anyone without the patient's written consent, unless it is legally required through a subpoena. A subpoena is a written order that commands someone to appear in court to give evidence. If a legal case is presented and a medical record is subpoenaed, be sure to only release the requested information.

Laws that affect medical records

HIPAA

HIPAA gives patients rights over their health care information. They have the right to get a copy of their information, ensure the medical record is correct, and know who has had access to the record. Covered entities that must adhere to HIPAA include health plans, providers, and health care clearinghouses. If a covered entity engages a business associate to provide health care functions, the covered entity must have a written business associate contract or other arrangement with the business associate that establishes in detail what the business associate has been requested to do and requires the business associate to comply with the HIPAA requirements to protect the privacy and security of protected health information. In addition to these contractual obligations, business associates are directly liable for compliance with certain provisions of the HIPAA rules.

HIPAA requires providers to explain patient rights. The law requires patients to sign a form indicating they have received a privacy notice from a doctor, hospital, or other provider. HIPAA requires written consent when sharing health care information. HIPAA does not require a provider or health plan to share information with a patient's family or friends, unless they are the patient's personal representatives.

HITECH Act

The Health Information Technology for Economic and Clinical Health (HITECH) Act of 2009 was created to improve health care quality, safety, and efficiency for information technology and electronic health records. The HITECH Act provides barriers to information exchange. The act dictates nationwide use of health information technology to encourage an effective marketplace, improved competition, and consumer choice.

Medical record storage and retention laws

The medical record contains documented medical information that may be used for many different reasons. Accurate documentation in health care is critical. The record is used to manage health care and acts as a legal document. The record must be stored and retained in compliance with state laws that will differ for each state. HIPAA requires that documentation be retained for a minimum of 6 years. However, some states require a longer period. In this case, state law overrides federal law.

LEGAL REQUIREMENTS REGARDING REPORTABLE VIOLATIONS OR INCIDENTS

Anyone can file a privacy complaint to the Office of Civil Rights (OCR) through email, fax, postal mail, or via the OCR portal. The complaint must be filed within 180 days of when the known privacy violation occurred, and the complaint cannot be in retaliation. OCR will only investigate covered entities, which include doctors, clinics, hospitals, psychologists, chiropractors, nursing homes, pharmacies, dentist, health insurance companies, company health plans, Medicare, Medicaid, and other government programs that pay for health care. OCR can impose fines from $100 to $250,000 and imprisonment based on the complaint.

Mandatory reporting laws

There might be an occasion in which a medical assistant witnesses a breach of privacy. A breach is an infraction or violation of a law, obligation, or standard. A breach of unsecured protected health information must be reported unless there is low probability that the health information has been compromised based on the following risk assessment.

- The nature and extent of the protected health information involved, including the types of identifiers and the likelihood of re-identification

- The unauthorized person who used the protected health information or to whom the disclosure was made

- Whether the protected health information was actually acquired or viewed

- The extent to which the risk to the protected health information has been mitigated

17.1 HIPAA complaint process

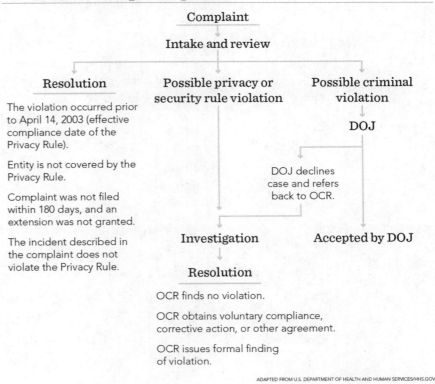

ADAPTED FROM U.S. DEPARTMENT OF HEALTH AND HUMAN SERVICES/HHS.GOV

There are three exceptions to the definition of breach.

- Unintentional acquisition, access, or use of the protected health information

- Unintentional disclosure of protected health information

- Good-faith belief that the unauthorized person to whom the impermissible disclosure was made would not have been able to retain the information.

PROFESSIONAL CODES OF ETHICS

Ethics is the discipline concerned with what is morally good and bad, or right and wrong. Ethics can be debated depending on a person's beliefs or way of thinking. An individual's personal morals and religious upbringing often contribute to their personal ethics. Professional ethics are a set of accepted behaviors and values that a person is expected to possess in a particular organization or profession.

Hippocratic Oath

Medical assistants work under the direct supervision of providers who take the Hippocratic Oath. Many doctors recite this oath during their graduation ceremony from medical school. The Hippocratic Oath sets the framework for ethical principles related to the practice of medicine.

Medical assisting code of ethics

Each credentialing organization has a code of ethics for the professionals they certify. The code of ethics is a pledge to guide members' behavior. Although organizations have different sets of ethics, they all are committed to abiding by all laws.

NHA Code of Ethics

As a certified professional through the NHA, I have a duty to:

- Use my best efforts for the betterment of society, the profession, and the members of the profession.

- Uphold the standards of professionalism and be honest in all professional interactions.

- Continue to learn, apply, and advance scientific and practical knowledge and skills; stay up to date on the latest research and its practical application.

- Participate in activities contributing to the improvement of personal health, our society, and the betterment of the allied health industry.

- Continuously act in the best interests of the general public.

- Protect and respect the dignity and privacy of all patients.

PERSONAL OR RELIGIOUS BELIEFS AND VALUES, AND UNBIASED CARE

Patients may have religious and personal beliefs and values that affect their decisions surrounding health care. Some current ethical issues surrounding health care include end-of-life care, resuscitation orders, euthanasia, abortion, birth control, and genetic testing. There are many areas of health care that can be tied to a person's religious or personal beliefs. Regardless of a patient's personal or religious beliefs, they must receive standard care.

In some cases, a medical assistants' religious or personal beliefs may be violated as a result of performing duties associated with employment. Examples include assisting same-sex couples with infertility treatments or performing phlebotomy procedures at a termination or abortion clinic. It is important to know responsibilities associated with a position prior to employment to avoid being placed in an ethical or moral dilemma. Whether medical assistants agree with a patient's or coworker's position on an ethical issue does not give them the right to ridicule or treat that individual differently.

MEDICAL DIRECTIVES

Working in the medical industry has many joyful moments, such as observing a couple that has tried to conceive for years find out they are going to be parents or the celebration of news that someone is no longer battling cancer. Unfortunately, the news isn't always good, such as when a patient finds out there are no treatment options left to treat a terminal disease. As patients come to terms with the prognosis, they often realize the importance of end-of-life planning. End-of-life planning includes determining what will happen if the patient is unable to speak for himself.

Medical directives consist of a set of requests that patients put in writing for their provider, family, and other health care professionals to carry out surrounding end-of-life medical treatment. The provider must obtain, review, and comply with the directives. A medical directive will indicate what medical treatment patients wish to have if they are dying or permanently unconscious, and identifies an *agent* for the patients. The health care agent will make decisions on the patient's behalf. The agent is someone that acts or exerts power.

In the ambulatory setting, the medical assistant is often the first health care worker to ask the patient about these forms. Patients often find it hard to accept the invitation to discuss these options because it might feel like the health care community is giving up on them or that they are giving up on themselves. This is why it is best to start these discussions as early in the process as possible. Patients who are hesitant to complete these forms should be told that they can always make changes if they change their mind. The medical assistant should alert the provider when the patient wants to learn more about these forms.

agent. Someone that acts or exerts power

Types of medical directives

Living will is a legal document stating what procedures the patient would want, which ones she wouldn't want, and under what conditions she would want the provider to do organ and tissue donation, dialysis, blood transfusions, and do-not-resuscitate orders.

Durable power of attorney for health care is a legal document naming a health care agent or proxy to make medical decisions for patients when they are not able to do so. The agent will be able to decide as the patient would when treatment decisions need to be made. A durable power of attorney for health care enables patients to be more specific about their medical treatment than a living will.

Do-not-resuscitate (DNR) orders indicate to the medical staff not to return the patient's heart to normal rhythm if it stops or is beating unevenly.

MOLST is a medical document that specifies which treatments will be allowed during end-of-life care. A provider must sign off on the MOLST orders. These orders move with the patient if the patient changes facilities, and the form is bright pink for easy identification.

Organ and tissue donation orders allow organs or body parts from a healthy person to be transferred to people who need them.

Obtaining, reviewing, and storing medical directives

Once the patient has completed a medical directive, a copy should be given to the family, hospital, and providers to review and have on file. The directive should be reviewed often and revised if necessary.

Storing medical directives is just as important as obtaining them. The document must be portable, available in a timely manner, and protected from theft, fire, or water damage. Several copies of the documents should be made, with the original kept in a safe, accessible place.

Complying with medical directives

Medical directives are legally valid throughout the United States as soon as the patient signs them in front of the required witnesses. The laws governing medical directives vary by state. Providers must fully evaluate the patient's condition before advance directives can be applied. Medical directives do not expire; they remain in effect until they are officially changed.

HEALTH CARE PROXIES AND AGENTS

A health care proxy or agent is the person assigned to make health care decisions for the patient if they are incapacitated. Determining the health care proxy or agent is an important decision when planning for the future. Once a documented proxy is in place, be sure the patient's family and providers have a copy of the documentation.

SUMMARY

The future of health care and health care laws is ever-changing. Laws will continue to guide the health care industry in response to a changing society. Patients will continue to be educated on medical directives and have a greater effect on their health care. Medical assistants must stay current with the laws and regulations related to health care to protect themselves as well as their patients.

IN PRACTICE
Quizzes

QUIZ 1: HEALTH CARE SYSTEMS AND SETTINGS

1. Which of the following professionals assists patients with improving mobility, strength, and range of motion?
   A. Occupational therapist
   B. Emergency medical technician
   C. Physical therapist
   D. Radiology technician

2. A medical assistant is preparing a referral slip for a patient who reports symptoms of vertigo. The medical assistant should refer the patient to which of the following specialists?
   A. Otolaryngologist
   B. Anesthesiologist
   C. Neurologist
   D. Ophthalmologist

3. Which of the following health care professionals is legally responsible for the outcomes of a medical assistant's duties and performance?
   A. Registered nurse
   B. Family practitioner
   C. Office manager
   D. Pharmacy technician

4. Which of the following duties is a medical assistant allowed to perform independently?
   A. Prescribe medication
   B. Record vital signs
   C. Give medical advice
   D. Provide medication samples

5. Which of the following providers specializes in the management and treatment of interstitial cystitis?
   A. Immunologist
   B. Cardiologist
   C. Pathologist
   D. Urologist

6. Which of the following professionals specializes in evaluating mental illness, physical illness, and disability through analyzing patient health needs and providing health education to patients of all ages?
   A. Physical medicine and rehabilitation specialist
   B. Pediatrician
   C. Pathologist
   D. Preventive medicine specialist

7. Which of the following roles provides an opportunity to obtain certification or registration based on state regulations but does not require a license to secure employment within the health care industry?
   A. Medical assistant
   B. Physician assistant
   C. Diagnostic radiologist
   D. Anesthesiologist

8. A provider requests that a patient see a specialist for hyperthyroidism. The assistant should expect to contact which of the following specialty clinics for this consultation?
   A. Gastroenterology
   B. Endocrinology
   C. Urology
   D. Cardiology

9. Which of the following health care delivery models emphasizes patients' involvement in organizing their own health care?
   A. Hospice
   B. Home health agency
   C. Accountable care organization (ACO)
   D. Patient-centered medical home (PCMH)

10. Which of the following insurance plan models requires a referral from a ' primary care provider to schedule an appointment with a dermatologist?
    A. Preferred provider organization (PPO)
    B. Pay-for-performance
    C. Health maintenance organization (HMO)
    D. Exclusive provider organization (EPO)

11. Which of the following types of providers is qualified to assess patients of all ages with a wide variety of acute to severe medical conditions?
    A. Internist
    B. Specialist
    C. Pediatrician
    D. Family practitioner

12. A patient has had a cerebrovascular accident (CVA). Which of the following types of therapy will assist the patient with regaining motor functions and independence?
    A. Respiratory therapy
    B. Massage therapy
    C. Physical therapy
    D. Behavioral therapy

13. A patient experiencing a subluxation should be treated by which of the following alternative medicine practices?
    A. Acupuncture
    B. Chiropractic care
    C. Biofeedback
    D. Herbal medicine

14. A medical assistant is reviewing charges for an in-office procedure. Which of the following terms describes the maximum reimbursement a third-party payer will provide?
    A. Deductible
    B. Coinsurance
    C. Fee schedule
    D. Allowable amount

15. Which of the following insurance providers is the oldest and largest system of independent health insurers in the U.S.?
    A. Tricare
    B. Medicare
    C. Blue Cross/Blue Shield
    D. Medicaid

QUIZ 2: MEDICAL TERMINOLOGY

1. A medical assistant is reviewing a patient's medical record. Which of the following acronyms should the medical assistant identify as the notation used when interpreting the correlation between the patient's body weight and height?
    A. KUB
    B. LMP
    C. PID
    D. BMI

2. When a medical assistant is documenting data in a patient's progress notes, which of the following abbreviations is acceptable for use?
    A. >
    B. O_2
    C. $MgSO_4$
    D. μg

3. Which of the following abbreviations is used in place of the word "prescription" in a patient's chart?
    A. Rx
    B. Tx
    C. Sx
    D. Hx

4. Which of the following abbreviations should a medical assistant use when documenting initial assessment data collected prior to a patient's wellness examination?
    A. HPI
    B. p/o
    C. VS
    D. f/u

5. Which of the following should a medical assistant identify as a diagnostic procedure that produces images of body structures?
   A. Audiometry
   B. Electromyography
   C. Computed tomography
   D. Holter monitoring

6. When processing a patient's referral, a medical assistant should identify which of the following as a laboratory test?
   A. Barium enema
   B. Blood urea nitrogen
   C. Computed tomography
   D. Benign prostatic hyperplasia

7. When reviewing a patient's medical history, a medical assistant should identify which of the following terms as a medical disorder that involves inflammation of the joints?
   A. Rheumatoid arthritis
   B. Multiple sclerosis
   C. Osteoporosis
   D. Carcinoma

8. A medical assistant is preparing to record a patient's heart rhythm. Which of the following devices should the medical assistant use to perform this recording?
   A. Stethoscope
   B. Electroencephalogram machine
   C. Sphygmomanometer
   D. Electrocardiogram machine

9. Using knowledge of roots and suffixes, a medical assistant should identify that the term "oophorectomy" has which of the following meanings?
   A. Brain disorder
   B. Breakdown of blood cells
   C. Opening in the windpipe
   D. Removal of the ovaries

10. Using knowledge of medical roots and suffixes, a medical assistant should identify which of the following terms as a procedure that involves an incision into the eardrum?
    A. Otodynia
    B. Rhinorrhea
    C. Myringotomy
    D. Lithotripsy

11. Using knowledge of prefixes and suffixes, a medical assistant should identify that the term "presbyopia" has which of the following meanings?
    A. Age-related vision loss
    B. Weakened bones
    C. Drooping eyelid
    D. Kidney infection

12. Using knowledge of prefixes and suffixes, a medical assistant should identify the term for slow breathing as which of the following?
    A. Oximetry
    B. Bradypnea
    C. Neuralgia
    D. Tachycardia

13. Using knowledge of positional and directional prefixes and terms, a medical assistant should identify that the term "contralateral" has which of the following meanings?
    A. Directed downward
    B. The opposite side
    C. Directed upward
    D. The same side

14. A medical assistant is preparing a patient for a rectal examination. The medical assistant should help the patient into which of the following positions?
    A. Fowler's
    B. Lithotomy
    C. Trendelenburg
    D. Sims'

15. A medical assistant is preparing to apply a compression bandage to a patient's extremity. The medical assistant begins applying the bandage at the farthest point from the patient's trunk and moves to the nearest point. Which of the following pairs of terms describes this progression?
    A. Distal to proximal
    B. Posterior to anterior
    C. Proximal to distal
    D. Anterior to posterior

QUIZ 3: BASIC PHARMACOLOGY

1. A medical assistant is preparing a patient for a physical examination. The patient reports difficulty falling asleep. The medical assistant should anticipate that the provider will prescribe which of the following medications?

   A. Esomeprazole

   B. Loperamide

   C. Metformin

   D. Zolpidem

2. A medical assistant is transcribing a prescription from a provider for a medication that must be taken hourly. Which of the following abbreviations should the medical assistant identify as the correct notation of when and how often the patient should take the medication?

   A. qd

   B. qh

   C. qs

   D. qid

3. A medical assistant is reviewing the medications for a patient who is undergoing chemotherapy to treat breast cancer. The medical assistant should identify that the provider prescribed ondansetron because it is in which of the following medication classifications?

   A. Antiemetic

   B. Antitussive

   C. Antilipemic

   D. Antipyretic

4. A medical assistant is transcribing a prescription for fentanyl patches for a patient. The medical assistant should identify that this medication has specific requirements because it is classified in which of the following schedules of controlled substances?

   A. Schedule I

   B. Schedule II

   C. Schedule III

   D. Schedule IV

5. A medical assistant is providing teaching to a patient who is starting lisinopril, a medication that helps lower blood pressure. The medical assistant should instruct the patient to report which of the following effects to the provider immediately?

   A. Nausea

   B. Orthostatic hypotension

   C. Facial swelling

   D. Taste disturbance

6. A medical assistant is converting a prescription for 30 mL of liquid medication from milliliters to tablespoons. The medical assistant should calculate that this amount of medication converts to how many tablespoons?

   A. 1 tbsp

   B. 1.5 tbsp

   C. 3 tbsp

   D. 2 tbsp

7. A medical assistant is reviewing a prescription for oral liquid medication. The prescription calls for 10 mg diazepam oral solution. Available is diazepam oral solution 5 mg/5 mL. How many mL of the solution are required for each dose?

   A. 4.5 mL

   B. 7.5 mL

   C. 10 mL

   D. 12.5 mL

8. A medical assistant is arranging medication in a storage cabinet according to the routes of administration. The medical assistant should categorize methyl salicylate liniment in which of the following routes?

   A. Oral

   B. Otic

   C. Topical

   D. Ophthalmic

9. A medical assistant is caring for a patient who is scheduled for a flexible sigmoidoscopy and will be self-administering an enema at home. The medical assistant should explain that the medication will be in which of the following forms?

   A. Suppository
   B. Solution
   C. Lotion
   D. Foam

10. A medical assistant should identify which of the following look-alike and sound-alike medications as an anticonvulsant?

    A. Clonazepam
    B. Chlorpropamide
    C. Amlodipine
    D. Alprazolam

11. A medical assistant is preparing to perform a Mantoux test. Which of the following routes should the medical assistant use for this injection?

    A. Intradermal
    B. Subcutaneous
    C. Intramuscular
    D. Intravenous

12. A medical assistant is explaining to an older adult patient that she will require a lower dosage of a medication than a younger adult. The medical assistant should explain that this difference in dosage is primarily because of the effect that aging has on which of the following pharmacokinetic processes?

    A. Absorption
    B. Distribution
    C. Metabolism
    D. Excretion

13. A patient tells a medical assistant that the provider said to take the prescribed antibiotic four times per day because of the medication's half-life. The patient wants to know what "half-life" means. Which of the following responses should the medical assistant make?

    A. "A medication's half-life is the time at which it will lose all of its effectiveness."
    B. "A medication's half-life is the time it takes for your body to absorb half of the dosage."
    C. "A medication's half-life occurs when the primary function of the medication is at its peak."
    D. "A medication's half-life is the time it takes for the body to process and eliminate half of the dosage."

14. A medical assistant is preparing to administer a vitamin injection to a patient. As part of verifying the right medication, which of the following actions should the medical assistant take?

    A. Calculate the medication's dosage.
    B. Check the medication label's expiration date.
    C. Ensure the patient has consented to receiving the injection.
    D. Find out why the provider prescribed the medication.

15. A medical assistant is preparing to administer a medication that should be taken at least 2 hr after a meal. The medical assistant asks when the patient last ate. Which of the following rights of medication administration is the medical assistant demonstrating?

    A. Right time
    B. Right route
    C. Right technique
    D. Right documentation

QUIZ 4: NUTRITION

1. A medical assistant is providing teaching to a patient about the importance of water intake. Which of the following information should the medical assistant include?
   A. It is important to drink at least 1 L of water daily.
   B. Water provides minimal nutritional value for the body.
   C. Severe dehydration can cause an increase in blood volume.
   D. Water helps regulate body temperature.

2. A medical assistant is reviewing nutritional guidelines with a patient who is following a high-protein diet. Which of the following statements should the medical assistant make?
   A. "An increased intake of sodium is necessary to metabolize protein."
   B. "Without sufficient carbohydrates and fat, the body will burn protein for energy."
   C. "The body uses dietary fiber to rebuild muscle."
   D. "Half of your daily caloric intake should consist of protein."

3. A medical assistant is encouraging a patient to increase fiber intake. Which of the following foods should the medical assistant recommend?
   A. Chicken breast
   B. Cottage cheese
   C. Eggs
   D. Apples

4. A medical assistant is reviewing a daily diet with a patient. Which of the following foods should the medical assistant recommend to help the patient increase intake of vitamin D?
   A. Beans
   B. Fish
   C. Rice
   D. Nuts

5. A medical assistant is reviewing the dietary intake of a patient who has lactose intolerance. Which of the following foods should the medical assistant remind the patient to limit?
   A. Cream cheese
   B. Green beans
   C. Grilled chicken
   D. Black coffee

6. A medical assistant is teaching a patient about the major food groups. Which of the following information about grains should the medical assistant include?
   A. Grains help with the absorption of fat-soluble vitamins.
   B. Grains help maintain body heat.
   C. Grains help regulate muscle activity and heart rhythm.
   D. Grains help prevent and manage constipation.

7. A medical assistant is providing patient education on bone loss and calcium regulation. Which of the following supplements should the medical assistant recommend?
   A. Vitamin A
   B. Vitamin C
   C. Vitamin D
   D. Vitamin E

8. Which of the following foods should a medical assistant recommend to a patient who needs to increase dietary intake of vitamin A?
   A. Blueberries
   B. Potatoes
   C. Oranges
   D. Cauliflower

9. A medical assistant is reviewing dietary minerals with a patient. Which of the following minerals is essential for blood coagulation?

   A. Iron

   B. Magnesium

   C. Calcium

   D. Potassium

10. A medical assistant is collecting information from a patient prior to a physical examination. Which of the following details disclosed by the patient should the medical assistant recognize as an indication of bulimia nervosa?

    A. Laxative use

    B. Ritualistic behavior

    C. Starvation

    D. Counting calories

11. A medical assistant is preparing a patient for an examination. Which of the following findings should the medical assistant recognize as an indication of anorexia nervosa?

    A. Protruding bones

    B. Reports of painful menstrual periods

    C. Reports of constant hunger

    D. Erosion of tooth enamel

12. A medical assistant should identify that which of the following manifestations differentiates binge-eating disorder from bulimia nervosa?

    A. Chronic overeating

    B. Avoiding self-induced vomiting

    C. Losing weight

    D. Buying large amounts of food

13. A medical assistant is explaining how to understand nutritional information on food labels to a patient. Which of the following statements should the medical assistant make?

    A. "Your standard calorie consumption per day should be less than 1,000 calories."

    B. "The ingredients are listed in ascending order of weight."

    C. "The amount of each nutrient is expressed in weight per serving and as a percentage of the daily value."

    D. "Sugar alcohol is a required component of a food label."

14. A medical assistant is educating a patient about how to interpret food labels. The medical assistant should inform the patient that the FDA requires nutrition labels to include measurements of which of the following nutritional elements?

    A. Cholesterol

    B. Xylitol

    C. Thiamine

    D. Polyunsaturated fat

15. To avoid having patients underestimate the amount of nutrients in a food product, a medical assistant should remind patients to check which of the following labeling components?

    A. Percent of daily value

    B. Total amounts of caloric intake per day

    C. Ingredient order

    D. Serving size

QUIZ 5: PSYCHOLOGY

1. A medical assistant is talking with an older adult patient who expresses frustration about having looked forward to retirement but now finding "too much time on my hands." Which of the following is one of the developmental tasks for this patient's age group?
   A. Serving the community
   B. Making good decisions
   C. Having a sense of self-worth
   D. Finding mutual self-respect

2. A medical assistant is talking with a young adult patient who says he has found a partner he loves but cannot seem to make a commitment to their relationship. The developmental crisis this patient is experiencing is which of the following?
   A. Ego integrity vs. despair
   B. Intimacy vs. isolation
   C. Generativity vs. stagnation
   D. Identity vs. role confusion

3. A medical assistant is talking with the parents of a 1-year-old infant about developmental achievements and milestones to expect. According to the infant's developmental stage, a lack of achievement of the tasks of that stage can result in which of the following negative outcomes?
   A. Suspiciousness
   B. Anger with self
   C. Inadequacy
   D. Guilt

4. A medical assistant is talking with a patient whose brother died of heart disease 1 month ago. The patient tells the medical assistant that she blames herself because she should have persuaded her brother to take better care of himself. The patient is in which of the following of Elisabeth Kübler-Ross's stages of grief?
   A. Denial
   B. Anger
   C. Bargaining
   D. Depression

5. A medical assistant is talking with a patient who just learned that she has advanced breast cancer. The patient says, "It's just an infection. I'm way too young to have cancer!" Which of the following actions should the medical assistant take to help this patient during this stage of grief?
   A. Encourage the patient to express sadness.
   B. Redirect the patient's attention away from angry feelings.
   C. Reinforce education about the patient's disease process.
   D. Refer the patient to a support group.

6. A patient who walks with difficulty as a result of nerve damage on one side of the body enters a clinic for a first visit. Which of the following statements should the medical assistant in the front office make?
   A. "Are you walking this way as the result of an accident?"
   B. "Would you prefer to wait in one of our inner offices?"
   C. "How can I make you more comfortable while you wait?"
   D. "I'm so sorry for what you must have gone through."

7. A patient who uses a wheelchair arrives at the office for an appointment and is visibly upset. Which of the following methods should the medical assistant use to establish positive therapeutic communication with the patient?
   A. Face the patient at eye level.
   B. Speak in a quiet voice.
   C. Hold the patient's hand.
   D. Maintain a closed posture.

8. Which of the following defense mechanisms is characterized by a patient's externalization of guilt, blame, or responsibility?
   A. Denial
   B. Apathy
   C. Undoing
   D. Projection

9. According to Erikson's psychosocial theory, an adolescent experiences which of the following stages?

   A. Initiative vs. guilt

   B. Industry vs. inferiority

   C. Autonomy vs. shame and doubt

   D. Identity vs. role confusion

10. A medical assistant is preparing a patient for a physical examination. The patient tells the medical assistant that she is having serious problems at work, and she feels so much stress that she cannot focus on anything at work or at home. Based on the patient's anxiety level, which of the following findings should the medical assistant expect?

    A. Drowsiness

    B. Dry skin

    C. Back pain

    D. Rapid respirations

11. A medical assistant is preparing a patient for the Mini-Mental State Examination. The examiner names three objects and asks the patient to repeat them. In doing so, the examiner is asking the patient to perform a task in which of the following areas?

    A. Orientation

    B. Registration

    C. Attention and calculation

    D. Language

12. A medical assistant is observing a patient who is undergoing the Mini-Mental State Examination. To test the patient's ability to perform tasks in the area of language, the examiner asks the patient to do which of the following?

    A. Copy a geometric design.

    B. Identify the city they are in.

    C. Spell their first name backward.

    D. Name the three objects stated earlier.

13. A medical assistant is collecting initial data for an older adult patient at a clinic visit. Which of the following should suggest to the medical assistant that the patient needs a mental status evaluation?

    A. The patient has lost a significant amount of weight.

    B. The patient reports a decrease in energy.

    C. The patient repeatedly asks the same question.

    D. The patient reports not sleeping well.

14. A medical assistant is discussing dietary concerns with a patient who has heart disease. The patient states, "I haven't been as careful about salt and fat as I should be, but I have been exercising more than usual." The medical assistant should identify that this patient is using which of the following defense mechanisms?

    A. Compensation

    B. Displacement

    C. Repression

    D. Reaction formation

15. The parent of a 5-year-old child tells a medical assistant that the child has begun sucking her thumb. The parent states, "She hasn't done this since she was a baby." The medical assistant should identify that the child is using which of the following defense mechanisms?

    A. Rationalization

    B. Regression

    C. Suppression

    D. Sublimation

QUIZ 6: BODY STRUCTURES AND ORGAN SYSTEMS

1. Which of the following is an example of connective tissue?
   A. Pancreas
   B. Blood
   C. Spinal cord
   D. Skin

2. A medical assistant is collecting data from a patient who reports back pain. Which of the following terms should the medical assistant use to describe the patient's pain in the intake notes?
   A. Caudal
   B. Cephalic
   C. Medial
   D. Dorsal

3. Which of the following planes divides the body into upper and lower portions?
   A. Transverse
   B. Coronal
   C. Sagittal
   D. Midsagittal

4. When considering the anatomy of the body, which of the following statements is correct?
   A. The heart is superficial to the ribs.
   B. The patella is distal to the tibia.
   C. The stomach is superior to the diaphragm.
   D. The thumb is lateral to the index finger.

5. Which of the following body structures is part of both the digestive and endocrine systems?
   A. Appendix
   B. Pancreas
   C. Liver
   D. Gallbladder

6. Which of the following glands in the endocrine system is located just below the larynx and consists of two lobes, one on each side of the trachea?
   A. Thyroid
   B. Hypothalamus
   C. Pituitary
   D. Adrenal

7. Which of the following organs produces vitamin D, provides protection, and helps regulate body temperature?
   A. Liver
   B. Lung
   C. Skin
   D. Brain

8. Which of the following systems provides the framework to protect the body from pathogenic organisms and maintain fluid balance?
   A. Musculoskeletal
   B. Gastrointestinal
   C. Integumentary
   D. Lymphatic

9. Which of the following body systems contains cardiac, skeletal, and smooth tissues?
   A. Lymphatic
   B. Integumentary
   C. Muscular
   D. Endocrine

10. Which of the following body systems works with the respiratory system to transport waste products from the body's cells?
    A. Peripheral nervous
    B. Endocrine
    C. Cardiovascular
    D. Reproductive

11. Which of the following organ structures within the digestive system is primarily responsible for the absorption of nutrients?
    A. Stomach
    B. Small intestine
    C. Bile duct
    D. Esophagus

12. Which of the following glands is part of both the immune and endocrine systems?
    A. Thyroid
    B. Pineal
    C. Thymus
    D. Pituitary

13. Which of the following is used to indicate homeostasis in the body?
    A. Height
    B. Weight
    C. Pulse oximetry
    D. Vital signs

14. When pain signals are received by the brain, which of the following body systems is alerted to initiate a movement response?
    A. Muscular
    B. Cardiovascular
    C. Digestive
    D. Integumentary

15. Which of the following body systems experiences a decrease in activity caused by the sympathetic branch of the nervous system during "fight-or-flight" response?
    A. Cardiovascular
    B. Respiratory
    C. Muscular
    D. Digestive

QUIZ 7: PATHOPHYSIOLOGY AND DISEASE PROCESSES

1. Which of the following conditions is defined as a loss of bone density?
    A. Osteoporosis
    B. Osteomyelitis
    C. Rheumatoid arthritis
    D. Scoliosis

2. Which of the following is a risk factor for the development of congestive heart failure (CHF)?
    A. Chronic hypertension
    B. Atherosclerosis
    C. Endocarditis
    D. Family history of CHF

3. A medical assistant is speaking with a patient who recently underwent a right-sided radical mastectomy and lymphadenectomy. The medical assistant should inform the patient that which of the following is a manifestation of lymphedema?
    A. Swelling of the right arm
    B. Palpable nodules in the left breast
    C. Scaly patches on the skin
    D. Migraine headaches

4. A medical assistant should recognize that which of the following is the purpose of contrast media in diagnostic imaging?
    A. Highlights the inner contours of body structures
    B. Makes body structures easier to see through
    C. Indicates the location of bones
    D. Protects internal organs from radiation

5. Which of the following is the medical assistant's primary role in magnetic resonance imaging (MRI) in the medical office setting?
    A. Instructing a patient about examination preparations
    B. Administering contrast media intravenously
    C. Communicating the results of the imaging to the patient
    D. Positioning the imaging equipment

6. A medical assistant recommends the rest, ice, compression, and elevation (RICE) method to a patient who calls the office to report an injury. Which of the following injuries is the patient likely to have sustained?
    A. Ankle sprain
    B. Shoulder dislocation
    C. Head contusion
    D. Restless leg syndrome

7. Which of the following hernias is characterized by the top portion of the stomach protruding through the diaphragm?
    A. Hiatal
    B. Umbilical
    C. Inguinal
    D. Incisional

8. Which of the following diseases affects about 9% of the population of the U.S. and is characterized by the body's inability to produce sufficient insulin?
   A. Diabetes mellitus
   B. Diabetes insipidus
   C. Coronary artery disease
   D. Polycystic kidney disease

9. A medical assistant is caring for a patient whose dietary choices have resulted in elevated uric acid levels. As a result of these risk factors, the patient is at risk for developing which of the following musculoskeletal disorders?
   A. Myasthenia gravis
   B. Rheumatoid arthritis
   C. Osteoporosis
   D. Gout

10. Which of the following factors puts a patient at high risk of developing coronary artery disease?
    A. Smoking
    B. Underweight
    C. High HDL cholesterol
    D. Cellulitis

11. Which of the following factors puts a patient at high risk of experiencing a cerebrovascular accident (CVA)?
    A. Hypoglycemia
    B. Hypotension
    C. Pyloric stenosis
    D. Sleep apnea

12. A low-fiber, high-fat diet is a risk factor for which of the following diseases?
    A. Colorectal cancer
    B. Crohn's disease
    C. Cholelithiasis
    D. Cirrhosis

13. A medical assistant should recognize that a worldwide, rapidly spreading novel infection can result in which of the following?
    A. Pandemic
    B. Prevalence
    C. Endemic
    D. Outbreak

14. Which of the following diseases caused a historical pandemic that led to the creation of the first vaccine?
    A. Smallpox
    B. Influenza
    C. Tetanus
    D. Malaria

15. Which of the following viral diseases resulted in an epidemic in the U.S. and presents with symptoms including weakness and paralysis of muscles, fever, and headache?
    A. Polio
    B. Measles
    C. Rubella
    D. Rabies

QUIZ 8: MICROBIOLOGY

1. Which of the following structures in a human cell contains the cell's genetic information?
   A. Nucleus
   B. Cytoplasm
   C. Plasma membrane
   D. Nucleolus

2. Which of the following components of the body's cells provides the energy the cell needs to perform its specific functions?
   A. Lysosome
   B. Centriole
   C. Mitochondrion
   D. Cilia

3. Which of the following structures in a human cell sorts and synthesizes glycoproteins?
   A. Ribosome
   B. Cytoskeleton
   C. Endoplasmic reticulum
   D. Golgi apparatus

4. Which of the following components of the body's cells helps propel substances through passageways in the body?
   A. Cilia
   B. Flagellum
   C. Cytoskeleton
   D. Microvilli

5. Which of the following components of the body's cells plays a part in cell division?
   A. Cytoplasm
   B. Centriole
   C. Golgi apparatus
   D. Endoplasmic reticulum

6. A medical assistant should identify which of the following micro-organisms as having a helpful function in the human body?
   A. *Clostridium botulinum*
   B. *Lactobacillus acidophilus*
   C. *Treponema pallidum*
   D. *Haemophilus influenzae*

7. A medical assistant is talking with a patient who has a new diagnosis of mononucleosis. Which of the following viruses causes this infection?
   A. Human papillomavirus
   B. Parvovirus
   C. Human immunodeficiency virus
   D. Epstein-Barr virus

8. A medical assistant is talking with a patient who has a new diagnosis of *Pediculus humanus capitis*. The medical assistant should explain that this is an infestation of which of the following multicellular parasites?
   A. Pubic lice
   B. Pinworms
   C. Head lice
   D. Tapeworms

9. A medical assistant is talking with a patient who has a vaginal yeast infection. Which of the following micro-organisms causes this type of infection?
   A. *Pneumocystis carinii*
   B. *Legionella pneumophila*
   C. *Helicobacter pylori*
   D. *Candida albicans*

10. Which of the following types of bacteria has a structure with a shape similar to a comma?
    A. Coccus
    B. Spirillum
    C. Vibrio
    D. Bacillus

11. A medical assistant is talking with a patient who has a new prescription for amoxicillin. The medical assistant should explain that this medication aids in the destruction of which of the following types of micro-organisms?
    A. Bacteria
    B. Viruses
    C. Fungi
    D. Protozoa

12. Which of the following types of micro-organisms is a mold when it is multicellular?
    A. Bacteria
    B. Viruses
    C. Fungi
    D. Protozoa

13. Which of the following links initiates the chain of infection?
    A. Portal of entry
    B. Infectious agent
    C. Susceptible host
    D. Mode of transmission

14. A medical assistant is talking with the parent of a child who has molluscum contagiosum warts. The medical assistant should explain that which of the following is the mode of transmission for this infection?
    A. Foodborne
    B. Droplet
    C. Fomite
    D. Contact

15. A medical assistant is talking with a patient who has Lyme disease. Which of the following is the means of transmission for this infection?
    A. Fomite
    B. Droplet
    C. Vector
    D. Airborne

QUIZ 9: GENERAL PATIENT CARE

1. Which of the following actions should a medical assistant take when closing the clinical area at the end of the day?
   - A. Restock medical supplies in the examination rooms.
   - B. Prepare and cover a sterile field for the next day.
   - C. Discard the biohazard bags from the examination rooms in the trash.
   - D. Refrigerate all collected blood specimens for retrieval the next day.

2. Which of the following actions should the medical assistant take to prevent patient accidents in the clinical setting?
   - A. Stand with feet together when transferring a patient.
   - B. Bundle computer cables that cross walkways with cable ties.
   - C. Clean a spill on the hallway floor using a towel.
   - D. Store cleaning supplies on top of cabinets.

3. A medical assistant is preparing a patient for an examination. Which of the following is a component of the patient's medical history?
   - A. Objective data
   - B. Treatment plan
   - C. Chief complaint
   - D. Informed consent form

4. A medical assistant is preparing to obtain vital signs from an adult patient during a routine physical examination. Which of the following arteries should the medical assistant use to palpate the patient's pulse?
   - A. Carotid
   - B. Brachial
   - C. Radial
   - D. Femoral

5. Which of the following is an anthropometric measurement that a medical assistant should collect from a 2-year-old child?
   - A. Tympanic temperature
   - B. Head circumference
   - C. Apical pulse
   - D. Blood pressure

6. A medical assistant notices that the patient is slurring speech and has developed a slight drooping of one side of the mouth. These manifestations are indications of which of the following emergent conditions?
   - A. Myocardial infarction
   - B. Syncope
   - C. Anxiety attack
   - D. Cerebrovascular accident

7. A provider instructs a medical assistant to position a patient for an examination of the patient's dorsal cavity. The medical assistant should place the patient in which of the following positions?
   - A. Lithotomy
   - B. Supine
   - C. Prone
   - D. Semi-Fowler's

8. A patient in a clinic is experiencing symptoms of a myocardial infarction. The provider prescribes sublingual nitroglycerin. Which of the following actions should the medical assistant take?
   - A. Apply the medication to the skin.
   - B. Place the medication under the tongue.
   - C. Insert the medication into the rectum.
   - D. Inject the medication into a muscle.

9. A medical assistant is performing suture removal. Which of the following actions should the medical assistant take?
   - A. Remove each suture after cutting next to the knot.
   - B. Remove sutures from the center of the wound moving outward.
   - C. Remove the sutures in the opposite order of insertion.
   - D. Remove the sutures after placing adhesive skin closures.

10. A medical assistant is caring for a patient who has conjunctivitis. Which of the following actions should the medical assistant take when performing an eye instillation?

    A. Ensure the medication is instilled in the upper conjunctiva.

    B. Instruct the patient to look down when instilling the medication.

    C. Use gloves when instilling the medication.

    D. Use a separate bottle of medication for each eye.

11. A medical assistant is performing an ear irrigation. The patient reports dizziness. These symptoms could be caused by which of the following?

    A. Pressure from the water has caused the cerumen to move.

    B. The speed at which the water is being introduced is too slow.

    C. Trapped air is increasing the pressure against the tympanic membrane.

    D. The temperature of the water is too cold.

12. A provider has instructed a medical assistant to prepare a wound for suturing. When performing basic wound care, which of the following steps should the medical assistant take to ensure proper cleansing of the wound area?

    A. Wipe the center of the wound with an antiseptic swab, moving toward the edges in a circular motion.

    B. Scrub the wound with an antiseptic swab in a back and forth motion for 5 min.

    C. Flood the wound with hydrogen peroxide prior to wiping it with sterile gauze.

    D. Cleanse the wound a minimum of three times using alcohol prep pads.

13. Which of the following patients should a medical assistant recognize as the top priority to receive immediate care?

    A. A patient has sustained an animal bite on the left leg and has a low-grade fever.

    B. A patient has had an episode of syncope but is are responsive and able to answer questions.

    C. A patient has a laceration on the right forearm and is bleeding from the site.

    D. A patient has epistaxis and is taking warfarin.

14. A medical assistant is assisting a provider with an adult patient who sustained a wound from a dirty metal object. Which of the following orders should the medical assistant expect the provider to give for the patient?

    A. "You do not need to receive a tetanus booster if you received the DTaP series as a child."

    B. "You should receive a tetanus booster if your last one was administered more than 2 years ago."

    C. "You should receive a tetanus booster if your last one was administered more than 5 years ago."

    D. "You should receive a tetanus booster every time a laceration occurs."

15. During a surgical procedure, a provider requests sterile solution from a medical assistant. Which of the following actions should the medical assistant take?

    A. Pick up the sterile solution bottle, remove the cap, and hand the bottle to the provider.

    B. Open the bottle, pour the contents into a container, and set the container on the sterile field.

    C. Place a sterile container on the field and pour a small amount of sterile solution into the container.

    D. Draw the sterile solution up in a syringe and place the syringe on the sterile field for the provider.

QUIZ 10: INFECTION CONTROL

1. A medical assistant receives a splash of potentially infectious material to the eyes while collecting a urine specimen. Which of the following actions should the medical assistant take to prevent the spread of infection?

    A. Rinse eyes with mild soap and water for 5 min.

    B. Flush eyes at an eyewash station for at least 15 min.

    C. Apply a cool compress to eyes for 1 hr.

    D. Massage eyes with a clean cloth for 10 min.

2. Which of the following concentrations of bleach solution should a medical assistant use as a disinfectant in a clinical setting?

    A. 1:10

    B. 1:5

    C. 1:20

    D. 1:1

3. Which of the following statements about alcohol-based hand sanitizer is correct?

    A. Hand sanitizer should be used when there is visible debris on the hands.

    B. Hand sanitizer should have at least 50% alcohol content.

    C. Hand sanitizer should be used in conjunction with a bleach solution.

    D. Hand sanitizer should be applied to dry hands.

4. Which of the following is recommended regarding fingernail care and hand hygiene?

    A. Wash hands under running water with the fingers pointing upward.

    B. Keep reusable cloth towels at handwashing stations.

    C. Trim natural fingernails to 1.3 cm (0.5 in) past the tip of the finger.

    D. Remove artificial nails when working with high-risk populations.

5. According to CDC recommendations, what is the minimum length of time a medical assistant should spend scrubbing hands with soap and water when performing hand hygiene?

    A. 10 seconds

    B. 15 seconds

    C. 20 seconds

    D. 25 seconds

6. A medical assistant is washing infectious debris off several sharp surgical instruments. Which of the following actions should the medical assistant take?

    A. Keep all hinged instruments closed.

    B. Use a soft-bristled brush to clean the surface of the instruments.

    C. Soak the instruments in a bleach solution to sterilize them prior to sanitization.

    D. Wear utility gloves while sanitizing the instruments.

7. Which of the following methods should a medical assistant use when storing a disinfected endoscope?

    A. Hang vertically

    B. Flat on a clean, dry surface

    C. An airtight container

    D. Its original container

8. A medical assistant is preparing to sterilize a vaginal speculum. Which of the following sterilization techniques should the medical assistant use?

    A. Ultrasonic

    B. Gas

    C. Autoclave

    D. Ionizing radiation

9. A medical assistant is loading prepackaged hemostats into an autoclave. Which of the following actions should the medical assistant take to ensure sterilization?

    A. Layer the packages so that they overlap one another.

    B. Alternate the packages with unwrapped instruments.

    C. Organize the packages loosely without touching the walls of the autoclave.

    D. Submerge the packages in disinfectant before placement in the autoclave.

10. A patient who is coughing and sneezing repeatedly enters the reception area at a clinic. Which of the following actions should a medical assistant take?

    A. Allow the patient to remain in the reception area.

    B. Assist the patient into an examination room.

    C. Notify the provider of the patient's condition immediately.

    D. Distribute masks to other patients in the reception area.

11. Which of the following steps should a medical assistant take to follow aseptic guidelines when administering injections?

    A. Don full personal protective equipment (PPE).

    B. Wipe the injection site with an alcohol pad.

    C. Dispose of the syringe with the needle pointed upward.

    D. Use the same needle for drawing and injecting.

12. Which of the following procedures requires a medical assistant to use aseptic technique?

    A. Cryosurgery

    B. Sonogram

    C. Sigmoidoscopy

    D. Suturing

13. Which of the following disposal methods should a medical assistant use in accordance with OSHA guidelines for handling biohazardous waste?

    A. Dispose of soiled bandages in a covered trash receptacle.

    B. Contact a local waste management company for disposal instructions.

    C. Label chemicals with their names and data before disposal.

    D. Place used syringes in a red biohazard bag.

14. A medical assistant is cleaning a room following a surgical procedure. Which of the following actions should the medical assistant take to ensure proper biohazardous waste handling of used gauze pads?

    A. Place the gauze pads in a red polyethylene bag.

    B. Dispose of the gauze pads in a covered trash bin.

    C. Soak the gauze pads in a sterilizing solution.

    D. Place the gauze pads in a sharps container.

15. A medical assistant is reviewing OSHA regulations regarding sharps container placement. In which of the following locations should the medical assistant place a sharps container?

    A. Reception area

    B. Centrally located between exam rooms

    C. Exam room

    D. Nurses' station

QUIZ 11: TESTING AND LABORATORY PROCEDURES

1. A medical assistant is instructing a patient on the collection of a clean-catch urine specimen for culture and sensitivity (C&S). Which of the following instructions should the medical assistant give the patient?

   A. "Void into a clean container and then transfer it into a sterile container."

   B. "Void into a sterile container directly after cleaning the perineum."

   C. "Void into a container from home and bring it to the office."

   D. "Void a small amount of urine into the toilet and then void the next portion into a sterile container."

2. A medical assistant is instructing a patient about collecting stool specimens at home for occult blood testing. Which of the following statements should the medical assistant make about the patient's medications?

   A. "Discontinue all your medications 72 hours before the test."

   B. "Take a laxative 24 hours prior to the test."

   C. "Discontinue any NSAIDs a week before the test."

   D. "Take 500 milligrams of a vitamin C supplement daily."

3. A medical assistant is preparing to perform a rapid strep test. Which of the following actions should the medical assistant take?

   A. Bring the reagents and devices to room temperature.

   B. Leave the swab in the solution for 5 min.

   C. Express the liquid from the swab with gloved fingers.

   D. Place the tip of the reagent bottle into the tube before dispensing.

4. A medical assistant reviews the results of a urine pregnancy test and sees that a blue line did not appear in the control area. This indicates which of the following?

   A. The pregnancy test is positive.

   B. The pregnancy test is not valid.

   C. The pregnancy test specimen is not concentrated.

   D. The pregnancy test is negative.

5. A medical assistant is performing a visual acuity test on an adult patient. The patient is able to read the 20/30 line with both eyes, but misses one letter. Which of the following results should the medical assistant document in the patient's medical record?

   A. 20/30-1 both eyes

   B. 20/30 left eye

   C. 20/30-1 right eye

   D. 20/20 both eyes

6. A medical assistant is performing a routine hearing test on a patient. Which of the following procedures measures a patient's hearing by using air and bone conduction?

   A. Audiometric test

   B. Otoscopic exam

   C. Tuning fork test

   D. Cerumen removal

7. A medical assistant is performing an allergen skin test. Which of the following actions should the medical assistant take?

   A. Notify the provider immediately if the patient demonstrates signs of anaphylaxis.

   B. Allow the patient to choose the thigh or stomach for the injection or application site.

   C. Stop the test immediately if the patient wheezes and sneezes.

   D. Continue allergen testing on areas where the patient has developed wheals or hives.

8. Which of the following sites should the medical assistant use for the administration of an intradermal skin test?

   A. Lateral thigh

   B. Lower abdomen

   C. Anterior forearm

   D. Inner heel

9. Which of the following instructions should a medical assistant provide to a patient prior to spirometry testing?

   A. "Use your inhaler prior to arriving for the test."

   B. "Avoid smoking for at least an hour prior to the test."

   C. "Wear tight clothing for the duration of the test."

   D. "Do not eat or drink anything at least 6 hours prior to the test."

10. A medical assistant is preparing to perform a pulmonary function test on a patient who is dressed in a suit and tie. When preparing the patient for the test, the medical assistant should instruct the patient to do which of the following?

    A. Sit with legs crossed.

    B. Undress from the waist up.

    C. Loosen the tie and top buttons.

    D. Point chin slightly toward the chest.

11. A medical assistant receives a call from a reference laboratory reporting a fasting blood glucose of 450 mg/dL for a patient. According to protocol, which of the following actions should the medical assistant take?

    A. Notify the provider of the test results.

    B. Place the results on the provider's desk for review.

    C. Have the provider speak to the laboratory.

    D. Contact the patient to have them come into the office.

12. A medical assistant is reviewing the results of a urine collection provided by an adult patient at the clinic. Which of the following laboratory results is outside of the expected reference range?

    A. pH 7.9

    B. pH 5.1

    C. Specific gravity 1.014

    D. Specific gravity 1.042

13. A medical assistant is collecting a specimen for testing. When is it appropriate for the medical assistant to label the specimen?

    A. Prior to collecting the specimen

    B. After collecting the specimen

    C. Prior to sending the specimen to a laboratory

    D. After laboratory processing of the specimen

14. A medical assistant is performing venipuncture. Which of the following pieces of information should be included on both the requisition form and the specimen label?

    A. Insurance information

    B. Patient's address

    C. Date of birth

    D. Provider's name

15. A medical assistant is assisting a provider with the collection of a fecal occult specimen. Which of the following statements about the collection is true?

    A. The specimen should be developed 1 min after collection.

    B. The results can be interpreted immediately after the developer is applied.

    C. Four drops of developer should be applied to the specimen.

    D. The result is positive if a trace of blue color is detected on the edge of the smear.

QUIZ 12: PHLEBOTOMY

1. Prior to performing a phlebotomy procedure, a medical assistant should ask the patient to verify which of the following information?

    A. Patient's account number

    B. Patient's power of attorney

    C. Patient's phone number

    D. Patient's date of birth

2. A medical assistant is obtaining samples for a CBC test. Which of the following tubes should the medical assistant select?

    A. Royal blue

    B. Lavender

    C. Yellow

    D. Gray

3. A medical assistant is obtaining a sample for a erythrocyte sedimentation rate (ESR) test. Which of the following tubes should the medical assistant use for blood collection?

    A. Serum separator

    B. Green

    C. Lavender

    D. Light blue

4. A medical assistant is performing phlebotomy on an 80-year-old patient who has small veins. Which of the following venipuncture methods should the medical assistant use for this patient?

    A. Finger puncture

    B. Evacuated tube

    C. Heel stick

    D. Butterfly needle

5. Which of the following veins is the preferred vein for routine phlebotomy?
   A. Basilic
   B. Cephalic
   C. Median cubital
   D. Median antebrachial

6. When drawing blood cultures, a medical assistant should prepare a patient's skin using which of the following products?
   A. Hydrogen peroxide
   B. Glutaraldehyde
   C. Sterile water
   D. Iodine solution

7. To avoid hemoconcentration during venipuncture, which of the following actions should a medical assistant take?
   A. Apply an ice pack to the area.
   B. Remove the tourniquet before 1 min has elapsed.
   C. Instruct the patient to keep the arm bent.
   D. Insert the needle into the vein with the bevel down.

8. Which of the following tubes should a medical assistant select first when adhering to the proper order of draw?
   A. Red
   B. Yellow
   C. Green
   D. Gray

9. Which of the following digits is the preferred site for capillary puncture on an adult patient?
   A. Fifth
   B. Fourth
   C. Second
   D. First

10. A medical assistant removes a needle from the antecubital space of a patient following a phlebotomy procedure and applies pressure. Which of the following steps should the medical assistant take next?
    A. Apply a bandage.
    B. Label the tubes.
    C. Dispose of the needle.
    D. Confirm the ordered tests.

11. A medical assistant should allow a serum specimen tube without an anticoagulant additive to stand for which of the following lengths of time prior to centrifuge?
    A. 2 hr
    B. 15 min
    C. 45 min
    D. 20 min

12. At which point during a venipuncture process should a medical assistant label the blood specimen tube?
    A. Before the patient is discharged
    B. After the patient is discharged
    C. Prior to venipuncture
    D. During venipuncture

13. A medical assistant has completed a blood collection. Which of the following actions should the medical assistant take to ensure proper specimen processing?
    A. Verify that the requisition form has been completed.
    B. Provide the patient with postprocedure instructions.
    C. Place all specimens in the refrigerator.
    D. Centrifuge all blood tubes collected.

14. When reviewing blood work results, a medical assistant notices a fasting blood glucose of 200 mg/dL. Which of the following actions should the medical assistant take?
    A. Notify the patient's provider of the results.
    B. Inform the patient that the results confirm diabetes.
    C. Schedule the patient for a same-day appointment.
    D. Send the provider an urgent alert.

15. After receiving blood test results from the reference laboratory, which of the following actions should the medical assistant take?
    A. Have a provider review the lab results.
    B. Have the medical records staff review the lab results.
    C. Interpret the lab results and contact the patient.
    D. Schedule the patient for a follow-up appointment.

QUIZ 13: EKG AND CARDIOVASCULAR TESTING

1. A medical assistant is preparing a patient who has shortness of breath for an EKG. In which of the following positions should the assistant place the patient?

   A. Prone

   B. Semi-Fowler's

   C. Supine

   D. Sims'

2. A medical assistant is preparing a patient for an EKG. Which of the following instructions should the medical assistant provide?

   A. "Avoid food or drink for 4 hours prior to the test."

   B. "Remove all clothing from the waist up."

   C. "Apply moisturizing lotion to the electrode placement sites."

   D. "Maintain a full bladder for the duration of the test."

3. A medical assistant is preparing to perform an EKG recording on a patient. Which of the following information is true of limb leads and electrodes?

   A. Limb leads are unipolar.

   B. Leads V1 through V6 are limb leads.

   C. Limb leads are placed on the fleshy areas of the skin.

   D. The left leg lead wire serves as the ground.

4. A medical assistant is calibrating an EKG machine. Which of the following should the assistant identify as the standard speed of the recording?

   A. 25 mm/second

   B. 50 mm/second

   C. 10 mm/second

   D. 5 mm/second

5. A medical assistant is preparing a patient for an EKG. In which of the following locations should the assistant place the V4 lead?

   A. 5th intercostal space at the anterior axillary line

   B. 5th intercostal space at the midaxillary line

   C. Midway between V3 and V5

   D. 5th intercostal space at the midclavicular line

6. A medical assistant notes a wandering baseline throughout an EKG tracing. Which of the following electrocardiograph issues could have resulted in this occurrence?

   A. The electrode pads were defective or poorly attached.

   B. The machine was missing the grounding prong for the outlet.

   C. The machine did not have the proper standardization settings set.

   D. The cable tips were loose or had become separated.

7. A medical assistant notices rhythmic sharp spikes throughout an EKG tracing. Which of the following artifacts is occurring?

   A. Wandering baseline

   B. Interrupted baseline

   C. Interference

   D. Somatic tremor

8. What is the ratio of applied leads to recorded leads for a standard EKG machine?

   A. 10:10

   B. 3:6

   C. 10:12

   D. 9:12

9. When performing an EKG, a medical assistant notices a widened QRS complex on the patient's EKG strip. Which of the following is a possible cause of this type of artifact?

   A. Atrial fibrillation

   B. Bradycardia

   C. Sinus dysrhythmia

   D. Premature ventricular contraction

10. Which of the following is a state of cellular rest and is represented by a flatline on an EKG strip?

    A. Myocardial infarction

    B. Polarization

    C. Premature atrial contraction

    D. Somatic tremor

11. An EKG tracing shows an expected P wave, QRS complex, and T wave configuration. There are five complete cardiac cycles on a 6-second strip. This represents which of the following cardiac rhythms?

    A. Sinus bradycardia

    B. Atrial fibrillation

    C. Ventricular fibrillation

    D. Sinus tachycardia

12. A medical assistant is providing instructions to a female patient prior to a stress test. Which of the following instructions should the medical assistant include?

    A. "Eat a large meal before coming to the test."

    B. "You should wear a dress on the day of the test."

    C. "Take your medications on the day of the test."

    D. "You can wear sandals when completing the test."

13. A medical assistant is providing teaching to a patient who is to undergo Holter monitoring. Which of the following information should the medical assistant include?

    A. "You can place a piece of tape over the electrode if it becomes loose."

    B. "You can wear the monitor while you take a shower."

    C. "You should refrain from doing your usual activities."

    D. "Your diary should focus on your food intake."

14. A provider requests a rhythm strip in addition to a regular EKG tracing for a patient. The medical assistant should identify that which of the following leads provides the clearest recording of the heart rhythm?

    A. I

    B. II

    C. III

    D. V2

15. A medical assistant is performing an EKG on a patient who has a heart rate of 105/min. The medical assistant should identify this finding as an indication of which of the following conditions?

    A. Sinus rhythm

    B. Atrial fibrillation

    C. Bradycardia

    D. Tachycardia

QUIZ 14: PATIENT CARE COORDINATION AND EDUCATION

1. Which of the following describes the purpose of a patient's discharge summary in a provider's office?

   A. Give a complete record of the patient's hospitalization

   B. Document information necessary for continuity of care

   C. Complete authorization requests for hospitalization

   D. Provide the patient with information about the diagnosis

2. A medical assistant is reviewing the chart of a patient who is scheduled for an appointment later that day. Which of the following tasks should the medical assistant complete prior to the patient's appointment?

   A. Verify the patient's known allergies.

   B. Refill any medications needed.

   C. Confirm all pertinent information is available.

   D. Pre-order tests for the follow-up visit.

3. Which of the following actions is important for a medical assistant to take to serve patients effectively?

   A. Avoid referencing patients' barriers to wellness.

   B. Instruct patients to refer to family members for assistance options.

   C. Work independently from the clinical staff.

   D. Assist patients with locating appropriate community resources.

4. Which of the following community resources should a medical assistant recommend to an older adult patient who lost his partner 3 months ago?

   A. Department of Health and Human Services

   B. Parks and recreation department

   C. Organized support groups

   D. Hospice care centers

5. A patient has a new diagnosis of malignant melanoma. When transitioning the patient's care from a primary care provider (PCP) to an oncologist, which of the following processes is the PCP taking part in?

   A. Quality control

   B. Audit

   C. Continuity of care

   D. Termination of care

6. A medical assistant is caring for a patient who has a new medication prescription from a provider. Which of the following actions should the medical assistant take to facilitate patient understanding and medication adherence?

   A. Instruct the patient to discontinue the medication once symptoms subside.

   B. Review the dosage and administration instructions with the patient.

   C. Recommend possible over-the-counter replacements for the medication.

   D. Inform the patient that side effects are expected and do not need to be reported.

7. Which of the following approaches should a medical assistant take when discussing a patient's adherence to dietary guidelines?

   A. Maintain an empathetic tone.

   B. Deliver the information quickly.

   C. Avoid providing written instructions.

   D. Maintain a closed posture.

8. Recognizing patients' needs and barriers, coordinating care, and identifying resources to meet those needs best describes the responsibilities of which of the following positions?

   A. Physician assistant

   B. Nurse practitioner

   C. Emergency provider

   D. Patient navigator

9. A patient-centered medical home (PCMH) has five core functions and attributes. Which of the following features is included in those functions?

   A. Ambulatory services

   B. Comprehensive care

   C. Electronic health records incentives

   D. Affordable health care

10. A medical assistant should identify which of the following features as part of the patient-centered medical home (PCMH) model of care?

    A. Focuses on evidence-based patient care and shared decision-making

    B. Adheres to a uniform plan of care for patients who have similar diagnoses

    C. Identifies the provider as the primary source of comprehensive care for the patient

    D. Provides stability by adhering to industry-standard office hours and accessibility

11. When reviewing a patient's medical record prior to an appointment with a primary care provider (PCP), it is important for a medical assistant to verify that which of the following items is in the chart?
    A. Current medication list
    B. Updated insurance card
    C. Specialist authorization form
    D. Diagnostic test results

12. Which of the following information should a medical assistant include when creating a list of community-based organizations related to a patient's physical health care needs?
    A. Board of directors
    B. Volunteer opportunities
    C. Physical addresses
    D. Cost of services

13. A medical assistant is reviewing the plan of care summary with the adult son of an 81-year-old patient who has dementia. The patient's son states he is feeling overwhelmed with his mother's care. Which of the following community-based organizations should the medical assistant recommend?
    A. Hospice services
    B. Grief support
    C. Rehabilitation services
    D. Adult day care

14. Which of the following actions involves health coaching?
    A. Helping patients find community resources related to health care needs
    B. Directing patients to an agency that can refer them to a specialist
    C. Encouraging patients to live a sedentary lifestyle
    D. Meeting Medicare's Meaningful Use criteria

15. A medical assistant is part of a team that is caring for a patient who is being discharged from the hospital. Which of the following actions would contribute to a successful transition of care?
    A. The provider discontinues all medications started in the hospital and relays the information to the rest of the team.
    B. The medical assistant schedules a meeting with the medical staff members of the team.
    C. The provider receives laboratory results and reviews them alone prior to filing.
    D. The medical assistant follows up with the patient 1 week after discharge from the hospital.

QUIZ 15: ADMINISTRATIVE ASSISTING

1. A medical assistant is helping a patient check out. Which of the following actions should the medical assistant take?
    A. Ask the patient for a photo ID.
    B. Have the patient fill out a registration form.
    C. Review the patient's medical record.
    D. Verify the patient's insurance policy.

2. Which of the following resources provides a standard language for services provided during a medical visit?
    A. Centers for Medicare and Medicaid Services
    B. International Classification of Diseases, Tenth Revision
    C. Centers for Disease Control and Prevention
    D. Current Procedural Terminology manual

3. A medical assistant receives instructions from a primary care provider to refer a patient to a dermatologist. Which of the following actions should the medical assistant take first?
    A. Complete a patient referral form.
    B. Give the patient a copy of the authorization code.
    C. Obtain prior authorization.
    D. Document the date of referral approval.

4. A medical assistant is posting charges to a patient's account. The medical assistant should obtain the necessary information from which of the following sources?
    A. Pegboard system
    B. Fee profile
    C. Fee schedule
    D. Itemized statement

5. Which of the following terms describes the act of unlawfully increasing the reimbursement amount from a third-party payer?
   A. Downcoding
   B. E/M codes
   C. Add-on codes
   D. Upcoding

6. A medical assistant is performing bookkeeping duties using the office's EHR software. For which of the following reasons should the medical assistant enter an adjustment on a patient's account?
   A. Nonsufficient funds check
   B. Duplicate payment
   C. Insurance refund
   D. Insurance disallowance

7. A medical assistant is performing claim submission for a medical office. Which of the following processes involves the electronic auditing and sorting of claims?
   A. Clearinghouse submission
   B. Direct billing
   C. Intelligent character recognition
   D. Universal claim form

8. Which of the following methods of filing paper medical records involves placing newer reports on top of older reports?
   A. Alphabetic
   B. Purging
   C. Shingling
   D. Numeric

9. Which of the following medical record content areas includes a patient's demographic data?
   A. Objective
   B. Assessment
   C. Subjective
   D. Plan

10. A provider notifies a medical assistant that she will be arriving 20 min late to the office. Which of the following actions should the medical assistant take?
    A. Cancel the next scheduled patient's appointment.
    B. Tell the next scheduled patient that she has to see a different provider.
    C. Notify the next scheduled patient about the delay.
    D. Have the next scheduled patient wait in an exam room.

11. Which of the following terms describes a collection of associated files that function as a basis for retrieving information?
    A. Cookies
    B. Cache
    C. Queries
    D. Database

12. Which the following resources provides information about the use of chemicals in a medical facility?
    A. Safety data sheet (SDS)
    B. OSHA Form 301
    C. Emergency action plan
    D. Code of Federal Regulations (CFR)

13. A medical assistant is performing inventory for a clinic. Which of the following actions should the medical assistant take?
    A. Prepare a purchase order.
    B. Dispose of all unused medical supplies.
    C. Review the clinic's overhead costs.
    D. Send an invoice to the supply vendor.

14. In which of the following categories would a medical assistant find a wheelchair listed?
    A. Consumable item
    B. Expendable item
    C. Intangible item
    D. Durable item

15. Which of the following allows a patient to confirm or cancel an appointment remotely?
    A. Automated call routing
    B. Appointment cards
    C. Wave scheduling
    D. Advanced booking

QUIZ 16: COMMUNICATION AND CUSTOMER SERVICE

1. A medical assistant is checking in a patient who does not speak the same language as the medical assistant. Which of the following actions should the medical assistant take?

    A. Ask a bilingual staff member to assist with communication.

    B. Address the patient by first name.

    C. Use medical terminology when speaking to the patient.

    D. Avoid using body gestures when communicating.

2. A medical assistant is speaking with a patient. Which of the following might occur as a barrier to communication?

    A. Empathy

    B. Rapport

    C. Active listening

    D. Stereotyping

3. A medical assistant is checking in a patient who has hearing loss. Which of the following actions should the medical assistant take?

    A. Speak loudly to the patient.

    B. Stand within the patient's field of vision.

    C. Use firm touch to get the patient's attention.

    D. Minimize hand gestures when speaking.

4. A medical assistant is providing discharge instructions for a patient who has visually impairment. Which of the following actions should the medical assistant take?

    A. Use a low tone when communicating.

    B. Notify the patient when entering the room.

    C. Use body gestures when communicating.

    D. Provide small-font printed material.

5. A patient calls into the office to report that a medication is not working. Which of the following responses should the medical assistant make?

    A. "I will notify the provider about your situation."

    B. "You should keep taking the medication until it works."

    C. "You should double the dose of the medication."

    D. "I will call the pharmacy to authorize a refill for your medication."

6. During the admission process, a patient explains manifestations of a chief complaint to a medical assistant. Which of the following actions should the medical assistant take?

    A. Provide advice about temporary relief measures.

    B. Document the patient's concerns in the medical record.

    C. Reassure the patient that there is no immediate cause for worry.

    D. Evaluate the relevance of the patient's concerns.

7. When communicating on the telephone with a patient, which of the following actions by a medical assistant demonstrates the use of appropriate technique for outgoing calls?

    A. Placing the patient on hold when accessing information

    B. Speaking with an unchanging pitch

    C. Holding the receiver a minimum 5 cm (2 in) from the mouth

    D. Allowing the patient to be the one to end the call

8. A medical assistant is preparing business correspondence. Which of the following is a characteristic of the modified block letter style?

    A. Each paragraph is indented.

    B. The signature is in all capital letters.

    C. All lines are flush with the left margin.

    D. The complimentary closing is centered on the page.

9. In which of the following locations should the inside address appear in a business letter?

    A. Between the letterhead and the dateline

    B. Between the dateline and the salutation

    C. Between the salutation and the subject line

    D. Between the signature block and the identification line

10. A medical assistant is caring for a patient who is frustrated and states, "My doctor doesn't have any idea how to treat my condition." Which of the following responses by the medical assistant is an example of therapeutic communication?

    A. "Your provider is doing everything she can to help you."

    B. "Don't you want your provider to keep trying to help you get better?"

    C. "Are you saying that you don't think your provider knows how to help you?"

    D. "If you don't remain calm, we'll have to ask you to leave the office."

11. A medical assistant is approached by a patient who is angry and yelling. Which of the following actions should the medical assistant take?

    A. Display emotion.

    B. Remain calm.

    C. Avoid apologizing.

    D. Speak loudly.

12. A patient in a waiting room approaches a medical assistant and states, "I've been waiting 30 minutes to see my doctor. Can't you do something?" Which of the following responses by the medical assistant is an example of active listening?

    A. "You sound frustrated about how long you've been waiting."

    B. "You won't have to wait much longer. I promise."

    C. "You don't want to leave and miss your appointment, do you?"

    D. "Maybe you should file a complaint and reschedule the appointment."

13. A medical assistant is engaging in conversation with a patient who was recently terminated from the practice. The patient has come to the office and is demanding an explanation. Which of the following actions should the medical assistant take?

    A. Dissociate from the conversation.

    B. Sympathize with the patient.

    C. Defend the provider's decision.

    D. Acknowledge the patient's concern.

14. To be a successful member of a team, which of the following actions should a medical assistant take?

    A. Include personal feelings in work decisions.

    B. Report all team conflict to the supervisor.

    C. Focus on achieving individual goals.

    D. Demonstrate willingness to perform extra duties.

15. Which of the following elements is essential for successful teamwork?

    A. Related short-term and long-term goals

    B. Large number of members

    C. Similar abilities and skill sets

    D. Suppression of negative information

QUIZ 17: MEDICAL LAW AND ETHICS

1. Employers are accountable for providing a safe and healthy workplace for employees by setting and enforcing standards. This environment is achieved by providing training, outreach, education, and assistance. Which of the following regulatory agencies oversees this standard?
   A. Centers for Disease Control and Prevention (CDC)
   B. Occupational Safety and Health Administration (OSHA)
   C. National Institutes of Health (NIH)
   D. Department of Health and Human Services (HHS)

2. A medical assistant witnesses a coworker knowingly commit an unlawful and wrongful act. The medical assistant should identify this act as which of the following types of negligence?
   A. Misfeasance
   B. Malpractice
   C. Malfeasance
   D. Misdemeanor

3. A medical assistant sees a coworker take a pain medication from a locked cabinet. The medical assistant knows that the coworker is a single parent who has a child who was recently injured. Which of the following types of ethical situations does this problem create for the medical assistant?
   A. Ethical dilemma
   B. Locus of authority issue
   C. Dilemma of justice
   D. Ethical distress

4. Which of the following moral codes should a medical assistant reference when facing an ethical dilemma?
   A. AMA Code of Ethics
   B. Hippocratic Oath
   C. Code of Hammurabi
   D. Percival's Code

5. Which of the following is the legal document that states the life-saving procedures a patient authorizes in the event he is incapable of verbalizing his desire for medical treatment?
   A. Organ and tissue donation consent
   B. Living will
   C. Durable power of attorney for health care
   D. Do-not-resuscitate order

6. Once advance directives are in place, they can be updated at which of the following times?
   A. Never
   B. Any time
   C. Every 10 years
   D. Annually

7. When designating a medical power of attorney, which of the following people is an acceptable choice for a health care proxy?
   A. Patient's provider
   B. Executor of the patient's will
   C. Member of the patient's faith community
   D. Patient's attorney

8. A patient expresses to a medical assistant that he would like to designate his daughter as his health care proxy. Which of the following is the minimum age to be eligible as a health care proxy?
   A. 14
   B. 16
   C. 21
   D. 18

9. Which of the following provides instructions for an emergency medical technician to follow when transporting an elderly or critically ill patient?
   A. Medical Order for Life-Sustaining Treatment
   B. Uniform Anatomical Gift Act
   C. Patient Self-Determination Act
   D. Patient's Bill of Rights

10. A medical assistant is assisting a provider with a gynecological examination. The patient says, "My religious beliefs do not allow me to use contraception." The medical assistant should expect the provider to make which of the following statements?

   A. "You have the right to make choices regarding your health."

   B. "You should reconsider your stance on contraception."

   C. "I am your provider, so you need to listen to my advice."

   D. "I am very concerned about the potential consequences to your health."

11. Which of the following gives patients the rights over their health care information, including the right to receive a copy of their information, the right to ensure their medical records are correct, and the right to know who had access to their records?

   A. Americans with Disabilities Act (ADA)

   B. Health Insurance Portability and Accountability Act (HIPAA)

   C. Family Medical Leave Act (FMLA)

   D. Protected health information (PHI)

12. Which of the following entities must adhere to HIPAA guidelines?

   A. Workers' compensation

   B. Public health authorities

   C. State agencies

   D. Health care clearinghouses

13. A medical assistant left a computer unlocked with a patient's chart visible. Which of the following actions should the medical assistant take in the future to prevent unauthorized viewing of patient information?

   A. Place privacy filters on the monitor screen.

   B. Set up encryption software.

   C. Install firewalls.

   D. Perform a records audit.

14. A patient believes that her health care privacy has been violated. The patient's complaint must be filed within how many days?

   A. 30

   B. 90

   C. 180

   D. 365

15. When measuring the vital signs of a 10-year-old child, a medical assistant recognizes indications of abuse. Which of the following actions should the medical assistant take?

   A. Notify the child's school counselor.

   B. Question the child.

   C. Question the child's parent.

   D. Notify the child's provider.

QUIZ ANSWERS

Quiz 1: Answer key

1. A. An occupational therapist assists patients who have loss of function resulting from an illness, injury, or disability to relearn activities of daily living.

   B. An emergency medical technician provides emergency medical care and transports patients to a hospital facility for treatment.

   C. CORRECT. A physical therapist assists patients with regaining mobility and improving strength and range of motion.

   D. A radiology technician uses equipment to help providers diagnose and treat some diseases.

2. A. CORRECT. An otolaryngologist specializes in diseases of the ear, nose, and throat, as well as conditions that affect the head and neck.

   B. An anesthesiologist specializes in pain management during medical procedures and surgeries.

   C. A neurologist specializes in disorders of the nervous system.

   D. An ophthalmologist specializes in the treatment and care of the eye and surrounding structures.

3. A. Registered nurses are required to maintain a license based on state requirements, but they are not legally responsible for the outcomes of the medical assistant's duties and performance.

   B. CORRECT. A licensed health care provider, such as a family practitioner, is legally responsible for the outcomes of the medical assistant's duties and performance.

   C. Office managers are not licensed health care professionals. They are not legally responsible for the outcomes of the medical assistant's duties and performance.

   D. Pharmacy technicians are required to maintain registration based on state requirements, but they are not legally responsible for the outcomes of the medical assistant's duties and performance.

4. A. Medical assistants cannot prescribe medication, but they can request medications or call in a refill request with the provider's prescription.

   B. CORRECT. Medical assistants can independently record vital signs.

   C. Giving medical advice is outside of the medical assistant's scope of practice.

   D. Medical assistants can provide medication samples only when the provider has prescribed them.

5. A. Immunologists specialize in diseases and disorders of the immune system.

   B. Cardiologists specialize in diagnosing and treating diseases or conditions of the heart and blood vessels.

   C. Pathologists specialize in the study of tissues, cells, and organs to help determine the etiology of diseases.

   D. CORRECT. Urologists specialize in the treatment of diseases and disorders of the urinary tract, including interstitial cystitis.

6. A. A physical medicine and rehabilitation specialist assists patients of all ages with restoring function after an injury.

   B. A pediatrician specializes in child development and treats children and adolescents.

   C. A pathologist studies the cause of various diseases. Many pathologists also perform autopsies to determine what might have caused a patient's death.

   D. CORRECT. Preventive medicine specialists evaluate mental illness, physical illness, and disability through analyzing patient health needs. They also provide health education to patients of all ages.

7. A. CORRECT. Medical assistants are eligible to obtain registration or certification on an optional basis, but it is not required to secure employment within the health care industry. The health care facility decides whether the medical assistant needs to be certified for the position.

   B. Physician assistants are required to have a master's degree and a state license to practice and secure employment within the health care industry.

   C. Diagnostic radiologists are required to have a doctorate's degree and a license to practice and secure employment within the health care industry.

   D. Anesthesiologists are required to have a doctorate's degree and a license to practice and secure employment within the health care industry.

8. A. The assistant should expect to contact a gastroenterologist for patients who have a disorder of the esophagus, stomach, or intestines. Hyperthyroidism is a disorder of the thyroid gland.

   B. CORRECT. An endocrinologist specializes in treating patients who have a hormonal disorder, such as diabetes mellitus or hyperthyroidism.

   C. The assistant should expect to contact a urologist for patients who have a disorder of the bladder or kidneys. Hyperthyroidism is a disorder of the thyroid gland.

   D. The assistant should expect to contact a cardiologist for patients who have a disorder of the heart or blood vessels. Hyperthyroidism is a disorder of the thyroid gland.

9. A. Hospice is organized care provided by nurses, nursing assistants, and volunteers to patients who have life-limiting illnesses and their families. Patients are not directly involved in the organization process of this health care delivery model.

   B. Home health agencies provide in-home services by skilled health care professionals to minimize the effects of disabilities or diseases and to restore patients' overall health. Patients are not directly involved in the organization process of this health care delivery model.

   C. ACOs are a collaboration of physicians and health care staff whose goal is to re-establish the cost and quality of health care to patients. Patients are not directly involved in the organization process of this health care delivery model.

   D. CORRECT. PCMHs are health care delivery models coordinated through a patient's primary care provider. The five core attributes of PCMHs are comprehensive care, patient-centered care, coordinated care, accessible services, and quality and safety.

10. A. The PPO model has more flexibility than the HMO model. Patients do not need a primary care provider's referral to see a specialist.

B. The pay-for-performance model ensures providers are only compensated if they meet certain measures for quality and efficiency.

C. CORRECT. The HMO model contracts with a medical center or group of providers to provide preventive and acute care for insured patients. HMOs require referrals for specialists, outpatient procedures, treatments, precertification, preauthorization, and hospital admissions.

D. The EPO model shares features of the HMO and PPO models. Patients can choose from a network of providers, but they do not need a referral to see a specialist.

11. A. Internists specialize in the treatment of adults.

B. Specialists diagnose and treat disorders of specific body systems, not a wide variety of illnesses.

C. Pediatricians specialize in the treatment of patients from infancy through adolescence.

D. CORRECT. Family practitioners treat patients of all ages for all types of illnesses.

12. A. Respiratory therapy assists patients who have respiratory illnesses and other cardiopulmonary conditions.

B. Massage therapy uses manual techniques to positively affect the health and well-being of a patient.

C. CORRECT. Physical therapy assists patients who need therapeutic intervention to regain motor functions and independence, such as patients who have had a CVA.

D. Behavioral therapy assists patients who have behavioral, emotional, or mental disorders, as well as disorders of the brain and central nervous system.

13. A. Acupuncture treatments involve pricking the skin or tissues with needles. Acupuncture might help relieve spinal pain, but it would not treat the subluxation.

B. CORRECT. Chiropractic care is a form of alternative medicine that diagnoses and treats disorders of the musculoskeletal system. Chiropractors treat subluxations, or misalignments, of the spine.

C. Biofeedback helps patients relax by recognizing bodily functions. It also teaches patients how to control their physiologic responses to stress.

D. Herbal medicine uses plant-based products to promote health and treat symptoms. Herbal medicine might help relieve spinal pain, but it would not treat the subluxation.

14. A. A deductible is the amount of money a patient must pay out of pocket before an insurance carrier begins paying.

B. Coinsurance is a policy provision frequently found in medical insurance where an insurance company and the policyholder share the cost of covered charges in a specified ratio, such as 80:20.

C. A fee schedule is a list of charges for procedures and services performed in the provider's office.

D. CORRECT. The allowable amount is the maximum reimbursement a third-party payer will provide for a particular procedure or service.

15. A. The Social Security Amendments of 1965 created Medicare and Medicaid, resulting in the development of CHAMPUS/CHAMPVA, now referred to as Tricare.

B. Medicare was established in 1965.

C. CORRECT. Blue Cross/Blue Shield was founded in 1929. It is the oldest and largest insurance entity in the U.S.

D. Medicaid was established in 1965.

Quiz 2: Answer key

1. A. KUB is an acronym that stands for kidneys, ureter, and bladder. This acronym is typically used on diagnostic imaging forms to identify the area to be imaged.

B. LMP is an abbreviation commonly used to refer to a patient's last menstrual period.

C. PID is an abbreviation for pelvic inflammatory disease, an infection of the female reproductive organs.

D. CORRECT. BMI is an abbreviation for body mass index. BMI is a measure of body fat that helps identify a patient's nutritional status and need for weight management. Besides using a BMI calculator or chart, the medical assistant can calculate this value by dividing a patient's weight in kilograms by height in meters squared.

2. A. The abbreviations for greater than (>) and less than (<) are on the error-prone abbreviation list and should not be used in medical chart notation. These symbols can be misinterpreted as the number 7 or the letter L.

B. CORRECT. O_2 is the abbreviation for oxygen and is approved for use in medical chart notation.

C. $MgSO_4$ is the abbreviation for magnesium sulfate and is on the error-prone abbreviation list. It should not be used in medical chart notation because it can be misinterpreted as the abbreviation for morphine sulfate.

D. μg is the abbreviation for microgram and is on the error-prone abbreviation list. It should not be used in medical chart notation because it can be misinterpreted as milligrams (mg).

3. A. CORRECT. The medical assistant should identify Rx as the abbreviation for prescription.

B. Tx is an abbreviation for treatment.

C. Sx is an abbreviation for symptoms.

D. Hx is an abbreviation for history.

4. A. The abbreviation HPI stands for history of present illness and would not pertain to a wellness visit. It is not used when documenting a patient's assessment data prior to a wellness examination.

B. The abbreviation p/o is used to refer to a patient's postoperative status and would not be used when documenting a patient's assessment data prior to a wellness examination.

C. CORRECT. The abbreviation VS stands for vital signs and is a notation that precedes measurements of physiological functioning, specifically temperature, heart rate, respiratory rate, and blood pressure. It can also include pain severity and oxygen saturation.

D. The abbreviation f/u stands for follow up. It would be used when a patient is seen for reevaluation for an illness or injury. This abbreviation would not be used when documenting a patient's assessment data prior to a wellness examination.

5. A. Audiometry measures a patient's ability to hear and does not produce images of body structures.

B. Electromyography detects nerve impulses and the electrical activity of muscle tissue. It does not produce images of body structures.

C. CORRECT. Computed tomography, commonly referred to as a CT scan, is a radiographic imaging procedure used to produce three-dimensional cross sections of body structures for diagnostic purposes.

D. A Holter monitor is a portable cardiac monitoring device used to record cardiac activity over 24 hr or longer. It does not produce images of body structures.

6. A. A barium enema is a diagnostic procedure that involves instilling a radiopaque contrast medium into the rectum and colon to help diagnose various disorders. This procedure takes place in the radiology department, not in the laboratory.

B. CORRECT. Blood urea nitrogen is a laboratory test that helps determine the adequacy of renal function by identifying the levels of urea nitrogen in the blood.

C. Computed tomography, commonly referred to as a CT scan, is a diagnostic procedure that takes place in the nuclear medicine department, not in the laboratory.

D. Benign prostatic hyperplasia is a medical condition, not a diagnostic test. It is a noncancerous enlargement of the prostate gland.

7. A. CORRECT. Rheumatoid arthritis is an inflammatory disease that causes pain, swelling, and deformity in the joints, especially in the hands and feet.

B. Multiple sclerosis is a disorder that involves the destruction of myelin, a fatty material that insulates nerve cells and helps them conduct impulses.

C. Osteoporosis is a loss of bone density that results in bones becoming porous and susceptible to fracture.

D. A carcinoma is a cancerous tumor, often found in glands or the skin.

8. A. With a stethoscope, a provider can determine a patient's heart rate and, to some extent, the rhythm, but this device does not record heart rhythm.

B. An electroencephalogram machine produces a record of the brain's electrical activity. It does not record a patient's heart rhythm.

C. A sphygmomanometer is used to measure blood pressure. It does not record a patient's heart rhythm.

D. CORRECT. An electrocardiogram machine produces a record of the heart's electrical impulses, rate, and rhythm. It detects dysrhythmias, which are abnormalities in cardiac rhythm.

9. A. The root "encephal" means brain, and the suffix "pathy" means disorder or disease. Adding a connecting vowel creates "encephalopathy," which means brain disorder.

B. The root "hem" means blood, and the suffix "lysis" means to loosen, dissolve, or disintegrate. Adding a connecting vowel creates "hemolysis," which is the breakdown or disintegration of blood cells.

C. The root "trache" means airway or windpipe, and the suffix "ostomy" means making an opening into. This combination creates tracheostomy, which is the creation of an opening into the trachea, or windpipe, to bypass a problem in the upper airway that is making it difficult or impossible for the patient to breathe.

D. CORRECT. The root "oophor" means ovary, and the suffix "ectomy" means removal or excision. Oophorectomy is the surgical removal of the ovaries.

10. A. The root "oto" means ear, and the suffix "dynia" means pain. Otodynia means pain in the ear.

B. The root "rhino" means nose, and the suffix "rrhea" means flow or discharge. Rhinorrhea means runny nose.

C. CORRECT. The root "myringo" means tympanic membrane (eardrum), and the suffix "otomy" means cutting into. Myringotomy is making an incision into the eardrum to drain fluid or relieve pressure that is causing ear pain or infection.

D. The root "lith" means stones, and the suffix "tripsy" means surgical crushing. Lithotripsy is a surgical procedure that breaks up stones, such as kidney stones or gallstones.

11. A. CORRECT. The prefix "presby" means old age, and the suffix "opia" means vision. Together, these word parts create presbyopia, which means the loss of near vision that develops with aging due to the loss of elasticity of the lens of the eye.

B. The prefix "osteo" means bone, and the suffix "malacia" means weakening or softening. Together, these word parts create osteomalacia, which means a weakening of the bones.

C. Ptosis is drooping of the upper eyelid. Ptosis can involve the upper eyelid covering the eye totally or partially.

D. The prefix "neph" means kidney, and the suffix "itis" means infection. Together, these word parts create nephritis, which means kidney infection.

12. A. The prefix "ox" means oxygen, and the suffix "metry" means measurement. Oximetry is the measurement of oxygen saturation.

B. CORRECT. The prefix "brady" means slow, and the suffix "pnea" means breathing. Bradypnea is slow breathing.

C. The prefix "neur" means nerve, and the suffix "algia" means pain. Neuralgia is nerve pain.

D. The prefix "tachy" means fast, and the suffix "cardi" refers to the heart. Tachycardia is a rapid heart rate.

13. A. Inferior means below or directed downward.

B. CORRECT. The prefix "contra" means against or in opposition to, and the suffix "lateral" means side. Contralateral means on the opposite side.

C. Superior means above or directed upward.

D. The prefix "ipsi" means same and the suffix "lateral" means side. Ipsilateral means on the same side.

14. A. In Fowler's position, the patient is sitting up. It would be difficult for the provider to perform a rectal examination with the patient in this position.

B. In the lithotomy position, the patient is lying on the back with knees bent. Although it is possible to perform a rectal examination with the patient in this position, another position is necessary for an efficient rectal examination.

C. In the Trendelenburg position, the patient is lying on the back with head lower than legs. This position does not facilitate a rectal examination.

D. CORRECT. In Sims' position, the patient is lying on one side with the upper leg drawn toward the abdomen. Sims' position is optimal for a rectal examination because it facilitates both physical examination and visualization.

15. A. CORRECT. Distal means situated away from the trunk of the body, and proximal means situated closer to the trunk of the body. The medical assistant should move from distal to proximal when applying a compression bandage to help decrease swelling.

B. A posterior point is behind or at the back of the body, and an anterior point is in front of or at the front of the body. The bandage that the medical assistant is applying is not described as being applied from back to front.

C. Proximal means closer to the trunk of the body, and distal means farthest from the trunk of the body. When a bandage application moves from the nearest point to the farthest point, the progression is proximal to distal.

D. A posterior point is behind or at the back of the body, and an anterior point is in front of or at the front of the body. The bandage that the medical assistant is applying is not described as being applied from front to back.

Quiz 3: Answer key

1. A. Esomeprazole reduces stomach acid. It is not a sedative and would not be prescribed for insomnia.

B. Loperamide relieves diarrhea. It is not a sedative and would not be prescribed for insomnia.

C. Metformin lowers blood glucose levels and is used to treat diabetes mellitus. It is not a sedative and would not be prescribed for insomnia.

D. CORRECT. Zolpidem is a sedative-hypnotic that is prescribed to treat insomnia by increasing relaxation and inducing sleep.

2. A. The "q" means every, and the "d" means daily, which is true for this prescription. However, it does not specify when during the day the patient should take the medication, which is hourly.

B. CORRECT. The "q" means every, and the "h" means hour. Combining these two letters correctly indicates how often the patient should take the medication.

C. The abbreviation "qs" means quantity sufficient, which does not indicate the time or frequency of the medication administration.

D. The abbreviation "qid" is from the Latin term "quater in die," which means four times per day. The patient should take this medication once each hour for an indicated period of time, not four times per day.

3. A. CORRECT. Antiemetics are used to reduce nausea and vomiting. Medications that destroy cancer cells, such as those used in chemotherapy, usually cause nausea and vomiting. Therefore, antiemetics like ondansetron are often prescribed in conjunction with chemotherapy treatment.

B. Antitussives, such as dextromethorphan and codeine, are used to control coughing. They are not a standard component of pharmacological treatment in conjunction with chemotherapy.

C. Antilipemics, such as atorvastatin and fenofibrate, are used to reduce cholesterol. They are not a standard component of pharmacological treatment in conjunction with chemotherapy.

D. Antipyretics, such as acetaminophen and aspirin, are used to reduce fever. They are not a standard component of pharmacological treatment in conjunction with chemotherapy.

4. A. Schedule I includes drugs that have a high potential for abuse and no medical use. They are illegal; providers cannot prescribe them. Schedule I drugs include heroin, mescaline, and lysergic acid diethylamide (LSD).

B. CORRECT. Schedule II includes medications that have a high potential for abuse, including morphine, oxycodone, and fentanyl. When prescribing Schedule II medications, providers must give patients a handwritten prescription with no refills.

C. Schedule III includes medications that have a moderate to low potential for physical and psychological dependence. Schedule III medications include ketamine, anabolic steroids, and testosterone.

D. Schedule IV includes medications that have a low potential for abuse and dependence. Schedule IV medications include diazepam, eszopiclone, and clonazepam.

5. A. The patient does not need to report nausea to the provider immediately. Nausea is a common side effect of lisinopril and can subside over time. Other common adverse effects of this medication include insomnia and fatigue.

B. The patient does not need to report orthostatic hypotension to the provider immediately. Orthostatic hypotension is a common side effect of lisinopril and can subside over time. Other common adverse effects of this medication include loss of appetite and diarrhea.

C. CORRECT. If the patient develops facial swelling or swelling of the eyes, lips, or tongue, the provider should be notified immediately because it can be an indication of a life-threatening allergic reaction to the medication.

D. The patient does not need to report taste disturbance to the provider immediately. Taste disturbance is a common side effect of lisinopril and can subside over time. Other common adverse effects of this medication include headache and a rapid heart rate.

6. A. This amount is equal to 14.8 mL.

B. This amount is equal to 22.2 mL.

C. This amount is equal to 44.4 mL.

D. CORRECT. The medical assistant should take the following steps to complete the conversion.

Step 1: What is the unit of measurement the medical assistant should convert? mL

Step 2: What is the ratio of mL to tbsp? 15 mL to 1 tbsp

Step 3: Set up an equation and solve for X.
15 mL / 1 tbsp = 30 mL / X tbsp
X = 2

Step 4: Reassess to determine if the amount makes sense. If there are 15 mL in 1 tbsp, it makes sense that 30 mL converts to 2 tbsp.

7. A. This amount of medication does not deliver the dosage required by the prescription. If the medical assistant administers 4.5 mL, the patient will only receive 4.5 mg of medication.

    B. This amount of medication does not deliver the dosage required by the prescription. If the medical assistant administers 7.5 mL, the patient will only receive 7.5 mg of medication.

    C. CORRECT. This is the correct amount of diazepam oral solution to give the patient. The medical assistant should take the following steps to complete the conversion.

    Step 1: What is the unit of measurement to calculate? mL

    Step 2: What is the dose to administer?
    Dose to administer = 10 mg (Desired)

    Step 3: What is the dose available?
    Dose available = 5 mg (Have)

    Step 4: Should the medical assistant convert the units of measurement? No

    Step 5: What is the quantity of the dose available? 5 mL

    Step 6: Set up an equation and solve for X.
    Desired/Have x Quantity = X
    10 mg / 5 mg x 5 mL = X mL
    10 = X

    Step 7: Round if necessary.

    Step 8: Reassess to determine whether the amount to administer makes sense. If there are 5 mg/5 mL and the amount prescribed is 10 mg, it makes sense to administer 10 mL. The medical assistant should identify that 10 mL of diazepam oral solution is required for each dose.

    D. This amount of medication does not deliver the dosage required by the prescription. If the medical assistant administers 12.5 mL, the patient will receive 12.5 mg of medication.

8. A. There are many oral dosage forms (capsules, buccal tablets, lozenges, emulsions). However, liniments are not administered orally.

    B. Otic medications are usually either liquid drops or ointments, not liniments. Liniments are not administered to the ear.

    C. CORRECT. A liniment is a liquid or semiliquid preparation that contains oil, alcohol, or water for application to the skin, often as a counterirritant or to relieve joint or muscle pain. Methyl salicylate liniment is a topical medication.

    D. Ophthalmic medications are usually liquid drops, not liniments. Liniments are not administered to or around the eye.

9. A. Suppositories are solid, dissolvable cylinders that contain medication and are for insertion into the rectum or vagina. A suppository is not as fast-acting as an enema solution. Therefore, an enema solution is preferable for preparation for a flexible sigmoidoscopy.

    B. CORRECT. An enema involves inserting a nozzle into the rectum and instilling a liquid solution, usually to relieve constipation or to prepare the patient for a procedure.

    C. Lotions are creamy liquids for topical application, not rectal instillation.

    D. Foams are frothy, bubbly liquids that are most commonly prescribed for vaginal use, not rectal instillation.

10. A. CORRECT. Clonazepam is an anticonvulsant that can be confused with clonidine.

    B. Chlorpropamide is an oral hypoglycemic that can be confused with chlorpromazine.

    C. Amlodipine is an antihypertensive that can be confused with amiloride.

    D. Alprazolam is an anxiolytic that can be confused with lorazepam.

11. A. CORRECT. The medical assistant should administer the Mantoux test intradermally at a 15° angle. For a Mantoux test, the forearm is the ideal site because of the ease in reading the result 48 to 72 hr later.

    B. A subcutaneous route would be too deep and would make the test results unreadable. Insulin is given via the subcutaneous route.

    C. An intramuscular route would be too deep and would make the test results unreadable. Tetanus vaccines are given via the intramuscular route.

    D. A medical assistant should not give medication intravenously. Also, it is not the appropriate route for a Mantoux test.

12. A. Absorption is the conversion of a medication into a form the body can use. Although aging can affect all physiologic processes, absorption depends more on the route and form of a medication than on a patient's age.

    B. Distribution is the transportation of a medication throughout the body. Although aging can affect all physiologic processes, distribution is affected more by specific disorders that impair circulation, such as heart disease, than by a patient's age.

    C. CORRECT. Metabolism is the process of breaking down a medication into a form that the body can use. How the body metabolizes a medication depends on many factors, including a patient's age. Infants and older adults have the least efficient metabolisms; thus, medication dosages must be lowered to compensate.

    D. Excretion is the removal of metabolites from the body. Although aging can affect all physiologic processes, excretion is affected more by specific disorders that impair kidney or bowel function than by a patient's age.

13. A. A medication might still have some effectiveness when it is at half-life.

    B. By the time of half-life, the body will have absorbed all of the medication.

    C. At half-life, a medication's peak action has passed.

    D. CORRECT. A medication's half-life is how long it takes for the processes of metabolism and excretion to eliminate half of the dose. Knowledge of medication half-lives helps determine dosing intervals.

14. A. This action is part of verifying the right dose. The medical assistant must perform the mathematical calculations for administering the right dosage or find a medication container with a dosage form that matches the provider's prescription.

    B. CORRECT. When verifying the right medication, the medical assistant must guarantee that the medication can be administered. The medication might be ineffective or dangerous if the expiration date has passed.

C. Checking for consent is associated with a patient's right to refuse. If a patient refuses a medication, the medical assistant should not coerce the patient into taking the medication. The medical assistant should document the refusal and notify the provider.

D. Learning the reason for the prescription is associated with the right reason. The medical assistant should confirm the purpose of the medication with the patient.

15. A. CORRECT. As part of the right time check, the medical assistant must make sure that medication administration adheres to any timing specifications.

B. As part of the right route check, the medical assistant must verify whether the medication should be taken orally or parenterally.

C. As part of the right technique check, the medical assistant must know how to prepare and administer medications of various types by various routes.

D. As part of the right documentation check, the medical assistant must accurately document how the medication was administered. The medication name, dose, route, and time should be documented.

Quiz 4: Answer key

1. A. Adults should drink 2 L water per day for optimal health.

B. Water is vital to all body processes. The body consists of 80% water, which provides high nutritional value for the body.

C. Hypovolemia is a loss of blood volume, which can lead to hypovolemic shock and organ malfunction. Severe dehydration can cause hypovolemia, not hypervolemia.

D. CORRECT. Water helps regulate body temperature through perspiration. Water also transports nutrients and oxygen throughout the body, lubricates many bodily structures, and helps remove waste from the body.

2. A. Sodium plays a key role in acid-base balance, aids in controlling muscle contractions, and transmits nerve impulses. Sodium is not involved in the process of metabolizing protein.

B. CORRECT. Primarily, the amino acids found in protein are used to repair and build tissues. To prevent using protein as a source of energy, the patient should include sufficient amounts of carbohydrates and fats in the diet.

C. Dietary fiber does not help rebuild muscle. It does help lower cholesterol, protect against heart disease, and promote bowel movements.

D. Protein-rich foods should make up 10% to 35% of the patient's daily caloric intake. A diet containing too much protein can result in adverse effects like increased risk of kidney stones, constipation, and dehydration.

3. A. Chicken breasts are protein-based and do not contain fiber.

B. Cottage cheese is a dairy product and does not contain fiber.

C. Eggs are protein-based and do not contain fiber.

D. CORRECT. One cup of chopped apple with peel provides 3 g fiber. The medical assistant should recommend this food.

4. A. Beans are a source of vitamin B_6, folate, and protein. Beans do not contain vitamin D.

B. CORRECT. Fish is a source of vitamin B_6, vitamin D, and protein. Other sources of vitamin D include fortified milk, eggs, and butter.

C. Rice contains vitamin B_1 and aids in the release of carbohydrates. However, it does not contain vitamin D.

D. Nuts are a source of vitamin B_6, vitamin E, and protein. However, nuts do not contain vitamin D.

5. A. CORRECT. Lactose sensitivity or intolerance is a reaction to foods that contain lactose, the sugar found in milk and milk products. Patients who have this sensitivity should reduce or avoid consuming dairy products.

B. The patient does not need to avoid consuming green beans. Lactose is the sugar found in milk and milk products.

C. The patient does not need to avoid consuming chicken. Lactose is the sugar found in milk and milk products.

D. The patient does not need to avoid consuming black coffee. Lactose is the sugar found in milk and milk products.

6. A. Oils help with the absorption of fat-soluble vitamins.

B. Protein-rich foods help maintain body heat.

C. Minerals and electrolytes help regulate muscle activity and heart rhythm.

D. CORRECT. Grain products, especially whole grains, provide fiber. Fiber adds bulk to the stool to promote regular bowel movements, which help to prevent and manage constipation.

7. A. Vitamin A is an antioxidant and a fat-soluble vitamin that helps with the maintenance of healthy skin and vision. It does not prevent bone loss or help regulate calcium absorption.

B. Vitamin C is an antioxidant and a water-soluble vitamin that helps the body to build and maintain strong tissues, as well as resist infection. It does not prevent bone loss or help regulate calcium absorption.

C. CORRECT. Vitamin D is a fat-soluble vitamin that regulates the absorption of calcium and aids in building strong bones and teeth.

D. Vitamin E is an antioxidant and a fat-soluble vitamin that aids in red blood cell protection. It does not prevent bone loss or help regulate calcium absorption.

8. A. Blueberries are a relatively poor source of vitamin A. One cup of blueberries provides 80 IU vitamin A.

B. Potatoes are a very poor source of vitamin A. One medium baked potato provides 4 IU vitamin A.

C. CORRECT. Good sources of vitamin A include yellow and orange fruits. One cup of orange slices provides 416 IU vitamin A.

D. Cauliflower does not contain vitamin A.

9. A. Iron forms hemoglobin in red blood cells for oxygen transport, and it contributes to the formation and function of enzymes and protein. Iron is not essential for blood coagulation.

B. Magnesium metabolizes carbohydrates and protein, and it assists with muscle contraction and structure. Magnesium is not essential for blood coagulation.

C. CORRECT. Calcium assists with blood coagulation and building healthy bones and teeth.

D. Potassium assists with muscle contraction and fluid balance as well as nerve, muscle, and heart function. Potassium is not essential for blood coagulation.

10. A. CORRECT. Patients who have bulimia nervosa consume large quantities of food and purge by vomiting, over-exercising, or using laxatives.

B. Ritualistic behavior is an indication of anorexia nervosa.

C. Starvation is an indication of anorexia nervosa.

D. Counting calories is a behavior associated with anorexia nervosa.

11. A. CORRECT. Patients who have anorexia nervosa demonstrate excessive weight and muscle loss, which allows bones to protrude.

B. Females who have anorexia nervosa experience amenorrhea, or absence of menstrual periods.

C. It is common for patients who have anorexia nervosa to deny feeling hungry.

D. Erosion of tooth enamel is an indication of bulimia nervosa, not anorexia nervosa.

12. A. Chronic overeating is a behavior that could indicate binge-eating disorder or bulimia nervosa.

B. CORRECT. Patients who have bulimia nervosa self-induce vomiting. Patients who have binge-eating disorder do not.

C. Patients who have binge-eating disorder or bulimia nervosa tend to maintain or gain weight.

D. Buying large amounts of food is a behavior that could indicate binge-eating disorder or bulimia nervosa.

13. A. For weight management, the standard calorie intake should be 2,000 to 2,500 calories per day.

B. The ingredients on a food label are listed in descending order of weight.

C. CORRECT. The medical assistant should explain that the amount of each nutrient is expressed in weight per serving and as a percentage of the daily value.

D. Sugar alcohol is a voluntary component and is not required information to be included on a food label.

14. A. CORRECT. Nutrition labels must contain the number of milligrams of cholesterol, sodium, and potassium per serving.

B. The amount of xylitol, a sugar substitute, can be included on the nutrition label, but it is not required by the FDA.

C. The amount of thiamine (vitamin B_1) per serving can be included voluntarily on the nutrition label, but it is not required by the FDA. It is mandatory to include the percent of daily value for vitamins A and C.

D. The amount of polyunsaturated and monounsaturated fats can be included voluntarily on the nutrition label. It is mandatory to include the number of grams of total fat, saturated fat, and trans fat.

15. A. Percent of daily value on the nutrition label is useful for determining if the food product will meet nutritional needs, but it will not help patients avoid underestimating the specific amount of nutrients in a food product.

B. This value on the nutrition label is useful for determining the amount of nutrients patients need if they consume a 2,000 or 2,500 calorie/day diet, but it will not help them avoid underestimating the specific amount of nutrients in a food product.

C. The nutrition label lists ingredient amounts in descending order by weight. It will not help patients avoid underestimating the specific amount of nutrients in a food product.

D. CORRECT. The medical assistant should remind patients to check the serving size and the number of servings in the package on the food label. It is common to mistake the list of calories and nutrients as the amount in the entire package, when it might only be a small percentage.

Quiz 5: Answer key

1. A. During middle adulthood, adults often raise children and some become grandparents. Achieving the developmental tasks associated with middle age results in professional and personal achievements and active participation in serving the community and society.

B. During adolescence, teenagers try to figure out where they fit in and what direction their lives should take. Achieving the developmental tasks associated with adolescence results in emotional stability, commitment, and sound decision-making.

C. CORRECT. During older adulthood, most people retire, which causes them to re-evaluate their usefulness. Achieving the developmental tasks associated with older adulthood results in self-acceptance, a sense of self-worth, and coming to terms with having achieved some goals and not others.

D. During young adulthood, people begin to think about family and career. Achieving the developmental tasks associated with young adulthood results in the ability to feel mutual self-respect and love toward others.

2. A. Ego integrity vs. despair is the developmental crisis typically seen in older adults (65 years and older).

B. CORRECT. Intimacy vs. isolation is the developmental crisis typically seen in young adults (20 to 35 years). During this stage, young adults begin to think about partnership, marriage, family, and career. Achieving the developmental tasks of this stage results in the ability to feel mutual self-respect and love, intimacy, and commitment to others and to a career.

C. Generativity vs. stagnation is the developmental crisis typically seen in middle adults (35 to 65 years).

D. Identity vs. role confusion is the developmental crisis typically seen in adolescents (12 to 20 years).

3. A. CORRECT. Trust vs. mistrust is the psychosocial crisis for infants. The developmental tasks for infants are to form attachments with and develop trust in their caregivers, and then generalize those bonds to others. Not achieving these tasks leads to suspiciousness and struggles with interpersonal relationships.

B. Anger with self is a negative outcome of the stage of autonomy vs. shame and doubt. Other negative outcomes include a lack of self-confidence and no pride in the ability to perform.

C. Inadequacy is a negative outcome of the stage of industry vs. inferiority. Another negative outcome is the inability to compromise and cooperate with others.

D. Guilt is a negative outcome of the stage of initiative vs. guilt. Other negative outcomes include feelings of inadequacy, defeat, and deserving punishment.

4. A. During this stage, the grieving person cannot or will not believe that the loss is happening or has happened.

B. During this stage, the grieving person might aim feelings of hostility at others, including health care staff, because they cannot cure the disease.

C. During this stage, the grieving person attempts to avoid the loss by making some kind of "deal," or wishing she had done so. Bargaining typically manifests before the loss has occurred.

D. CORRECT. During this stage, the reality of the situation takes hold, and the grieving person feels sad, lonely, and helpless. She might have feelings of regret and self-blame for not taking better care of herself or, in this case, not encouraging her brother to take better care of himself.

5. A. This patient is in the first stage of the grief process, denial. She might not be able to express sadness until she reaches the fourth stage, depression.

B. This patient is in the first stage of the grief process, denial. She is more likely to express anger in the second stage, anger.

C. CORRECT. This patient is in the first stage of the grief process, denial. She is expressing disbelief that she has breast cancer. Helpful interventions at this stage are to verbally reinforce information about the disease and to give her written information about breast cancer that she can refer to when she is ready to find out more. It is also helpful at this stage to involve close family members or loved ones in her care.

D. Although this is a helpful intervention, the patient is not yet ready to accept the services of others who understand or are dealing with a disease the patient is still denying that she has.

6. A. Unless the medical assistant is collecting data for the patient's medical history, it is inappropriate and unprofessional to ask questions out of curiosity.

B. With this question, the medical assistant is singling out the patient for being different, which is inappropriate. The question could also imply that other people in the waiting room shouldn't have to look at the patient, which could be offensive.

C. CORRECT. This response shows concern without asking probing or unnecessary questions about the patient's disability. When working with patients who have physical challenges, the medical assistant should make every effort to make them feel comfortable.

D. The medical assistant should show concern and empathy, but remarks like this can seem insincere. The patient could perceive this as the medical assistant making assumptions or pretending to understand what he is feeling.

7. A. CORRECT. This action by the medical assistant makes the patient more comfortable and demonstrates sensitivity and empathy.

B. Speaking too quietly or too loudly does not promote therapeutic communication.

C. Intimate contact can make the patient uncomfortable. The medical assistant should be sensitive and respect the patient's boundaries.

D. A closed posture indicates that the medical assistant is not open to or interested in what the patient is saying or feeling.

8. A. Denial is a defense mechanism characterized by a patient's avoidance of reality. This can include the patient's refusal to discuss a problem or receive any teaching about it.

B. Apathy is a defense mechanism characterized by a patient's lack of emotion, interest, feeling, or concern. It is a pretense of an indifference to the situation.

C. Undoing is a defense mechanism characterized by a patient's expression of the feeling that is opposite of what she is actually experiencing.

D. CORRECT. Projection is a defense mechanism characterized by a patient's externalization of feelings of guilt, blame, or responsibility. Patients can project their ideas, feelings, or attitudes onto objects or other people.

9. A. In this stage, preschoolers actively try out new skills but, if ignored or reprimanded, they might feel guilty or afraid to show initiative.

B. In this stage, school-age children find satisfaction in completing projects and being recognized for their accomplishments. If they feel they are unable to please their parents or get approval from their peers, they can develop feelings of inferiority.

C. In this stage, toddlers are beginning to show independence. Shame and doubt might occur if parental expectations are not met or parents are overprotective.

D. CORRECT. In this stage, adolescents experience hormonal and physical changes and are trying to figure out who they are. If identity and sense of direction are not established, they suffer role confusion.

10. A. A patient who has moderate to severe anxiety is more likely to exhibit hypervigilance and have difficulty sleeping.

B. A patient who has moderate to severe anxiety is more likely to experience profuse sweating, including in the palms of the hands.

C. A patient who has moderate to severe anxiety is more likely to experience chest pain than back pain.

D. CORRECT. A patient who has moderate to severe anxiety usually has increased heart and respiratory rates.

11. A. To test orientation, the examiner asks the patient to identify the present time and place.

B. CORRECT. To test registration, the examiner names three unrelated objects and asks the patient to repeat all three of them.

C. To test attention and calculation, the examiner asks the patient to count backward from 100 by intervals of 7 or spell the word "world" backward.

D. To test language, the examiner asks the patient to perform a series of actions, including following a three-step command.

12. A. CORRECT. When testing language, the examiner asks the patient to copy a design, such as overlapping pentagons.

B. When testing orientation, the examiner asks the patient for specific location information, such as the city or state.

C. When testing attention and calculation, the examiner asks the patient to count backward by intervals of 7, starting at 100, or to spell the word "world" backward.

D. When testing recall, the examiner asks the patient to name the three objects that the examiner named earlier in the test.

13. A. Significant weight loss can be caused by a variety of conditions, including several medical conditions. Because weight loss is a symptom of depression, it might prompt a depression screening, but it should not prompt a mental status evaluation.

B. Decreased energy can be caused by a variety of conditions, including several medical conditions. Because decreased energy is also a symptom of depression, it might prompt a depression screening, but it should not prompt a mental status evaluation.

C. CORRECT. Repetition can be a sign of memory impairment; the patient does not remember having already asked that question. This could indicate a cognitive condition, such as Alzheimer's disease or dementia, and should prompt a mental status evaluation.

D. Reduced or disrupted sleep can be caused by a variety of conditions, including several medical conditions. Because difficulty sleeping is also a symptom of depression, it might prompt a depression screening, but it should not prompt a mental status evaluation.

14. A. CORRECT. Compensation is a method of balancing a failure or inadequacy with an accomplishment. The patient is using extra exercise as an accomplishment to compensate for not following dietary guidelines.

B. Displacement is a shift in emotion or behavior that copes with a situation by substituting it with a more desirable alternative. The patient's actions are not an example of displacement.

C. Repression is the exclusion of unpleasant emotions, desires, or problems from the conscious mind as a coping strategy. The patient's actions are not an example of repression.

D. Reaction formation is the outward presentation of a patient's beliefs or emotions as their opposites. The patient's actions are not an example of reaction formation.

15. A. Rationalization is an explanation that makes something negative or unacceptable seem justifiable or acceptable.

B. CORRECT. Regression is a return to an earlier, more childlike developmental behavior. It is not unusual for children who are facing a stressful situation to revert to more infantile behaviors, such as thumb-sucking and bedwetting.

C. Suppression is the voluntary blocking of an unpleasant experience from one's awareness.

D. Sublimation is rechanneling unacceptable urges or drives into something constructive or acceptable.

Quiz 6: Answer key

1. A. The pancreas is an example of epithelial tissue and is part of the endocrine system.

B. CORRECT. Blood is a type of connective tissue. It transports substances throughout the body. Connective tissue is the most frequently occurring type of tissue in the body.

C. The spinal cord is an example of nervous tissue and is part of the nervous system.

D. The skin is an example of epithelial tissue and is part of the integumentary system.

2. A. Caudal describes locations toward the tail of the body.

B. Cephalic describes locations pertaining to the head.

C. Medial describes locations that are toward the middle of the body.

D. CORRECT. Dorsal describes locations that are toward the back of, or posterior to, the body.

3. A. CORRECT. The transverse plane divides the body into upper and lower portions.

B. The coronal plane divides the body into equal front and back portions.

C. The sagittal plane divides the body into asymmetrical left and right sides.

D. The midsagittal plane divides the body into bilaterally symmetrical left and right sides.

4. A. Superficial means on or near the surface. The heart is located in the thoracic cavity and away from the surface, which means it is deep to the ribs, not superficial to it.

B. Distal means farther away from the point of attachment. The patella is proximal to the tibia, which means it is closer to the tibia, not distal to it.

C. Superior means above another part. The stomach is inferior to the diaphragm, which means the stomach is below the diaphragm, not superior to it.

D. CORRECT. Lateral means toward, near, or from the midline. The thumb is lateral to the index finger.

5. A. The appendix is part of the digestive system, but it is not part of the endocrine system.

B. CORRECT. The pancreas is part of both the digestive and endocrine systems. It functions in the endocrine system by producing insulin and glucagon, which maintain blood glucose levels and store glucose for energy. It also functions in the digestive system by contributing to the breakdown of enzymes.

C. The liver is part of the digestive system, but it is not part of the endocrine system.

D. The gallbladder is part of the digestive system, but it is not part of the endocrine system.

6. A. CORRECT. The thyroid gland is located in the neck just below the larynx and consists of two lobes, one on each side of the trachea.

B. The hypothalamus gland is located in the inferior midportion of the brain.

C. The pituitary gland is located below the hypothalamus in the brain.

D. The adrenal glands are located in the upper portions of each kidney.

7. A. The liver is a major organ of the digestive system. It performs filtering, metabolism, storage, and synthesis.

B. The lungs are major organs of the respiratory system. They aid in the process of respiration.

C. CORRECT. The skin is a major organ of the integumentary system. It produces vitamin D, provides protection, and helps regulate body temperature.

D. The brain is a major organ of the nervous system that is the center of all mental activity. It monitors and interprets stimuli and responds accordingly.

8. A. The primary function of the musculoskeletal system is to provide support, posture, and heat production.

B. The primary function of the gastrointestinal system is to break down food into small molecules that can be absorbed by the cells of the body.

C. The primary functions of the integumentary system are to help regulate body temperature, aid in the synthesis of vitamin D, and provide sensory input.

D. CORRECT. The primary function of the lymphatic system is to defend the body against foreign cells and diseases, provide immunity, and maintain fluid balance.

9. A. The lymphatic system is a series of vessels. It does not contain cardiac, skeletal, or smooth tissues.

B. The integumentary system is comprised of skin and accessory structures. It does not contain cardiac, skeletal, or smooth tissues.

C. CORRECT. Cardiac tissue, skeletal tissue, and smooth tissue are all parts of the muscular system.

D. The endocrine system is comprised of glands that secrete hormones. It does not contain cardiac, skeletal, or smooth tissues.

10. A. The peripheral nervous system consists of spinal nerves that transmit information to and from the brain, but it does not aid in cellular elimination.

B. The endocrine system regulates metabolic activity, but it does not aid in cellular elimination.

C. CORRECT. The cardiovascular system works with the respiratory system to remove waste from the body's cells.

D. The reproductive system produces hormones and facilitates reproduction, but it does not aid in cellular elimination.

11. A. The stomach functions to produce secretions and digest proteins. It is not active in the absorption of nutrients.

B. CORRECT. The small intestine is primarily responsible for the absorption of nutrients, which is the final process of digestion.

C. The primary function of the bile duct is to deliver bile from the gallbladder to the duodenum. It is not active in the absorption of nutrients.

D. The esophagus is primarily a passageway for food with a mucus lining that eases the passage of food. It is not active in the absorption of nutrients.

12. A. The thyroid is part of the endocrine system, but it is not part of the immune system.

B. The pineal gland is part of the endocrine system. It is involved with circadian cycles in the body and influences the onset of puberty, but it is not part of the immune system.

C. CORRECT. The thymus is part of both the endocrine system and the immune system.

D. The pituitary gland is part of the endocrine system and helps control growth, blood pressure, and metabolism, but it is not part of the immune system.

13. A. The patient's height is measured in meters, inches, or feet and is not a factor to consider when maintaining homeostasis.

B. The patient's weight determines the patient's mass in kilograms or pounds and is not a factor to consider when maintaining homeostasis.

C. The patient's oxygenation status is assessed by performing a pulse oximetry and is not a factor to consider when maintaining homeostasis.

D. CORRECT. Vital signs are indicators of the body's ability to maintain homeostasis. Vital signs include temperature, heart rate, respirations, and blood pressure.

14. A. CORRECT. The muscular system receives signals from the nervous system in response to pain, which causes the muscles to contract or move.

B. The cardiovascular system does not control movement responses and would not be alerted.

C. The digestive system does not control movement responses and would not be alerted.

D. The integumentary system does not control movement responses and would not be alerted.

15. A. The cardiovascular system experiences an increase in heart rate during a fight-or-flight response.

B. The respiratory system experiences a widening of the bronchioles to increase the flow of oxygen during a fight-or-flight response.

C. The muscular system experiences an increase in blood flow to the skeletal muscles during a fight-or-flight response.

D. CORRECT. The digestive system experiences a decrease in peristalsis during a fight-or-flight response. The movement of food is slowed down as it passes through the digestive system, preventing vomiting or defecation as a response to fear or trauma. The system will remain in this state until the individual feels safe.

Quiz 7: Answer key

1. A. CORRECT. Osteoporosis is defined as a loss of bone density. This condition has a variety of causes, including a lack of calcium intake. Osteoporosis is most commonly identified through a bone density scan.

   B. Osteomyelitis is an inflammation of the bone caused by bacteria.

   C. Rheumatoid arthritis is an autoimmune disorder that causes the immune system to destroy the lining of the joints, leading to swelling and joint pain.

   D. Scoliosis is a lateral curvature of the spine that can result in a variety of complications.

2. A. CORRECT. Chronic hypertension can lead to weakness in the left ventricle of the heart. This weakness in the heart can progress to CHF when the ventricle fails.

   B. Atherosclerosis is caused by the formation of plaque in the arteries leading to the heart. Although this condition can lead to a myocardial infarction, it is not a cause of CHF.

   C. Endocarditis can cause scarring of the cardiac tissue, which can lead to mitral valve prolapse. It does not cause CHF.

   D. CHF is a secondary diagnosis that develops as a result of other preexisting conditions. Although these other pre-existing conditions can be hereditary, CHF itself is not a hereditary condition.

3. A. CORRECT. Following removal of lymph tissue, lymphedema can cause tissue in the affected extremity to swell with fluid due to inhibited reabsorption by the lymphatic system.

   B. Palpable nodules in the unaffected breast are not a manifestation of lymphedema. Nodules in breast tissue can be an indication of fibrocystic breast disease.

   C. Scaly patches are not a manifestation of lymphedema. Thick, silvery scales on the skin are an indication of psoriasis.

   D. Migraine headaches are not a manifestation of lymphedema. Causes of migraine headaches vary, but manifestations include photophobia, nausea, vomiting, and visual disturbances.

4. A. CORRECT. Contrast media is used to highlight the inner contours of body structures and to enhance visibility for diagnostic imaging of less-dense body structures.

   B. Contrast media has a higher density than what normally fills the gastrointestinal tract or blood vessels. Therefore, it serves to make body structures more radiopaque, or dense, not more radiolucent, or easier to see through.

   C. Bones are already one of the highest-density structures in the body. Contrast media is used to enhance visibility of less-dense body structures for diagnostic imaging. For the purposes of imaging, bones are not affected by contrast media.

   D. Although radioactive elements and radiation are used in diagnostic imaging, the primary use of contrast media is not to protect internal organs from radiation.

5. A. CORRECT. The medical assistant is responsible for instructing patients about necessary preparations for an MRI. This action is within the scope of practice of the medical assistant.

   B. Only licensed health care personnel are allowed to practice radiography, which includes administering contrast media IV as indicated by testing requirements. This action is outside the scope of practice of the medical assistant.

   C. The provider is responsible for communicating the results of the imaging to the patient. This action is outside the scope of practice of the medical assistant.

   D. Only licensed health care personnel are allowed to practice radiography, which includes positioning of the imaging equipment and the patient. This action is outside the scope of practice of the medical assistant.

6. A. CORRECT. The medical assistant should recommend the RICE method to a patient who reports an ankle sprain. This method helps to reduce swelling, inflammation, and pain.

   B. A joint dislocation requires reduction, which involves placing the bones of the joint back into alignment. RICE is not an appropriate treatment modality for this injury.

   C. A head injury can cause life-threatening intracranial pressure that might require treatment to reduce pressure within the skull. RICE is not an appropriate treatment modality for this injury.

   D. A patient who has restless leg syndrome should adhere to a treatment plan including relaxation exercises, caffeine intake reduction, and moderate exercise. RICE is not an appropriate treatment modality for this syndrome.

7. A. CORRECT. A hiatal hernia occurs when part of the top of the stomach protrudes through the diaphragm. Risk factors for a hiatal hernia include middle age and obesity.

   B. An umbilical hernia occurs when part of the bowel protrudes through the abdominal muscle wall.

   C. An inguinal hernia occurs when a portion of the bowel protrudes into the inguinal canal.

   D. An incisional hernia occurs when tissue protrudes at a surgical site.

8. A. CORRECT. Diabetes mellitus affects about 9% of the U.S. population and is characterized by chronic hyperglycemia and lack of insulin production or resistance to insulin at the cellular level.

   B. Diabetes insipidus is a pituitary gland disorder characterized by a lack of ADH production. It does not affect insulin production.

   C. Coronary artery disease is characterized by the formation of atherosclerotic plaque, which narrows the arteries and prevents blood flow. It does not affect insulin production.

   D. Polycystic kidney disease is characterized by the formation of benign, fluid-filled cysts in the kidneys. It does not affect insulin production.

9. A. Myasthenia gravis is a chronic neuromuscular disease that causes muscle contractions and weakness involving any voluntary muscles. This is considered an autoimmune disease with an unknown origin. Elevated uric acid levels are not a risk factor.

B. Rheumatoid arthritis is an autoimmune disorder that leads to severe joint pain and deformity, causing synovitis. Elevated uric acid levels are not a risk factor.

C. Osteoporosis is a progressive decrease in bone density and strength due to a decline in calcium deposits. Elevated uric acid levels are not a risk factor.

D. CORRECT. Gout is a musculoskeletal disorder caused by a buildup of uric acid in the joints, primarily the big toes and the knees. Risk factors include dietary choices that result in the overproduction or improper elimination of uric acid from the body.

10. A. CORRECT. A history of smoking is a risk factor for coronary artery disease.

B. Being underweight is not a risk factor for coronary artery disease. Excess body fat is a risk factor.

C. HDL cholesterol is considered good cholesterol. High LDL levels are a risk factor for developing coronary artery disease.

D. Cellulitis is an inflammation of the cellular or connective tissue and is not a risk factor of coronary artery disease.

11. A. Hypoglycemia is a condition in which a patient has too much insulin and is not a risk factor for CVA. Hyperglycemia, or insufficient insulin, is a risk factor for CVA.

B. Hypotension is a condition in which a patient has low blood pressure and is not a risk factor for CVA. Hypertension, or high blood pressure, is a risk factor for CVA.

C. Pyloric stenosis is a condition in which a patient has hardening and narrowing of the pyloric sphincter at the lower end of the stomach. It is typically seen as a congenital defect in infants and is not a risk factor for CVA.

D. CORRECT. Sleep apnea is a condition that causes the trachea to narrow or close during sleep, which temporarily causes breathing to stop. It is a risk factor for CVA.

12. A. CORRECT. Risk factors for colorectal cancer include a low-fiber, high-fat diet; genetic or family history; and being 55 years of age or older.

B. Crohn's disease is an inflammation in the ileum that reduces the small intestine's ability to absorb nutrients. A low-fiber, high-fat diet is not a risk factor for this disease.

C. Cholelithiasis, or gallstones, are formed in the gallbladder from insoluble cholesterol and bile salt. Reasons for gallstone formation are not always clear. A low-fiber, high-fat diet is not a risk factor for this disease.

D. Cirrhosis is a chronic liver disease caused by alcohol use disorder, hepatitis C, and chronic hepatitis B. A low-fiber, high-fat diet is not a risk factor for this disease.

13. A. CORRECT. A pandemic is an outbreak of a rapidly spreading novel infection that affects a large number of people across several countries or continents.

B. Prevalence is the existing number of cases of a particular disease in a specific population.

C. An endemic illness is always present in a given population.

D. An outbreak is a suddenly occurring disease in a limited geographic area in unexpected numbers.

14. A. CORRECT. The development of the first vaccine was a result of a smallpox pandemic in the 18th century.

B. The influenza vaccine is readily available, but it was not the first vaccine created.

C. The tetanus vaccine is readily available, but it was not the first vaccine created.

D. Malaria is a fatal parasitic disease that is treated using a combination of oral antimalarial medications.

15. A. CORRECT. The polio virus affected thousands of people in the U.S. A vaccine was developed in 1952 that greatly reduced the incidence of the disease on a national scale.

B. Measles presents with fever, nasal discharge, rash, and red eyes. A vaccine series is readily available.

C. Rubella presents with rash and swollen lymph glands. A vaccine series is readily available.

D. Rabies presents with fever, throat spasms, profuse salivation, and uncontrollable excitement. A vaccine series is readily available for humans and animals.

Quiz 8: Answer key

1. A. CORRECT. The nucleus contains chromosomes, the thread-like structures made of deoxyribonucleic acid, which are the structures that contain the body's genetic information.

B. Cytoplasm is the gel-like fluid inside of the cell that contains organelles, such as mitochondria, that perform the functions of the cell.

C. The plasma membrane, or cell membrane, is the thin, outermost structure of human cells.

D. The nucleolus is a dense region of the nucleus that assists with forming proteins. It does not contain chromosomes.

2. A. A lysosome is an organelle that destroys and cleans out all cellular waste.

B. A centriole is an organelle that divides the chromosomes equally into the cells that result from the reproduction process.

C. CORRECT. A mitochondrion is an organelle that provides the cell with the energy needed to rebuild, transport, and reproduce cells.

D. Cilia are hair-like projections that create movement in a wavelike motion across the cell's surface.

3. A. Ribosomes contribute to protein synthesis by supporting the protein chains as ribonucleic acid builds them.

B. The cytoskeleton is a network of microtubules and microfilaments that help maintain the cell's shape and mobility.

C. The endoplasmic reticulum is a structure that provides networks of passageways for moving substances within the cytoplasm.

D. CORRECT. The Golgi apparatus sorts and combines carbohydrates and proteins to form glycoproteins.

4. A. CORRECT. Cilia are hair-like projections that help move substances through tracts and paths in the body. Some mucous membranes, such as those in the respiratory tract, have cilia.

B. A flagellum is a long projection that allows the cell to move in a swimming-like motion. Sperm cells have this organelle.

C. The cytoskeleton maintains the cell's shape and protects it.

D. The microvilli are tiny surface extensions that increase the cell's surface area.

5. A. Cytoplasm is the material inside the cell that contains organelles, such as mitochondria, that perform the functions of the cell.

B. CORRECT. Centrioles are cylindrical-shaped organelles that work in pairs and play a role in cell division.

C. The Golgi apparatus sorts and combines carbohydrates and proteins to form glycoproteins.

D. The endoplasmic reticulum provides networks of passageways for moving substances within the cytoplasm.

6. A. *C. botulinum* causes botulism, a type of food poisoning. It does not have any helpful functions in the human body.

B. CORRECT. *L. acidophilus* aids with digestion and is a common ingredient in probiotic supplements.

C. *T. pallidum* causes syphilis. It does not have any helpful functions in the human body.

D. *H. influenzae* causes bacterial meningitis and is found in the throat. It does not have any helpful functions in the human body.

7. A. The human papillomavirus causes genital warts and cancer.

B. The parvovirus causes fifth disease.

C. The human immunodeficiency virus causes AIDS.

D. CORRECT. The Epstein-Barr virus causes mononucleosis. The virus spreads via contact with saliva from an infected person.

8. A. *Pthirus pubis*, or the crab louse, is also known as pubic lice.

B. *Enterobius vermicularis* is also known as pinworms. It is the most common worm infestation in the U.S.

C. CORRECT. *Pediculus humanus capitis* is also known as head lice. It spreads by direct contact.

D. *Diphyllobothrium latum* is also known as tapeworms.

9. A. *P. carinii* causes *Pneumocystis pneumonia*, which is a lung infection.

B. *L. pneumophila* is a bacterium found in contaminated air conditioning systems that causes pneumonia.

C. *H. pylori* is a bacterium that is involved in peptic ulcer disease.

D. CORRECT. *C. albicans* is a fungus that causes vaginal yeast infections and also thrush, a yeast infection in the mouth.

10. A. Cocci are round, spherical, or oval in shape.

B. Spirilla are spiral-shaped.

C. CORRECT. Vibrios are comma-shaped.

D. Bacilli are rod-shaped.

11. A. CORRECT. Amoxicillin is a form of antibiotic that kills bacteria, so it is a major component of treatment plans for bacterial infections.

B. Antiviral medications are used to treat symptoms of viral infections.

C. Antifungal medications are used to kill fungi.

D. Antiprotozoal medications are used to kill protozoa.

12. A. Bacteria are single-cell micro-organisms.

B. Viruses consist of genetic material and require a host to survive.

C. CORRECT. Fungi are unicellular yeasts, and multicellular fungi are molds.

D. Protozoa are single-cell parasites.

13. A. The portal of entry is the manner in which the infectious agent enters a new host following the link of transmission.

B. CORRECT. The chain of infection starts with an infectious agent in its reservoir.

C. The susceptible host is the final link in the chain of infection, where the infectious agent can multiply depending on the host's state of health.

D. Mode of transmission is either direct or indirect and occurs after the infectious agent exits the reservoir.

14. A. Foodborne infections are transmitted by the oral ingestion of infected food products.

B. A droplet is an indirect mode of transmission via a cough or a sneeze.

C. Nonliving objects are fomites. When contaminated, they can transmit infectious organisms.

D. CORRECT. Direct contact with a person who has molluscum contagiosum warts spreads the molluscipoxvirus, which causes these warts.

15. A. Nonliving objects are fomites. When contaminated, they can transmit infectious organisms.

B. A droplet is an indirect mode of transmission via a cough or a sneeze.

C. CORRECT. A vector, in this case a tick, spreads *Borrelia burgdorferi*, the bacterium that causes Lyme disease.

D. A pathogenic organism can be spread via airborne transmission, or inhalation through the nose or mouth.

Quiz 9: Answer key

1. A. CORRECT. The medical assistant should restock medical supplies in each examination room to prepare the rooms for use the next day.

    B. The medical assistant should not prepare a sterile field a day in advance of a procedure because the field is not considered sterile once it is left unattended.

    C. The medical assistant might perform trash removal. However, the medical assistant should not discard biohazard trash bags in standard trash bins. Biohazard bags are collected by a separate, specialized disposal company, based on state, local, and federal guidelines.

    D. The medical assistant should not refrigerate all blood specimens overnight. Each blood specimen has specific requirements for storage and transportation. The medical assistant should communicate with the laboratory that will be receiving the specimen to determine the correct handling procedure for each specimen.

2. A. This is an example of poor body mechanics. The medical assistant should stand with feet shoulder-width apart during patient transfers. The use of proper body mechanics helps protect both the medical assistant and the patient when performing tasks involving lifting and patient transfer.

    B. The medical assistant should recognize that computer and telephone cables should not be arranged to cross walkways. Cables that are loose or bundled together present a tripping hazard to patients and staff.

    C. CORRECT. A spill on the floor could cause the walkway to become wet and slippery, which might result in a patient or staff member falling. The medical assistant should use a towel to clean the spill to prevent an accident.

    D. The medical assistant should store cleaning supplies in cabinets, not on top of them. Supplies stored on top of cabinets pose a risk of falling onto patients and staff.

3. A. Objective data is information collected about the patient through diagnostic testing, collection of vital signs, or patient observation. It is not a part of the patient's medical history.

    B. The treatment plan is recommended by the provider and includes patient instructions. It is not a part of the patient's medical history.

    C. CORRECT. The chief complaint is the reason for the patient's visit, stated in the patient's own words. It is a component of the patient's medical history.

    D. An informed consent form is necessary when a patient requires an invasive procedure as a part of diagnostic testing or treatment. An informed consent form is not a part of the patient's medical history.

4. A. The medical assistant should use the carotid artery for palpating pulses in emergency situations.

    B. The medical assistant should palpate and auscultate the brachial artery when measuring blood pressure.

    C. CORRECT. The radial artery is the most commonly used site for counting the heart rate in healthy adult patients.

    D. The medical assistant should use the femoral artery to measure heart rate for adults who are experiencing cardiac arrest or circulatory issues.

5. A. Tympanic temperature is a vital sign, not an anthropometric measurement.

    B. CORRECT. Head circumference is measure for children younger than 3 years old and is recorded on a growth chart. Commonly collected anthropometric measurements also include height or length and weight.

    C. Apical pulse is a vital sign, not an anthropometric measurement.

    D. Blood pressure is a vital sign, not an anthropometric measurement.

6. A. Myocardial infarction is caused by a blockage of the coronary artery and manifests with chest pain and cyanosis. However, slurred speech and a drooping mouth are not manifestations of this condition.

    B. Syncope is fainting caused by a temporary loss of blood flow to parts of the brain. It manifests as a loss of consciousness, not slurred speech and drooping of the mouth.

    C. An anxiety attack can manifest with multiple symptoms. However, slurred speech and a drooping mouth are not manifestations of this condition.

    D. CORRECT. A cerebrovascular accident (CVA) is an emergency situation and requires immediate action. A CVA can manifest with slurred speech, tinnitus, and partial paralysis due to loss of blood flow to parts of the brain.

7. A. Lithotomy position is used for rectal, vaginal, and pelvic examinations. In the lithotomy position, the patient lies supine with legs raised, separated, and supported in stirrups.

    B. Supine position is used for examination of the front of the patient's body, including the chest, abdomen, and breasts. In the supine position, the patient lies flat, facing up.

    C. CORRECT. Prone position is used for examination of the back of the patient's body, or dorsal cavity, and for some surgical procedures. In the prone position, the patient lies flat, facing down.

    D. Semi-Fowler's position is used for postoperative examination of the head, neck, and chest. It can also be used for patients who are having trouble breathing. In semi-Fowler's position, the patient lies supine with the head of the bed between 30° and 45°.

8. A. Applying medication to the patient's skin would be using topical application. The medical assistant should administer the medication sublingually, by placing it under the patient's tongue.

    B. CORRECT. Sublingual medication is absorbed through the oral cavity when it is placed under the tongue. Sublingual medication administration provides a rapid route of absorption into the blood stream.

    C. Inserting medication into the patient's rectum would be using rectal application. The medical assistant should administer the medication sublingually, by placing it under the patient's tongue.

    D. Injecting medication into a muscle would be using the intramuscular route of administration. The medical assistant should administer the medication sublingually, by placing it under the patient's tongue.

9. A. CORRECT. The medical assistant should grasp the knot using forceps and cut next to the knot to remove each suture.

   B. The medical assistant should start at one end of the wound and move to other end, removing all suture fragments to prevent irritation or infection.

   C. The order of insertion does not affect the suture removal process.

   D. Adhesive skin closures are used in place of sutures or applied after the sutures have been removed.

10. A. The medical assistant should instill the medication into the lower conjunctiva.

    B. The medical assistant should instruct the patient to look up when the medication is being instilled.

    C. CORRECT. When instilling medication into the eyes, the medical assistant should wear gloves to prevent introducing pathogens into the patient's eyes. Wearing gloves will also help prevent the medical assistant from being exposed to potentially pathogenic organisms.

    D. The patient should only have one bottle of medication. The medical assistant should avoid touching the tip of the bottle to the patient's lashes or conjunctiva, as this would contaminate the bottle.

11. A. Ear irrigation removes cerumen from the auditory canal. Removing the cerumen should relieve the patient's discomfort; it should not cause pain or dizziness.

    B. Too much water pressure or rapid instillation could cause pain or dizziness, but this symptom would not occur if the water is introduced slowly.

    C. The water should displace any air in the ear canal, so there is no air to be trapped against the tympanic membrane.

    D. CORRECT. Using water that is too cold for an ear irrigation can lead to dizziness. The medical assistant should use water at body temperature for ear irrigation.

12. A. CORRECT. The medical assistant should wipe the center of the wound with an antiseptic swab, moving toward the edges in a circular motion.

    B. The medical assistant should not scrub the wound or move the swab back and forth once the cleansing process has begun.

    C. The medical assistant should not flood the wound with hydrogen peroxide because this delays healing.

    D. The medical assistant should not use alcohol on open wounds, as it will cause the patient pain.

13. A. The patient should be treated on the same day that they sustained the animal bite. However, the patient is not in a crisis situation that requires immediate care.

    B. The cause of the episode of syncope should be investigated. However, the patient is not in a crisis situation that requires immediate care.

    C. This patient should be seen quickly, but this is not an emergent situation.

    D. CORRECT. This patient is at risk for hemorrhage and needs to be seen by the provider immediately.

14. A. Tetanus boosters should be administered routinely every 5 to 10 years.

    B. Tetanus boosters should be administered routinely every 5 to 10 years.

    C. CORRECT. Tetanus boosters should be administered routinely every 5 to 10 years. If the patient does not remember the date they received their last tetanus booster, then one should be administered.

    D. Tetanus boosters should be administered routinely every 5 to 10 years.

15. A. The outside of the bottle is not sterile. The medical assistant will cause the provider to contaminate their own gloves if they touch the bottle.

    B. The outside of the container is not sterile. Placing it on the sterile field will contaminate the sterile field.

    C. CORRECT. The medical assistant should pour the sterile solution into a sterile container or onto gauze that is on the sterile field.

    D. The outside of the syringe is not sterile. The medical assistant will cause the provider to contaminate their own gloves if they touch the syringe.

Quiz 10: Answer key

1. A. Soap applied to the eyes can cause eye irritation.

   B. CORRECT. The medical assistant should flush their eyes with water at an eyewash station for at least 15 min following exposure to potentially infectious material. Flushing eyes with water is the recommended method for preventing the spread of infection.

   C. A cool compress will not remove the material from the eyes and will not prevent the spread of infection.

   D. Massaging the eyes will not remove the material from the eyes and will not prevent the spread of infection.

2. A. CORRECT. A 1:10 bleach solution is recommended for use as a disinfectant in a clinical setting.

   B. A 1:5 bleach solution is too strong of a concentration for clinical use.

   C. A 1:20 bleach solution is too weak of a concentration for clinical use.

   D. A 1:1 bleach solution is too strong of a concentration for clinical use.

3. A. If visible debris is present, the medical assistant should wash hands with soap and water rather than using hand sanitizer.

   B. The alcohol content of hand sanitizer should be at least 60%.

   C. Hand sanitizer alone is enough to provide disinfection.

   D. CORRECT. Hands should be dry when sanitizer is applied.

4. A. When performing hand hygiene, the medical assistant should wash hands under running water with hands lower than the elbows and with fingers pointing downward to direct water away from the rest of the arm.

   B. The medical assistant should use paper towels when performing hand hygiene. Cloth towels are more likely to collect and develop bacteria and micro-organisms.

C. The CDC recommends that natural fingernails not be longer than 0.64 cm (0.25 in) past the tip of the finger.

D. CORRECT. The medical assistant should not wear artificial nails or nail extensions when working with high-risk populations due to the higher percentage of gram-negative bacteria found on artificial nails than on natural fingernails.

5. A. Scrubbing the hands for only 10 seconds is not sufficient to remove bacteria.

B. The CDC recommends scrubbing the hands with soap and water for a minimum of 20 seconds.

C. CORRECT. Scrubbing the hands for 20 seconds would remove bacteria. This is the minimum length of time that the CDC recommends.

D. Scrubbing the hands for 25 seconds would remove bacteria. However, the minimum length of time that the CDC recommends is 20 seconds.

6. A. Hinged instruments should be open so that all grooves, crevices, and serrations can be scrubbed with a firm-bristled brush.

B. The medical assistant should use a firm-bristled, stiff nylon brush when scrubbing the surface of the instruments to guarantee that all infectious debris is removed during cleaning.

C. Sterilization is performed after sanitization. Bleach would not be used to sterilize the instruments.

D. CORRECT. The medical assistant should wear utility gloves when sanitizing sharp objects to be protected from instrument penetration or laceration, which could transmit infections. Utility gloves also protect the medical assistant from the harsh effects of chemical solutions.

7. A. CORRECT. The medical assistant should store the endoscope vertically so that any residual fluid can drain and the equipment can dry.

B. Storing the endoscope flat can cause moisture to pool within the tube.

C. Storing the endoscope in an airtight container does not allow the endoscope to dry properly and could cause contamination and bacteria growth.

D. The medical assistant should not place the endoscope in its original container because this could cause contamination and bacteria growth.

8. A. Ultrasonic sterilization uses sound waves to sanitize delicate instruments. A vaginal speculum is not a delicate instrument.

B. Gas sterilization uses gas to sterilize sensitive equipment that can be damaged by heat and moisture and, due to size, cannot be sterilized by other methods. A vaginal speculum is heat- and moisture-resistant.

C. CORRECT. Autoclave sterilization is a quick and effective method that uses steam under pressure to sterilize on-site medical equipment. The medical assistant should use this method to sterilize a vaginal speculum.

D. Ionizing radiation is a method of sterilization that is not used in health care facilities.

9. A. When loading an autoclave, the medical assistant should organize the packages so there is enough room for the flow of steam to allow for proper steam penetration. Steam penetration is compromised when packages are crowded together.

B. Unwrapped instruments should be placed on a perforated stainless steel tray and stored in a clean area. Unpackaged items are not considered sterile.

C. CORRECT. To ensure optimal sterilization of all surfaces, the packaged instruments should be spread out and organized as loosely as possible within the autoclave. Steam penetration is optimized when there is sufficient space between packages.

D. A disinfectant is not necessary when an instrument is to be autoclaved. This would be a redundant step in the sterilization process. To ensure sterilization of all surfaces, the packaged instruments should be spread out and organized loosely within the autoclave.

10. A. The medical assistant should take action to ensure the other patients are protected from infection.

B. CORRECT. If a patient is visibly sick and potentially spreading the infection, the medical assistant should move the patient to a separate area or into an examination room to wait.

C. The patient has an appointment to see the provider, so it is not necessary to notify the provider of the patient's condition.

D. This might cause the other patients to become concerned about contracting the illness. It can also cause the coughing and sneezing patient to feel singled-out.

11. A. The medical assistant does not need to wear full PPE for injections.

B. CORRECT. The medical assistant should wipe the patient's skin with an alcohol pad prior to an injection when following aseptic guidelines.

C. When disposing of the syringe, the medical assistant should point the needle downward.

D. The medical assistant should use separate, sterile needles for drawing from a vial and for injecting.

12. A. Aseptic technique is not necessary for cryosurgery because this procedure is less invasive than traditional surgery. The extremely low temperatures involved in cryosurgery prevent colonization by bacteria.

B. Aseptic technique is not necessary for a sonogram because the procedure is noninvasive.

C. Aseptic technique is not necessary for a sigmoidoscopy because the rectum and colon are colonized by bacteria.

D. CORRECT. Suturing requires surgical aseptic technique. The procedure is invasive, and the risk for infection is higher than it is during noninvasive procedures.

13. A. The medical assistant should discard biomedical waste in leak-proof containers that are labeled with the biohazard symbol.

B. A trained, OSHA-certified company should be contacted for biomedical waste collection.

C. CORRECT. The medical assistant should label chemicals with their names and any applicable data before disposal. Biohazard waste disposal companies need this information to dispose of the chemicals safely.

D. The medical assistant should place used syringes in a puncture-proof sharps container.

14. A. CORRECT. The medical assistant should discard materials contaminated with blood or bodily fluid in a red polyethylene bag.

B. Only items that are noninfectious, such as patient gowns, should be disposed of in a regular garbage bin.

C. Gauze pads are disposable and cannot be sterilized after use.

D. The medical assistant should only place items that are sharp in sharps containers.

15. A. Sharps containers should be placed in locations closest to patient treatment areas. The reception area is not used for patient treatment.

B. Sharps containers should be placed in locations closest to patient treatment areas. Patient treatment occurs inside the exam rooms.

C. CORRECT. Sharps containers should be placed in locations closest to patient treatment areas. The medical assistant should place the sharps container in the exam room.

D. Sharps containers should be placed in locations closest to patient treatment areas. The nurses' station is not used for patient treatment.

Quiz 11: Answer key

1. A. A clean-catch specimen for C&S requires a sterile specimen. Using a transfer device could contaminate the specimen.

B. TA clean-catch specimen for C&S requires the patient to void a small amount of urine into the toilet before voiding into a sterile container.

C. A clean-catch specimen for C&S requires a sterile specimen. Using a nonsterile container could contaminate the specimen.

D. CORRECT. A clean-catch specimen for C&S requires the patient to void a small amount of urine into the toilet before voiding into a sterile container.

2. A. The medical assistant should instruct the patient to stop taking certain medications before the stool collection test. However, the patient should not stop taking maintenance medications, such as a vasodilator.

B. The medical assistant should not instruct the patient to take a laxative prior to the exam.

C. CORRECT. The medical assistant should instruct the patient to stop taking NSAIDs 1 week before the test, as NSAIDs can cause a false positive test result.

D. The medical assistant should not instruct the patient to take 500 mg vitamin C supplement daily, as taking more than 250 mg vitamin C daily can cause a false positive test result.

3. A. CORRECT. The medical assistant should bring all reagents and devices to room temperature for a minimum of 30 min before the test.

B. The medical assistant should leave the swab in the tube for exactly 1 min.

C. The medical assistant should express the liquid from the swab by squeezing the tube, not squeezing the swab directly.

D. The medical assistant should dispense the reagents as free-falling drops. The reagent bottle should not come into contact with the tube.

4. A. If a blue line appears in the control and test areas, the result of the pregnancy test is positive.

B. CORRECT. The medical assistant should recognize that the color of the control line must change to validate quality control. The pregnancy test is not valid.

C. The concentration of the specimen would not affect the results.

D. A negative pregnancy test is characterized by a blue line in the control area, but not in the test area.

5. A. CORRECT. The medical assistant should use this notation to document the results of the patient's visual acuity test. The medical assistant should use 20/30-1 both eyes to document what line the patient read, any letters the patient missed, and which eyes the patient used.

B. This notation does not correctly represent the results of the patient's visual acuity test.

C. This notation does not correctly represent the results of the patient's visual acuity test.

D. This notation does not correctly represent the results of the patient's visual acuity test.

6. A. An audiometric test measures the lowest decibel of sound that an individual can hear by delivering a variety of sound frequencies through headphones.

B. An otoscopic exam is used to view the inner part of the ear canal.

C. CORRECT. A tuning fork test measures hearing using air and bone conduction.

D. A cerumen removal procedure uses wax-softening drops and irrigation to remove cerumen from the ear.

7. A. CORRECT. Patients exposed to potential allergens are at risk for a severe allergic reaction. A provider should always be on site when a test is administered and the medical assistant should notify the provider immediately if signs of anaphylaxis develop.

B. The medical assistant should choose the injection or application site based on space availability. They should ensure there is enough room for the control injection and the actual allergen injection.

C. The allergy test can cause a mild reaction, such as wheezing and sneezing. The medical assistant should continue the test unless a severe reaction occurs.

D. If the allergen test causes wheals or hives to form, the test result is positive. The medical assistant should administer additional injections or applications in an area that is free of wheals or hives.

8. A. The lateral thigh is not an appropriate site for this test.

B. The lower abdomen is not an appropriate site for this test.

C. CORRECT. The medical assistant should perform an intradermal skin test on the forearm or back.

D. The inner heel is not an appropriate site for this test.

9. A. The patient should refrain from using an inhaler at least 6 hr before spirometry testing.

B. CORRECT. Smoking causes constriction and can interfere with the accuracy of spirometry testing and should be stopped at least 1 hr prior to the test.

C. Tight clothing can restrict breathing, which can affect the patient's performance during spirometry testing.

D. The patient should avoid eating a large meal 2 hr prior to the test.

10. A. If the patient is sitting, their legs should be uncrossed with their feet on the floor.

B. The patient should loosen any clothing that is tight, but the clothing does not need to be fully removed.

C. CORRECT. The patient should remove their jacket and loosen any clothing that is tight to avoid restricting breathing capacity.

D. The patient should slightly elevate their chin for the procedure.

11. A. CORRECT. An abnormal fasting blood glucose is between 300 to 750 mg/dL. According to these results, the medical assistant should notify the provider.

B. The medical assistant should recognize these results as an abnormal fasting blood glucose. According to these results, the provider should be notified.

C. The medical assistant is authorized to take laboratory reports over the phone. The medical assistant should notify the provider after the results are confirmed.

D. The medical assistant should recognize these results as an abnormal fasting blood glucose. According to these results, the medical assistant should notify the provider before contacting the patient.

12. A. The expected reference range for the pH of an adult patient's urine is 4.5 to 8.0.

B. The expected reference range for the pH of an adult patient's urine is 4.5 to 8.0.

C. The expected reference range for the specific gravity of an adult patient's urine is from 1.005 to 1.030.

D. CORRECT. This value is outside of the expected reference range for an adult patient's urine.

13. A. The medical assistant should label the specimen immediately after collecting it to avoid processing errors.

B. CORRECT. The medical assistant should label the specimen immediately after collecting it to avoid processing errors.

C. The medical assistant should label the specimen immediately after collecting it to avoid processing errors.

D. The medical assistant should label the specimen immediately after collecting it to avoid processing errors.

14. A. Insurance information is necessary on the requisition form but not on the specimen label.

B. The patient's address is necessary on the requisition form but not on the specimen label.

C. CORRECT. The patient's date of birth is necessary on both the requisition form and the specimen label.

D. The provider's name is necessary on the requisition form but not on the specimen label.

15. A. The medical assistant should wait 3 to 5 min before developing the specimen.

B. The medical assistant should interpret the results 1 min after the developer is applied.

C. The medical assistant should apply two drops of developer to the back of the card, not directly onto the specimen.

D. CORRECT. The medical assistant should recognize that the test result is positive if a trace of blue color is detected on or at the edge of the smear.

Quiz 12: Answer key

1. A. The patient's account number is internal information that is provided on the requisition form. The patient is not required to verify this information.

B. The patient's power of attorney is not required information for a phlebotomy procedure.

C. The patient's phone number is not required information for a phlebotomy procedure.

D. CORRECT. The patient's date of birth must be verified for proper identification prior to the phlebotomy procedure.

2. A. A royal blue tube is used for chemistry trace elements tests.

B. CORRECT. A lavender tube is used for hematology tests. It is the appropriate tube for a CBC test.

C. A yellow tube is used for blood or bodily fluid tests.

D. A gray tube is used for chemistry tests, specifically glucose and alcohol level tests.

3. A. A serum separator tube is not the proper tube for an ESR test.

B. Green tubes contain the additive heparin, which helps prevent coagulation.

C. CORRECT. A sedimentation rate test requires the use of a lavender tube for proper processing. The lavender tube contains EDTA, which helps to remove calcium and prevent coagulation.

D. Light blue tubes are used for pediatric specimen collection.

4. A. A finger puncture is a form of capillary puncture. It is performed when the test requires a very small sample and as a last resort for older adult patients who have no acceptable veins to use.

B. Small veins tend to collapse when using the evacuated tube method. This method is not preferred for use on a patient who has small veins.

C. A heel stick is a form of capillary puncture. It is performed when the test requires a very small sample and is typically used on infants who are younger than 1 year old and not walking.

D. CORRECT. For better control and less pressure, the medical assistant should use the butterfly needle method for an older adult patient who has small veins.

5. A. The basilic vein is located on the little finger side of the antecubital space. Basilic veins tend to roll or move away from needles.

B. The cephalic vein is located on the thumb side of the antecubital space. Cephalic veins tend to roll or move away from needles.

C. CORRECT. The median cubital vein is a prominent vein located in the antecubital space, and it does not roll or move away from needles. The median cubital vein is the preferred vein due to accessibility.

D. The median antebrachial vein is located in the forearm. It should be used as an alternative site if the antecubital area is inaccessible, but it is not the preferred vein for routine phlebotomy.

6. A. Hydrogen peroxide is used as an oxidizer or disinfectant. It does not inhibit the reproduction of bacteria that might contaminate the sample.

B. Glutaraldehyde is a disinfectant used to clean medical equipment and should never be used on the skin.

C. Sterile water is not used as a cleaning agent and would not properly decontaminate the site.

D. CORRECT. The medical assistant should cleanse the patient's skin with an iodine solution, which inhibits the reproduction of bacteria that might contaminate the sample.

7. A. Applying an ice pack to the area does not aid in the avoidance of hemoconcentration.

B. CORRECT. A tourniquet impedes blood flow. Applying a tourniquet to a patient for longer than 1 min increases the possibility of hemoconcentration and can alter test results.

C. Instructing the patient to bend their arm does not help to avoid hemoconcentration.

D. Inserting the needle into the vein with the bevel down does not help to avoid hemoconcentration.

8. A. The red tube is drawn after the yellow tube. It is used for collecting serum specimens.

B. CORRECT. The yellow tube is the first tube in the order of draw. It is used for collecting sterile blood cultures.

C. The green tube is drawn after the yellow tube. It is used for collecting specimens for chemistry tests.

D. The gray tube is drawn after the yellow tube. It is used for collecting specimens for chemistry tests, especially glucose and alcohol levels.

9. A. The fifth digit has too little tissue for a successful capillary puncture.

B. CORRECT. The fourth digit is the preferred capillary puncture site for adults and children.

C. The second digit has extra nerve endings that make capillary puncture more painful.

D. The first digit is usually too callused for a successful capillary puncture.

10. A. The medical assistant should apply a bandage after disposing of the needle.

B. The medical assistant should label the tubes after applying a bandage.

C. CORRECT. Per OSHA standards and precautions, the medical assistant should discard the needle immediately after applying pressure to the puncture site.

D. The medical assistant should confirm the ordered tests prior to performing the phlebotomy procedure.

11. A. When collecting a serum specimen without an anticoagulant, 2 hr exceeds the maximum time the tube should stand prior to centrifuge. The assistant should let it stand for 30 to 60 min.

B. When collecting a serum specimen without an anticoagulant, 15 min is not enough time for the tube to stand prior to centrifuge. The assistant should let it stand for 30 to 60 min.

C. CORRECT. When collecting a serum specimen without an anticoagulant, the assistant should let it stand for 30 to 60 min.

D. When collecting a serum specimen without an anticoagulant, 20 min is not enough time for the tube to stand prior to centrifuge. The assistant should let it stand for 30 to 60 min.

12. A. CORRECT. The medical assistant should label the blood specimen tubes after the venipuncture procedure is completed, but prior to the patient being discharged.

B. Blood specimen tubes should never be labeled after the patient is discharged due to an increased risk of processing error.

C. The medical assistant should not label the tubes prior to the venipuncture due to an increased risk of processing error.

D. The medical assistant should not label the tubes during the venipuncture. If the medical assistant's attention is shifted away from the procedure, there is an increased risk of needlestick injury.

13. A. CORRECT. The medical assistant should submit a completed requisition form in accordance with the provider's prescription.

B. Although the medical assistant should provide the patient with postprocedure instructions, it is not part of the specimen handling process.

C. Storage requirements vary depending on the purpose of the specimen. Refrigeration is not appropriate for all specimens.

D. Centrifuge requirements vary depending on the purpose of the specimen. It is not appropriate to centrifuge all specimens.

14. A. CORRECT. The medical assistant must maintain scope of practice and notify the provider that the patient's fasting blood glucose is outside the expected reference range.

B. It is outside of the medical assistant's scope of practice to diagnose. It is the provider's responsibility to review and confirm the diagnosis.

C. Based on the results, the fasting blood glucose is above the expected reference range, but it is not within the critical value range. The provider will determine when a follow-up appointment should be scheduled.

D. Based on the results, the fasting blood glucose is above the expected reference range, but it is not within the critical value range. The medical assistant should contact the provider about the patient's results; however, this finding does not require urgent notification.

15. A. CORRECT. After receiving a patient's blood test results from the reference laboratory, the medical assistant should have the provider review the results.

B. Providers are responsible for reviewing and interpreting laboratory test results prior to filing them in the patient's medical record.

C. Providers are responsible for interpreting laboratory test results.

D. Providers are responsible for interpreting laboratory test results prior to determining if a patient requires a follow-up appointment.

Quiz 13: Answer key

1. A. The medical assistant should not place the patient in a prone (face-down) position for an EKG.

B. CORRECT. The medical assistant should place the patient in semi-Fowler's position. The medical assistant can elevate the head of the bed up to 45° if the patient is experiencing dyspnea.

C. The medical assistant should place patients who do not have difficulty breathing in a supine position (lying flat). However, this patient is experiencing difficulty breathing, so supine position would not be appropriate.

D. Sims' position is a side-lying position and is not appropriate for an EKG.

2. A. There are no food or drink restrictions prior to an EKG recording.

B. CORRECT. Due to the placement of necessary electrodes for the EKG recording, the patient will need to disrobe from the waist up and expose the lower legs.

C. The patient should avoid applying lotions, powders, oils, ointments, or topical medications to the electrode placement sites to avoid possible artifacts due to impeded lead attachment.

D. There is no requirement for a full bladder during an EKG recording. The medical assistant should encourage the patient to empty their bladder prior to the recording for comfort.

3. A. Limb leads are bipolar.

B. V1 through V6 are precordial leads that are unipolar. Limb leads are bipolar.

C. CORRECT. The medical assistant should place the limb leads on fleshy areas of the patient's skin to promote conductivity and obtain an accurate EKG recording.

D. The right leg lead wire serves as the ground and helps to avoid artifacts in the EKG recording.

4. A. CORRECT. The medical assistant should identify that the standard speed for an EKG recording is 25 mm/second.

B. The medical assistant can change the paper speed to 50 mm/second to spread out the cycles. However, the standard speed for an EKG recording is 25 mm/second.

C. Although this is a possible speed selection, the standard speed for an EKG recording is 25 mm/second.

D. Although this is a possible speed selection, the standard speed for an EKG recording is 25 mm/second.

5. A. This is the proper placement for V5.

B. This is the proper placement for V6.

C. The only lead placed midway between two leads is V3, and it is placed midway between V2 and V4.

D. CORRECT. The medical assistant should use the patient's clavicle as a landmark to assist in the placement of V4.

6. A. CORRECT. Any interference in the transmission of impulses, either through poor skin contact or lead wire issues, can cause a wandering baseline in the tracing.

B. This would result in AC interference, not a wandering baseline.

C. This would result in an inaccurate tracing that could lead to misinterpretation of the results, not a wandering baseline.

D. This would result in an inaccurate tracing. It would create an up-and-down tracing on the paper, not a wandering baseline.

7. A. Wandering baseline occurs when the patient is not remaining still and can be recognized by a stylus shift away from the baseline of the recording.

B. Interrupted baseline occurs when there is a break in the connection due to a lead wire becoming detached, frayed, or broken. Interrupted baseline is characterized by breaks in the recording.

C. CORRECT. The medical assistant should identify that AC interference is occurring. To avoid this artifact, the medical assistant should check the lead wires, move the patient's bed away from the wall, turn off other electronics in the room, and ensure proper grounding of the right leg electrode.

D. Somatic tremor, also known as a muscle artifact, is caused by an involuntary muscle movement. Somatic tremor is characterized by an erratic, fuzzy baseline.

8. A. Even though there are 10 electrodes applied to the patient, the EKG machine records 12 leads. Therefore, the ratio of applied leads to recorded leads is 10:12.

B. In a multichannel EKG machine, three to six leads are recorded at once. For a standard EKG machine, the ratio of applied leads to recorded leads is 10:12.

C. CORRECT. A standard EKG machine records 12 leads. For a standard EKG machine, the ratio of applied leads to recorded leads is 10:12.

D. Nine of the electrodes are responsible for the recording, and the tenth electrode (on the right leg) is a ground, but 12 leads are recorded in an EKG.

9. A. Atrial fibrillation is an example of a cardiac dysrhythmia. This dysrhythmia would result in a variably irregular QRS complex, not a widened QRS complex.

B. Bradycardia is slowed heart rate, which would result in a normal P wave with a ventricular rate of less than 60/min. This would not result in a widened QRS complex.

C. Sinus dysrhythmia is a variable change in heart rate that alternates from fast to slow in correlation with breathing patterns. The waves will have normal configurations.

D. CORRECT. An abnormally widened QRS complex should alert the medical assistant to a ventricular dysrhythmia, such as premature ventricular contraction (PVC). A PVC is caused by an early contraction of the ventricles, which produces a widened QRS complex artifact.

10. A. Myocardial infarction is caused by oxygen deprivation of the heart muscle, leading to muscle death. This would result in a larger than normal Q wave and an elevated ST segment.

B. CORRECT. Polarization is the resting state of the myocardial wall, resulting in a flatline or pause on the EKG pattern. This is a normal phase of the EKG cycle and represents a state of cellular rest with a positively charged outside and negatively charged inside.

C. Premature atrial contraction is an increase in the SA node excitability, resulting in premature atrial beats and does not result in a flatline on the EKG pattern.

D. Somatic tremor is caused by involuntary muscle movement and does not result in a flatline on the EKG pattern. It will result in a fuzzy, irregular baseline on the EKG pattern.

11. A. CORRECT. This patient would have a heart rate of 50/min. A heart rate less than 60/min is considered bradycardia. This patient's cardiac waves are all within the expected reference range, so this is a sinus bradycardia.

B. Atrial fibrillation is an irregular heart rate that does not present as an expected P wave, QRS complex, and T wave configuration on the patient's EKG tracing.

C. Ventricular fibrillation is a state of cardiac dysfunction in which the heart is ineffective in pumping blood and does not provide a consistent heart rhythm. It would not present as an expected P wave, QRS complex, and T wave configuration on the EKG tracing.

D. Sinus tachycardia is indicated by a heart rate greater than 100/min. However, this patient's EKG tracing indicates a heart rate of 50/min.

12. A. The patient should avoid eating heavy meals within 2 hr prior to the test because it may make it more difficult to complete the test.

B. The patient should wear clothing that is easy to exercise in to allow for electrode placement.

C. CORRECT. The patient should continue to take prescribed medications unless instructed otherwise by the provider.

D. The patient should wear comfortable athletic shoes for the test.

13. A. CORRECT. For the Holter monitor to detect the electrical activity of the heart, the electrodes must be securely attached to the skin at all times.

B. The patient should be instructed to avoid baths and showers during the monitoring period.

C. The patient should continue with activities of daily living during the monitoring period. The Holter monitor is designed to be worn with minimal inconvenience during daily activities.

D. The patient should record all activities during the monitoring period, including emotional symptoms, food intake, sleep schedule, sexual activity, and bowel movements.

14. A. Although lead I records the heart rhythm, another option provides a clearer recording.

B. CORRECT. Lead II provides the clearest recording of the heart rhythm and is the standard lead used for a rhythm strip.

C. Although lead III records the heart rhythm, another option provides a clearer recording.

D. Although lead V2 records the heart rhythm, another option provides a clearer recording.

15. A. Sinus rhythm is a heart rate and rhythm within the expected reference range of 60 to 100/min.

B. Atrial fibrillation is an irregular heart beat.

C. A heart rate of 60/min or less indicates bradycardia.

D. CORRECT. A heart rate greater than 100/min indicates tachycardia.

Quiz 14: Answer key

1. A. Only a brief description of the patient's hospitalization is necessary for the provider to give continuous care.

B. CORRECT. The purpose of a discharge summary is to give the provider a brief description of the patient's illness, treatment, and condition during hospitalization.

C. The discharge summary is not used to obtain authorization for hospitalization.

D. The discharge summary is not used to provide the patient with information about the diagnosis.

2. A. The medical assistant should verify allergies during the patient's appointment.

B. Medications are reviewed and authorized by the provider during the patient's visit.

C. CORRECT. Prior to the patient's appointment, the medical assistant will obtain the patient's medical record. The medical record includes treatment results and patient progress notes. The medical assistant should ensure that all pertinent information is available for the provider prior to the appointment.

D. The provider should authorize and order any further tests during the patient's visit.

3. A. The medical assistant should treat patients according to their specific needs.

B. The medical assistant should help the patient with finding assistance options.

C. The medical assistant should be a team player and coordinate with multiple health care community resources.

D. CORRECT. The medical assistant should serve patients by helping them locate the appropriate community resources for their needs.

4. A. The Department of Health and Human Services is a department of the federal government that provides essential human services and protects the health of Americans.

B. The parks and recreation department works in conjunction with public health to provide individuals with the highest possible quality of life through parks and recreation-based physical activity.

C. CORRECT. Medical assistants serve as patient advocates to recommend organized support groups based on the needs of patients and their family members.

D. Hospice care centers provide personal care and palliative care for comfort and pain relief for patients who are dying.

5.   A. Quality control is a combination of activities designed to ensure adequate quality, especially in manufactured products. It is not used when a PCP is transitioning a patient's care to a specialist.

B. An audit is a formal examination of an organization's or individual's accounts. It is not used when a PCP is transitioning a patient's care to a specialist.

C. CORRECT. Services rendered from one provider to another, including data transfer and patient care, demonstrates the process of continuity of care.

D. Termination of care involves ending the provider-patient relationship. It is not used when a PCP is transitioning a patient's care to a specialist.

6.   A. The medical assistant should instruct the patient to take all of the provided medication as prescribed. Medication nonadherence can lead to a shortfall in the treatment objective and can be detrimental to the desired outcomes.

B. CORRECT. To facilitate patient understanding and medication compliance, the medical assistant should review all instructions concerning medication administration and dosage with the patient.

C. It is outside of the medical assistant's scope of practice to make medication recommendations. The patient should adhere to the provider's prescription to achieve treatment objectives.

D. The medical assistant should inform the patient to report any side effects experienced while taking the medication to the provider. In some cases, side effects can indicate an adverse reaction to the medication.

7.   A. CORRECT. Maintaining an empathetic tone promotes respect between the medical assistant and the patient.

B. The medical assistant should deliver the information clearly and at a speed the patient can easily comprehend.

C. The medical assistant should provide both verbal and written instructions for the patient.

D. Maintaining a closed posture, with the arms and legs crossed, can indicate disinterest toward the patient.

8.   A. The primary responsibility of a physician assistant is the overall care of patients.

B. The primary responsibility of a nurse practitioner is the overall care of patients.

C. The primary responsibility of an emergency provider is to assess patients and provide immediate care.

D. CORRECT. A patient navigator recognizes patients' needs and barriers and assists by coordinating care and identifying the community and health care resources to meet those needs.

9.   A. Ambulatory services are an attribute of various facilities that offer health care services to patients, including occupational health and surgical centers.

B. CORRECT. Comprehensive care is one of the five core functions and attributes of a PCMH. It is all-encompassing and includes a patient's physical and mental health care. A team of providers works together to care for the patient at a PCMH.

C. The HITECH Act provides financial incentives to health care facilities for the meaningful use of electronic health records technology to achieve efficiency and health goals.

D. The Affordable Care Act was implemented to increase the quality, availability, and affordability of private and public health insurance for individuals.

10.   A. CORRECT. The PCMH model of care is committed to providing safe, quality health care by relying on evidence-based medicine, information sharing, and shared decision making.

B. The PCMH model of care focuses on individualized, holistic patient care.

C. The PCMH model of care relies on a team of care providers to administer holistic, individualized patient care. The primary care provider is not expected to be the sole provider of comprehensive care for the patient.

D. The PCMH model of care focuses on providing accessible care through extended office hours, shortened wait times, and alternative routes of communication, such as email.

11.   A. The medical assistant will verify the patient's current medication list at the time of the visit, along with an update of any allergies and over-the-counter medications.

B. The medical assistant will place an updated insurance card in the patient's chart at the time of check-in.

C. A specialist authorization form is not necessary for an appointment with the PCP.

D. CORRECT. The PCP will need to review any diagnostic tests performed since the last appointment to determine whether current treatments are effective. The medical assistant should verify that the diagnostic test results are available in the patient's chart.

12.   A. The organization's board of directors is not necessary information to provide when making a list of community resources.

B. It is not necessary to provide volunteer opportunity information when creating a list of community-based organizations because the list is intended to help patients find resources for their physical health care needs.

C. CORRECT. Physical addresses of the organizations are important to provide, especially for patients who have difficulty with transportation and want local resources.

D. Community-based organizations have varied costs for services and would be difficult to provide in a list of community resources.

13.   A. Hospice services are for patients who have a terminal illness. This service would not be the best community resource to offer.

B. Grief support groups are beneficial for family members of the deceased. This service would not be the best community resource to offer.

C. Rehabilitation services provide assistance to patients who have physical disabilities that include injuries or trauma. This service would not be the best community resource to offer.

D. CORRECT. Adult day care provides supervision for older adults during the day who have family members providing care in the evening. This service would be the best community resource to offer respite care.

14. A. CORRECT. Meeting the patient's needs is the primary reason the medical assistant should refer the patient to community resources. This action demonstrates health coaching.

B. Referring patients to a specialist is completed internally by the medical office, but does not demonstrate health coaching.

C. A medical assistant should encourage a patient to make appropriate choices to maintain an active, healthy lifestyle.

D. Meeting Medicare's Meaningful Use criteria is not an example of health coaching

15. A. CORRECT. Communication between all members is imperative for a successful transition of care. All parties must be aware of what is being done for the patient and communicate that information to the patient and family members.

B. To achieve a successful transition of care, the patient should be included in planning and decision-making. Exclusion can lead to a lack of understanding and nonadherence to the care plan.

C. To ensure the patient's successful transition of care, every team member should have access to the same information regarding the patient.

D. The patient should be contacted within 24 to 48 hr after being discharged. Timely follow-up is imperative to achieve a successful transition of care.

Quiz 15: Answer key

1. A. The medical assistant should ask for a photo ID when checking in a patient.

B. The medical assistant should have the patient fill out a registration form when checking in.

C. CORRECT. The medical assistant should review the patient's medical record to check for further instructions from the provider. This information helps the medical assistant to schedule a follow-up appointment for the patient if necessary.

D. The medical assistant should verify the patient's insurance when checking in a patient.

2. A. The CMS provides regulations for the billing of Medicare and Medicaid services.

B. The ICD-10 coding manual provides a list of diagnostic coding for insurance and research purposes.

C. The CDC provides education and guidance about disease control and prevention to the public.

D. CORRECT. The CPT manual provides a standard language for reporting services provided during a medical visit.

3. A. CORRECT. The first action the medical assistant should take is to complete a patient referral form.

B. The third step the medical assistant should take is to give the patient a copy of the authorization code.

C. The second action the medical assistant should take is to obtain prior authorization to receive approval for the referral to a specialist.

D. The final step the medical assistant should take is to document the date of referral approval for tracking purposes.

4. A. A pegboard system is a method of tracking patient accounts. This an older method used for mathematical calculations.

B. A fee profile is used to compile an average of provider's fees over a given period of time.

C. CORRECT. Charges posted to a patient's account should be taken from a pre-established list of fee allowances based on a fee schedule.

D. An itemized statement is a confirmation of the patient's responsibility for services billed after charges have been posted.

5. A. Downcoding describes the unlawful act of a third-party payer paying for services at a lower rate than the contract agreement.

B. Evaluation and management codes are CPT codes that comprehensively cover services rendered by outpatient and inpatient care facilities.

C. Add-on codes are a type of CPT code that is added to describe category codes in further detail.

D. CORRECT. Upcoding describes the unlawful act of billing services at a higher rate than contracted to receive a larger reimbursement from a third-party payer. This is also known as overcoding, code creep, and overbilling.

6. A. When the office receives a returned check marked NSF (nonsufficient funds), the medical assistant should add the amount back to the patient's account balance.

B. When the office receives a duplicate payment for services, a credit balance is added to the patient's account.

C. When the office receives overpayment from an insurance company, the medical assistant should reimburse the insurance company and balance the patient's account accordingly.

D. CORRECT. An insurance disallowance results in an adjustment on the patient's account. The provider's usual charge is often more than the established allowed amount. The provider is not allowed to bill the patient for the difference, so the provider should write off the difference, resulting in an adjustment.

7. A. CORRECT. A clearinghouse submission allows a provider to submit multiple insurance claims electronically in batches for a small fee. The clearinghouse uses software to audit and sort claims for various insurance carriers.

B. Direct billing is a process where the insurance carrier allows the provider to submit claims electronically directly to the carrier. This does not involve the electronic auditing and sorting of claims.

C. Intelligent character recognition is a system that scans documents and captures claims information from CMS-1500 forms. This does not involve the electronic auditing and sorting of claims.

D. A universal claim form is used for submitting all government-sponsored claims. This form is not used to audit or sort claims.

8. A. Alphabetic filing involves organizing patient files in alphabetical order by patient name.

B. Purging is the process of moving active files to an inactive status.

C. CORRECT. Shingling is a method of filing in which a new report is laid on top of an older report, resembling the shingles on a roof.

D. Numeric filing involves organizing patient files by an established numbering system.

9. A. The objective content area includes physical examination findings and test results.

B. The assessment content area includes the provider's diagnosis based on findings from the objective and subjective content areas.

C. CORRECT. The subjective content area includes personal demographics, along with medical, family, and social history.

D. The plan content area includes the provider's documentation of how the patient will be treated.

10. A. The medical assistant should notify the next scheduled patient about the delay and give the patient the option to wait or reschedule.

B. The medical assistant should recognize that the patient can choose to wait, reschedule, or see a different provider.

C. CORRECT. The medical assistant should notify the next scheduled patient about the delay by calling the patient or informing the patient upon arrival at the office.

D. The medical assistant should take the next scheduled patient to an exam room only if the provider is available at that time to see the patient.

11. A. Cookies track browser history to identify users and personalize their online experience.

B. The cache tracks the websites that users visit to increase browser speed.

C. Queries are used to process the information that a database documents, tracks, and stores.

D. CORRECT. Databases are used in health care settings to document, track, and store patient information.

12. A. CORRECT. The SDS provides information regarding chemicals used in a medical facility and how to respond to a spill or exposure.

B. The OSHA Form 301 is used for incident reporting in the case of work-related injury or illness.

C. The emergency action plan provides procedures regarding natural disasters and other emergencies that can occur in a medical office.

D. The CFR contains the regulations laid out by various department and agencies of the federal government concerning a wide variety of subjects, including medical law.

13. A. CORRECT. The medical assistant should prepare a list of all supplies that require replacement and prepare a purchase order for those supplies.

B. Although some medical supplies have expiration dates, not all medical supplies have a date by which they should be used. Disposing of all unused supplies is a waste of resources and can be detrimental to a clinic's budget.

C. The overhead costs of the clinic include staff wages and business expenses. These are not relevant when performing an inventory of medical supplies.

D. The medical assistant should create a purchase order and send it to the vendor. After receipt of the purchase order, the vendor creates and sends invoices to the clinic.

14. A. A consumable item is a supply that can be emptied or used up, such as gauze, bandages, and alcohol pads.

B. An expendable item is an important and commonly used supply, such as pens, pencils, and paper.

C. An intangible item does not have a physical presence and cannot be touched. Examples include a positive attitude, enthusiasm, and initiative.

D. CORRECT. A durable item is a piece of equipment that is used repeatedly. Examples include crutches, wheelchairs, and walkers.

15. A. CORRECT. Automated call routing allows patients to confirm or cancel appointment times with keystrokes on a telephone.

B. Appointment cards are reminders given to patients at an appointment or sent to the patient prior to an appointment. They are not a method for the patient to confirm or cancel an appointment remotely.

C. Wave scheduling is a method of appointment scheduling in which multiple patients are scheduled for the same time and are seen in the order of their arrival to the clinic.

D. Advanced booking involves scheduling an appointment in advance. It is not a method for the patient to confirm or cancel an appointment remotely.

Quiz 16: Answer key

1. A. CORRECT. If there is a staff member present who speaks the same language as the patient, the medical assistant should ask that staff member to assist with communication.

B. The medical assistant should address the patient by their title and last name, unless the patient gives the medical assistant permission to use their first name.

C. The medical assistant should avoid using medical terminology with any patient, regardless of the presence of a language barrier.

D. The medical assistant should use body gestures to help enhance the patient's understanding of the information.

2. A. Empathy occurs when a medical assistant tries to view a patient's situation from the patient's perspective.

B. Rapport occurs when a relationship between a medical assistant and a patient is harmonious.

C. Active listening is two-way communication that involves paraphrasing information, asking questions, and providing feedback.

D. CORRECT. Stereotyping occurs when a medical assistant makes incorrect assumptions about a patient based on personal prejudices.

3. A. The medical assistant should speak in a low tone to help a patient who has hearing loss understand the information.

B. CORRECT. The medical assistant should stand within the patient's field of vision to communicate with a patient who has hearing loss.

C. The medical assistant should use gentle touch to get the patient's attention.

D. The medical assistant should use hand gestures when speaking with a patient who has hearing loss to enhance understanding.

4. A. The medical assistant should use a regular tone when communicating with a patient who has vision impairment.

B. CORRECT. The medical assistant should notify the patient upon entering the room to prevent startling the patient.

C. The medical assistant should avoid using body gestures when communicating with a patient who has vision impairment.

D. The medical assistant should provide large-font printed material for a patient who has vision impairment.

5. A. CORRECT. The medical assistant should notify the provider about the patient's situation.

B. This statement is not within the medical assistant's scope of practice.

C. This statement is not within the medical assistant's scope of practice.

D. This statement is not within the medical assistant's scope of practice.

6. A. Providing medical advice to a patient is outside the medical assistant's scope of practice.

B. CORRECT. The medical assistant should document all patient concerns in the medical record to properly communicate the information to the provider.

C. Although the medical assistant should acknowledge the emotions and concerns expressed by a patient to better communicate the patient's needs to the provider, false reassurance can be misleading and counterproductive to the communication process.

D. The medical assistant should document all patient concerns in the medical record. Evaluating whether a concern is valid is not within the medical assistant's scope of practice.

7. A. The medical assistant should have all information that is necessary for an outgoing call ready and available before calling the patient.

B. Speaking with varying pitch allows for emphasis when communicating. Speaking with an unchanging pitch can make it difficult for the patient to understand what is being said.

C. The medical assistant should hold the receiver of the telephone no more than 2.5 cm (1 in) from the mouth.

D. CORRECT. The medical assistant should allow the patient to end the call. This allows the patient the opportunity to ask clarifying questions before ending the call.

8. A. In a modified block letter style with indented paragraphs, each paragraph is indented.

B. In a simplified letter style, the signature is in all capital letters.

C. In a block letter style, all lines start flush with the left margin.

D. CORRECT. In a modified block letter style, the complimentary closing, date line, and signature are centered on the page.

9. A. In a properly formatted business letter, there is blank space between the letterhead and the dateline.

B. CORRECT. A properly formatted business letter is organized with the inside address falling between the dateline and the salutation.

C. In a properly formatted business letter, there is blank space between the salutation and the subject line.

D. In a properly formatted business letter, there is blank space between the signature block and the identification line.

10. A. The medical assistant should not contradict the patient's statement because this can be counterproductive to communication and intensify the patient's negative emotional reaction.

B. The medical assistant should not use leading questions because these types of questions direct the patient to answer in the way the medical assistant wants, which suppresses the patient's ability to answer honestly and express their emotions.

C. CORRECT. Recognizing and acknowledging a patient's emotions and their sources allows for effective communication and is a key step in redirecting those emotions to solving any perceived problems.

D. The medical assistant should try to communicate openly with the patient and understand what is causing the patient's emotional distress. Threatening the patient with removal from the clinic is a barrier to open communication.

11. A. The medical assistant should avoid displaying emotion and focus on calming the angry patient.

B. CORRECT. The medical assistant should remain calm and offer to help the patient.

C. The medical assistant should be willing to apologize and admit if a mistake has been made.

D. The medical assistant should avoid speaking loudly and gradually lower the volume of their voice. As a result, the patient will likely lower their volume to hear what the medical assistant is saying.

12. A. CORRECT. One aspect of active listening is reflection, which involves the medical assistant identifying the main idea of a patient's statements and acknowledging the patient's feelings.

B. This statement is providing the patient with false reassurance. The medical assistant should acknowledge the patient's feelings.

C. By asking the patient a leading question, the medical assistant is trying to indicate the preferred response for the patient to make. This does not acknowledge the patient's feelings.

D. The medical assistant should not provide unwanted advice because it does not acknowledge the patient's feelings and indicates that the feelings are invalid.

13. A. The medical assistant should not dissociate from the conversation. This could cause the patient to become more upset.

    B. The medical assistant should not interject the thoughts and feelings of the patient.

    C. The medical assistant should not argue with the patient, as this will not resolve the situation. This could cause the patient to become more upset.

    D. CORRECT. The medical assistant should display active listening and empathy for the patient by acknowledging their concern.

14. A. The medical assistant should set aside personal feelings when making decisions.

    B. Team members should discuss conflicts privately with each other before involving a supervisor.

    C. Team members should work toward a common goal while maintaining mutual accountability.

    D. CORRECT. For teamwork to be successful, team members should work together and be willing to perform duties outside of their formal job descriptions.

15. A. CORRECT. One of the essential elements of successful teamwork is having short-term and intermediate goals that relate to the team's long-term goals.

    B. One of the essential elements of successful teamwork is having a small team of less than 10 members.

    C. One of the essential elements of successful teamwork is having team members with a variety of abilities, skills, and talents.

    D. One of the essential elements of successful teamwork is the addressing of negative information with the team, as suppression of negative information can cause circulation of rumors.

Quiz 17: Answer key

1. A. The primary focus of the CDC is to be a reference for information and statistics associated with health care and to conduct research on health-related issues.

    B. CORRECT. OSHA is an agency of the Department of Labor and has a primary focus of protecting individuals in the workplace by establishing and enforcing safety regulations through training, outreach, education, and assistance.

    C. NIH is a division of HHS and has a primary focus of conducting biomedical research concerning the causes and prevention of disease. NIH also provides telehealth information to the health care industry.

    D. HHS is a department that protects the health of Americans and has a primary focus of offering multiple programs, which include free immunizations and financial assistance for low-income families, as well as overseeing Medicare and Medicaid.

2. A. Misfeasance is the performance of a legal act in an improper manner.

    B. Malpractice occurs when treatment provided to a patient does not meet expected levels of care. It is also known as medical professional liability, and it includes all liability that can occur during medical care.

C. CORRECT. Malfeasance is performed when a person knowingly commits an unlawful and wrongful act.

D. A misdemeanor is a minor criminal offense that is considered less serious than a felony and carries a lesser penalty.

3. A. Ethical dilemmas occur when there are two or more acceptable solutions, and only one option can be chosen.

    B. Locus of authority issues occur when two or more authority figures disagree on how a situation should be handled.

    C. Dilemmas of justice occur when benefits cannot be fairly distributed to health care consumers.

    D. CORRECT. Ethical distress occurs when the ethically correct action is indicated, but some type of barrier prevents the medical assistant from following through with that action. The medical assistant knows they should report their coworker, but they feel they cannot because it could lead to their coworker losing her job and being charged for theft.

4. A. CORRECT. The AMA Code of Ethics was written in 1846 and includes nine separate categories of ethical dilemmas concerning allied health professionals.

    B. The Hippocratic Oath is an oath taken by a provider when beginning the practice of medicine.

    C. The Code of Hammurabi is the earliest written code that included rules for medical practice involving ethical conduct, but it is no longer relevant.

    D. Percival's Code was written in 1803 and is concerned with sociologic matters. Percival's Code was acknowledged in the AMA Code of Ethics.

5. A. This legal document will allow healthy organs or tissues to be harvested from a donor and transferred to patients who are in need of organ or tissue donations.

    B. CORRECT. A living will is a legal document that states the life-saving procedures a patient authorizes in the event they are incapable of verbalizing their desire for medical treatment.

    C. This legal document names a health care advocate to make medical decisions for a patient when he is unable to do so.

    D. Do-not-resuscitate orders indicate to the medical staff that a patient refuses any life-saving interventions.

6. A. Advance directives can be updated at any time, as long as the instructions are received by the patient's primary provider.

    B. CORRECT. Advance directives can be updated whenever a patient wants, as long as the instructions are received by the patient's primary provider.

    C. Advance directives can be updated at any time, as long as the instructions are received by the patient's primary provider.

    D. Advance directives can be updated at any time, as long as the instructions are received by the patient's primary provider.

7. A. A member of the patient's medical team cannot be designated as the patient's health care proxy.

    B. It would be a conflict of interest and not conducive to the patient's best care to designate the executor of the will as the health care proxy.

    C. CORRECT. A member of a faith community whom the patient trusts is an acceptable choice to make decisions for end-of-life care.

    D. It would be a conflict of interest and not conducive to the patient's best care to designate the patient's attorney as the health care proxy.

8. A. A 14-year-old adolescent is considered a minor and does not meet the age requirements for a health care proxy.

    B. A 16-year-old adolescent is considered a minor and does not meet the age requirements for a health care proxy.

    C. A 21-year-old adult is eligible to become a health care proxy. However, 21 is not the minimum age to become a health care proxy.

    D. CORRECT. An individual becomes eligible as a health care proxy at age 18.

9. A. CORRECT. A Medical Order for Life-Sustaining Treatment form provides medical orders from the patient's provider regarding the patient's wishes for life-sustaining treatment. This form will be moved from one facility to another when the patient is transferred.

    B. The Uniform Anatomical Gift Act establishes the right of patients to document their wishes concerning organ donation in case of death.

    C. The Patient Self-Determination Act establishes the right of patients to determine what care they receive in case of medical need.

    D. The Patient's Bill of Rights ensures and clarifies the various rights of a patient receiving medical care.

10. A. CORRECT. The Patient's Bill of Rights establishes that patients have the right to determine which treatments they receive.

    B. This statement is biased and does not respect the patient's right to make decisions regarding her care.

    C. This statement is confrontational and does not promote a healthy patient-provider relationship. The patient has a right to make decisions regarding her care.

    D. This statement shows consideration for the patient's well-being, but it does not respect the patient's right to make decisions regarding her care.

11. A. The ADA forbids discrimination based on disability against any applicant or employee who could perform a job.

    B. CORRECT. The HIPAA Privacy Rule grants patients the right to access, review, and receive a copy of their health care information.

    C. FMLA requires some employers to give time off to employees.

    D. PHI includes the patient's demographic information, medical history, and insurance information, which is regulated through HIPAA.

12. A. Workers' compensation does not require the patient's authorization to disclose information to insurers, employers, or others involved in the workers' compensation system.

    B. Public health authorities include federal, tribal, and local law enforcement agencies. They are responsible for public safety within a community, and information gathered can affect the health of the population. These entities are required to report some diseases and injuries.

    C. State agencies are responsible for public safety, and information gathered can affect the health of a population. Therefore, state agencies are required to report certain diseases and injuries, along with births and deaths.

    D. CORRECT. Health care clearinghouses must adhere to HIPAA guidelines due to handling insurance claims, which contain protected health information.

13. A. CORRECT. Computers should never be left open or unlocked. However, if this does occur, using a privacy filter diminishes the viewing angle and blurs the content on the screen.

    B. Encryption software encodes the information to make it unreadable to users who are not authorized to view the material. This is not done at the user level.

    C. Firewalls are programs used by the facility to block and filter communication between the network and the Internet. They are not at the user level.

    D. An audit is used to track activity and identify the specific information a user is viewing. This involves the facility's information technology department, and it is not at the user level.

14. A. The complaint must be filed within 180 days of when the perceived privacy violation occurred.

    B. The complaint must be filed within 180 days of when the perceived privacy violation occurred.

    C. CORRECT. The complaint must be filed within 180 days of when the perceived privacy violation occurred.

    D. The complaint must be filed within 180 days of when the perceived privacy violation occurred.

15. A. It is not appropriate to notify the child's school counselor.

    B. It is not within the assistant's scope of practice to question the patient.

    C. It is not within the assistant's scope of practice to question the child's parent.

    D. CORRECT. The assistant should notify the child's provider. The provider will conduct a medical examination of the child to further investigate the indications of abuse.

IN PRACTICE
Case Studies

CASE STUDY 1: HEALTH CARE SYSTEMS AND SETTINGS

Meghan, a medical assistant, is taking medical history from Mr. Martin. Mr. Martin explains that he took his morning medication as usual and then went outside to prune his hedges. Upon going inside for lunch, he noticed a red, itchy rash on his lower right leg. Meghan documents this in the chart for the provider.

QUESTION 1 *What are some additional questions that the medical assistant should ask to document the history of this episode a little more?*

Answers will vary.

- "What medications did you take this morning?"
- "Have you experienced similar reactions in the past after taking your medications or when working in your garden?"
- "Did you notice any additional symptoms other than the itchy rash on your lower right leg, such as swelling, hives, or breathing difficulties?"

Following the screening, Mr. Martin asks if Meghan can suggest an over-the-counter medication to help with his rash. Meghan knows that the doctor normally prescribes diphenhydramine for local reactions.

QUESTION 2 *What response would be most appropriate based on this scenario?*

- **A.** "The doctor normally prescribes over-the-counter diphenhydramine for these types of rashes."
- **B.** "The doctor should be able to provide an answer to your question following her examination."
- **C.** "I can't prescribe medications because I am only a medical assistant."
- **D.** "You will need to have extensive testing to determine the cause of your rash before a treatment can be established."

The correct answer is B. Prescribing and recommending medications is outside the scope of practice of the medical assistant.

After thinking about his symptoms and possible contributors to his symptoms, Mr. Martin states that he has never had any previous reactions to his current medications but has had similar reactions when working in the garden. The provider thinks the patient would be best served by seeing a specialist.

QUESTION 3 *Which of the following specialists is the provider likely to recommend in this case?*

A. Dermatologist

B. Endocrinologist

C. Infectious disease specialist

D. Allergist

The correct answer is D. The provider will most likely refer the patient to an allergist for further care.

QUESTION 4 *The provider orders the medical assistant to administer a shot of diphenhydramine to the patient. What dictates whether a medical assistant can administer this type of medication?*

State medical board regulations and the medical office's organizational policies dictate who can administer medications.

CASE STUDY 2: BODY STRUCTURES AND ORGAN SYSTEMS

Kelly, a medical assistant, is taking a medical history from Ms. Stevens. Ms. Stevens explains that she has lower abdominal pain that starts in the center of her abdomen, well below her belly button, and radiates to the left side of her lower abdomen. She also reports lower back pain on the left side. The pain has been present for 2 days. The patient goes on to say that she has frequent and painful urination and a fever.

QUESTION 1 *In medical terms, which abdominal regions are involved?*

The hypogastric region and left iliac region.

QUESTION 2 *What body systems might be involved, based on the patient's symptoms?*

Urogenital

QUESTION 3 *What other questions should the medical assistant ask the patient?*

Answers will vary. "Do you have any vaginal symptoms, such as vaginal discharge, odor, or pain?"

After obtaining the chief complaint, Kelly needs to think ahead about what the provider will need during the examination and how to have Ms. Stevens disrobe.

QUESTION 4 *What type of exams or diagnostic testing should the medical assistant anticipate?*

If vaginal symptoms are involved, the medical assistant should set up a pelvic tray and gather the appropriate swabs for possible STI testing. The medical assistant should also collect a clean catch urine specimen for dipstick testing, and a possible urine culture and sensitivity.

QUESTION 5 *Should the medical assistant perform any testing before the provider examines the patient?*

In most cases no testing should be performed unless a direct order is given. However, some offices have a protocol to perform a chemical analysis of urine of any patient who has urinary symptoms.

CASE STUDY 3: PATHOPHYSIOLOGY AND DISEASE PROCESSES

Mr. Swanson comes into the office reporting wheezing, coughing, and a feeling of tightness across his chest. He states that he has a history of hay fever but never experienced any wheezing or chest tightness until after moving to an apartment in the city 6 months ago. He states that he has been to the Emergency Department (ED) at least three times since moving to the new apartment. The medical assistant, Darren, references the history section of Mr. Swanson's chart and notes that he is a smoker and also has hypertension.

QUESTION 1 *What body systems might be involved in the patient's symptoms?*

Respiratory, cardiovascular, and immune systems

After additional questioning, Darren learns that Mr. Swanson experienced similar symptoms each time he went to the ED. He received a diagnosis of asthma during each ED visit. Mr. Swanson used his inhaler earlier but just says he can't get full relief and didn't go back to the ED this evening because of the high deductible. He doesn't think that this attack is severe as previous attacks, but he is uncomfortable.

QUESTION 2 *What types of testing might the provider prescribe, and what should be the medical assistant's next step?*

Answers will vary. The provider will probably want spirometry testing, pulse oximetry testing, and possibly an EKG to rule out cardiac involvement. If the medical assistant identifies a possible breathing emergency, he should notify the provider right away and set up supplies needed in the event of a respiratory emergency. No testing should be performed until the provider gives an order.

The provider prescribes a breathing treatment, and the patient's symptoms subside. The provider would like the patient set up to have allergy testing and prescribes steroids.

QUESTION 3 *Why did the provider prescribe allergy testing?*

Because the patient's wheezing started once he moved into the apartment, there could be something in the apartment that is aggravating symptoms.

QUESTION 4 *What is the purpose of the steroid?*

The steroid will help to reduce airway inflammation.

QUESTION 5 *What lifestyle changes should the patient make to help reduce the risk of future attacks?*

Answers will vary. The patient should start a smoking cessation program because smoking worsens symptoms. The patient needs to identify environmental factors in the apartment (dust mites, roach infestation) that might be provoking the attacks.

CASE STUDY 4: PATIENT CARE COORDINATION AND EDUCATION

Ryan, a medical assistant, works for Dr. Tancred in a very prominent patient–centered medical home (PCMH). During a patient huddle, Ryan shared with Dr. Tancred that Ms. Grover, who has diabetes and heart disease, never showed up for her follow-up appointment after being in the hospital. Ryan tried to reach Ms. Grover on her cell phone several times, but the call went straight to her voicemail each time. Dr. Tancred asks Ryan to call the transitional care coordinator from the hospital, Maria, to see if she can assist in any way.

QUESTION 1 *Why is it important to get the patient into the office for a follow-up visit following hospitalization?*

Answers will vary. The patient might need wound care, blood work, or medication adjustments. Nonadherence of home instructions is more prevalent when the patient does not follow up with the primary care provider for postdischarge care, and as a result can lead to additional hospitalizations.

QUESTION 2 *What is the term for health care professionals from different teams working together to make sure that the patients receive comprehensive care and don't fall through the cracks?*

Collaborative care

Ryan contacts Maria, who is able to connect with Ms. Grover. Maria instructs Ms. Grover to call Ryan to reschedule the appointment. Ms. Grover states that she is unable to drive and doesn't have anyone to transport her to the doctor. She says she can't afford her copays on her medications and just feels like giving up.

QUESTION 3 *How should the medical assistant respond to the patient?*

Answers will vary. The medical assistant should be empathetic and professional. The medical assistant should let the patient know that he will see if he can connect her with health care personnel that can assist with her concerns.

QUESTION 4: *Who should the medical assistant consult regarding this new information?*

Answers will vary. The medical assistant should consult with the provider and the transitional care nurse from the hospital. The provider needs to be aware of what is going on to relay information to the patient until a solution can be determined. The transitional care coordinator already has an established relationship with the patient and has resources that the office doesn't have to assist the patient with transportation and medication costs.

Maria arranges for Ms. Grover to get transportation to her first appointment and works with the medication companies to get her medications at no cost for the first 3 months.

QUESTION 5 *What records will the medical assistant need to have available for the first appointment?*

The medical assistant will need the discharge summary from the hospital and any other relevant findings (laboratory results, x-ray reports).

CASE STUDY 5: MEDICAL LAW AND ETHICS

Ms. Yikes has a new diagnosis of an aggressive type of brain cancer for which there is no cure. She has an appointment today to meet with Dr. Singh, the oncologist, to discuss palliative measures to control pain. Tasia, the medical assistant, notices that there are no documents in the advance directives section of the medical record. Tasia asks Ms. Yikes if she has a living will or any other advance directives. Ms. Yikes lowers her head, sobs, and starts yelling that everyone is giving up on her and can't wait for her to die.

QUESTION 1 *How should the medical assistant respond to the patient?*

Answers will vary. The medical assistant should give the patient a tissue and allow her to talk out her frustrations. She should gently tell the patient that no one is giving up on her, nor wants her to die, and clarify that she asked just to make certain that the patient's wishes were known. The medical assistant should go on to say that the provider is available to explain all options (including the option of not signing advance directives) when Ms. Yikes is ready to discuss the topic in more depth.

Ms. Yikes discusses the topic with Dr. Singh and agrees to have an answer regarding an advanced directive during her next visit. When Tasia re-enters the exam room, Ms. Yikes apologizes for yelling at her during the initial part of the visit. Tasia tells her not to worry. Ms. Yikes smiles and thanks Tasia for understanding. Tasia hands Ms. Yikes a brochure that describes all of her options. Ms. Yikes asks Tasia if she can change her mind after signing an advanced directive.

QUESTION 2 *How should Tasia respond?*

Yes. Advanced directives can be reviewed at any time and updated to reflect current wishes.

The next week, Ms. Yikes brings her adult daughter with her to the visit. She would like to appoint her daughter as her health care advocate to make decisions for her in the event she is unable to so herself.

QUESTION 3 *Which medical directive would be most appropriate in this case?*

Durable power of attorney for health care

APPENDIX
References

Adams, A. P. (2014). *Kinn's the administrative medical assistant: An applied learning approach* (8th ed.). St. Louis, MO: Elsevier Saunders.

Administrative law definition, examples, cases, processes. (2016). *Legal dictionary.* Retrieved from http://legaldictionary.net/administrative-law/

AHC Media. (2016). *Case management, advocacy, and the Affordable Care Act.* Retrieved from https://www.ahcmedia.com/articles/134452-case-management-and-advocacy-in-the-era-of-the-affordable-care-act

American Academy of Family Physicians. (2016). *Physician expert witness in medical liability suits.* Retrieved from http://www.aafp.org/about/policies/all/physician-expert.html

American College of Asthma, Allergy, and Immunology. (2014). *Allergy testing.* Retrieved from http://acaai.org/allergies/treatment/allergy-testing

American Medical Association. (2001). *Principles of medical ethics.* Retrieved from http://www.ama-assn.org/ama/pub/physician-resources/medical-ethics/code-medical-ethics/principles-medical-ethics.page

American Medical Association. (2015). 6 simple ways to master patient communication. *AMA Wire.* Retrieved from http://www.ama-assn.org/ama/ama-wire/post/6-simple-ways-master-patient-communication

American Speech-Language-Hearing Association. (2016). *Speech testing.* Retrieved from http://www.asha.org/public/hearing/Speech-Testing/

Avis, E. (2016, February 10). *Population health: The "upstream effort."* Retrieved from http://www.hfma.org/Leadership/Archives/2016/Winter/Population_Health___The_%E2%80%9CUpstream_Effort%E2%80%9D/

Berman, A., Snyder, S. J., & Frandsen, G. (2016). *Kozier & Erb's fundamentals of nursing: Concepts, process, and practice* (10th ed.). Boston, MA: Pearson.

BlueCross BlueShield North Carolina. (n.d.). *CMS – 1500 (08/05) claim filing instructions.* Retrieved from https://www.bcbsnc.com/assets/providers/public/pdfs/CMS-1500-Filing-Inst.pdf

Booth, K., & O'Brien, T. (2012). *Electrocardiography for healthcare professionals* (3rd ed.). New York, NY: McGraw Hill.

Booth, K., Whicker, L., & Wyman, T. (2014). *Medical assisting: Administrative and clinical procedures with anatomy and physiology* (5th ed.). New York, NY: McGraw Hill.

Brooks, M. (2015, August 13). 100 Best-selling, most prescribed branded drugs through June. *Medscape Nurses.* Retrieved from http://www.medscape.com/viewarticle/849457

Buppert, C. (2008). Understanding medical assistant practice liability issues. *Dermatology Nursing, 20*(4), 327–329. Retrieved from http://www.medscape.com/viewarticle/580647_2

Burchum, J. R., & Rosenthal, L. D. (2016). *Lehne's pharmacology for nursing care* (9th ed.). Atlanta, GA: Elsevier.

Bureau of Labor Statistics. (2015). *Occupational outlook handbook*. Retrieved from http://www.bls.gov/ooh/healthcare/medical-assistants.htm#tab-6

Centers for Disease Control and Prevention. (2003). Slide 8: Chain of infection. In *Guidelines for Infection Control in Dental Health-Care Settings—2003*. Retrieved from https://www.cdc.gov/oralhealth/infectioncontrol/guidelines/slides/008.htm

Centers for Disease Control and Prevention. (2012). *Effective practices for the timely and accurate reporting of laboratory testing critical values*. Retrieved from https://wwwn.cdc.gov/futurelabmedicine/pdfs/CDC_ReportingCriticalValuesSummary.pdf

Centers for Disease Control and Prevention. (2015). *About adult BMI*. Retrieved from https://www.cdc.gov/healthyweight/assessing/bmi/adult_bmi/index.html

Centers for Disease Control and Prevention. (2015). *Clinical Laboratory Improvement Amendments (CLIA)*. Retrieved from http://wwwn.cdc.gov/clia/Default.aspx

Centers for Disease Control and Prevention. (2015). *Comorbidities*. Retrieved from http://www.cdc.gov/arthritis/data_statistics/comorbidities.htm

Centers for Disease Control and Prevention. (2015, September 4). *Handwashing: Clean hands save lives*. Retrieved from http://www.cdc.gov/handwashing/when-how-handwashing.html

Centers for Medicare & Medicaid Services. (2014). *HCAHPS: Patients' perspectives of care survey*. Retrieved from https://www.cms.gov/Medicare/Quality-Initiatives-Patient-Assessment-instruments/HospitalQualityInits/HospitalHCAHPS.html

Centers for Medicare & Medicaid Services. (2014). *Medicare Billing: 837P and Form CMS-1500*. Retrieved from https://www.cms.gov/Outreach-and-Education/Medicare-Learning-Network-MLN/MLNProducts/Downloads/837P-CMS-1500.pdf

Centers for Medicare & Medicaid Services. (2015). *Accountable care organization (ACO)*. Retrieved from https://www.cms.gov/Medicare/Medicare-Fee-for-Service-Payment/ACO/index.html?redirect=/aco/

Centers for Medicare & Medicaid Services. (2015). *Better care, smarter spending, healthier people: improving our health care delivery system*. Retrieved from https://www.cms.gov/Newsroom/MediaReleaseDatabase/Fact-sheets/2015-Fact-sheets-items/2015-01-26.html

Cohen, R. A., & Martinez, M. E. (2015). *Health insurance coverage: Early release of estimates from the National Health Interview Survey, 2014*. Retrieved from http://www.cdc.gov/nchs/data/nhis/earlyrelease/insur201506.pdf

Commission on Office Laboratory Accreditation. (2015). *About COLA*. Retrieved from http://www.cola.org/about-cola/

Compassion and Support at the End of Life. (2009). *Medical orders for life sustaining treatment - Patients & families*. Retrieved from https://www.compassionandsupport.org/index.php/for_patients_families/molst/molst_forms

Costich, J. F., Scutchfield, F. D., & Ingram, R. C. (2015). Population health, public health, and accountable care: Emerging roles and relationships. *American Journal of Public Health, 105*(5), 846–850. doi:10.2105/ajph.2014.302484

Delamare, L. (2015, July 17). *25 most prescribed drugs in the U.S.* Retrieved from http://drugs.healthgrove. com/stories/5221/25-most-prescribed-drugs-in-the-u-s

Dingley, C., Daugherty, K., & Derieg, M. K. (2008). Improving patient safety through provider communication strategy enhancements. In *Advances in Patient Safety: New Directions and Alternative Approaches.* Retrieved from http://www.ahrq.gov/downloads/pub/advances2/vol3/ advances-dingley_14.pdf

Doskow, E. (2016). *Defamation law made simple.* Retrieved from http://www.nolo.com/ legal-encyclopedia/defamation-law-made-simple-29718.html

Dudek, S. G. (2014). *Nutrition essentials for nursing practice* (7th ed.). Philadelphia, PA: Wolters Kluwer.

Edlin, G., & Golanty, E. (2010). *Health and wellness* (10th ed.). Sudbury, MA: Jones and Bartlett.

Ernst, D. J., & Ballance, L. O. (2008). *Blood specimen collection FAQs: Answers to hundreds of the most frequently asked questions on specimen collection.* Ramsey, IN: Center For Phlebotomy Education.

Farrington, C. (2014). *Lost in translation: The impact of medical jargon on patient-centred care.* Retrieved from https://www.theguardian.com/healthcare-network/2014/jul/01/ impact-medical-jargon-patient-centred-care

FindLaw. (2013). *The Americans with Disabilities Act – Overview.* Retrieved from http://civilrights. findlaw.com/discrimination/the-americans-with-disabilities-act-overview.html

FindLaw. (2016). *The Controlled Substances Act (CSA): Overview.* Retrieved from http://criminal.findlaw. com/criminal-charges/controlled-substances-act-csa-overview.html

FindLaw. (2013). *Employment discrimination: Overview.* Retrieved from http://employment.findlaw.com/ employment-discrimination/employment-discrimination-overview.html

FindLaw. (2013). *FMLA leave law: In-depth.* Retrieved from http://employment.findlaw.com/ family-medical-leave/fmla-leave-law-in-depth.html

FindLaw. (2013). *What are Advance Directives?* Retrieved from http://elder.findlaw.com/ what-is-elder-law/what-are-advance-directives-.html

FindLaw. (2016). *Health care power of attorney.* Retrieved from http://estate.findlaw.com/living-will/ healthcare-power-of-attorney.html

Fordney, M. T. (2016). *Insurance handbook for the medical office* (14th ed.). St. Louis, MO: Elsevier Saunders.

Fremgen, B. F., & Frucht, S. S. (2009). *Medical terminology: A living language* (4th ed.). Upper Saddle River, NJ: Pearson Prentice Hall.

Garza, D., & Becan-McBride, K. (2015). *Phlebotomy handbook: Blood specimen collection from basic to advanced* (9th ed.). Upper Saddle River, NJ: Pearson.

Ghaedi, M., & El-Khoury, J. M. (2016, July 1.) *Pre-analytical variation: The leading cause of error in laboratory medicine. Clinical laboratory news.* Retrieved from https://www.aacc.org/publications/cln/articles/2016/july/preanalytical-variation-the-leading-cause-of-error-in-laboratory-medicine

Goguen, D. (2016). *What is the "medical standard of care" in a malpractice case?* Retrieved from http://www.nolo.com/legal-encyclopedia/what-the-medical-standard-care-malpractice-case.html

Green, M. (2016). *Understanding health insurance* (13th ed.). Boston, MA: Cengage.

Grodner, M., Escott-Stump, S., & Dorner, S. (2016). *Nutritional foundations and clinical applications: A nursing approach* (6th ed.). St. Louis, MO: Elsevier Mosby.

Hacker, K., & Walker, D. K. (2013). Achieving population health in accountable care organizations. *American Journal of Public Health, 103*(7), 1163–1167. doi:10.2105/ajph.2013.301254

Halter, M. J. (2014). *Varcarolis' foundations of psychiatric mental health nursing* (7th ed.). Atlanta, GA: Elsevier.

Health IT. (2014). *Computerized physician order entry (CPOE) for medication, laboratory, and radiology orders.* Retrieved from https://www.healthit.gov/providers-professionals/achieve-meaningful-use/core-measures-2/computerized-physician-order-entry-cpoe-medication-laboratory-and-radiology

Health IT. (2014). *Health IT legislation and regulations.* Retrieved from https://www.healthit.gov/policy-researchers-implementers/health-it-legislation-and-regulations

Health IT. (2015). *What is a patient portal?* Retrieved from https://www.healthit.gov/providers-professionals/faqs/what-patient-portal

Hoeltke, L. B. (2012). *The complete textbook of phlebotomy* (4th ed.). Clinton Park, NY: Delmar Cengage Learning.

Hollard, K. (2012). *Crossing the line: Professional boundaries in nursing.* Retrieved from http://www.nursetogether.com/professional-boundaries-nursing

Institute for Healthcare Improvement. (n.d.). *Delivering great care: Engaging patients and families as partners.* Retrieved from http://www.ihi.org/resources/Pages/ImprovementStories/DeliveringGreatCareEngagingPatientsandFamiliesasPartners.aspx

Institute for Health Improvement. (2016). *Accuracy at every step: The challenge of medication reconciliation.* Retrieved from http://www.ihi.org/resources/pages/improvementstories/accuracyateverystep.aspx

Johns Hopkins Medicine. (2016). *Specimen collection.* Retrieved from http://www.hopkinsmedicine.org/microbiology/specimen/

Joint Commission. (2016). *Ambulatory care national patient safety goals.* Retrieved from https://www.jointcommission.org/assets/1/6/2016_NPSG_AHC_ER.pdf

Joseph, C. (2010). *What are the benefits of delivering excellent customer service?* Retrieved from http://smallbusiness.chron.com/benefits-delivering-excellent-customer-service-2086.html

LaTour, K., Maki, S., & Oachs, P. (2013). *Health information management concepts, principles, and practice* (4th ed.). Chicago, IL: AHIMA Press.

Leinbach-Reyhle, N. (2014). *3 tips to deal with difficult customers.* Retrieved from http://www.forbes.com/sites/nicoleleinbachreyhle/2014/07/28/dealing-with-difficult-customers/#7c018bec507a

Life Labs. (2016). *Laboratory requisitions.* Retrieved from http://www.bcbio.com/physicians/lab-requisitions/best-practices-for-solpr-in-emrphysician-practice-systems

Lindh, W. Q., Pooler, M. S., Tamparo, C. D., Dahl, B. M., Morris, J. A., & Rein, A.P. (2014). *Delmar's comprehensive medical assisting: Administrative and clinical competencies* (5th ed.). Clifton Park, NY: Delmar Cengage Learning.

Lorette, K. (2010). *The use of email in business communication.* Retrieved from http://smallbusiness.chron.com/use-email-business-communication-118.html

McDonald, K. M., Schultz, E., Albin, L., Pineda, N., Lonhart, J., Sundaram, V., Smith-Spangler, C., Brustrom, J., Malcolm, E., Rohn, L., & Davies, S. (2014). What is care coordination? In *Care coordination measures atlas update.* Retrieved from http://www.ahrq.gov/professionals/prevention-chronic-care/improve/coordination/atlas2014/chapter2.html

MedlinePlus. (2010). *Medical ethics.* Retrieved https://medlineplus.gov/medicalethics.html

Meyers, D., Peikes, D., Genevro, J., Peterson, G., Taylor, E. F., Lake, T., Smith, K., & Grumbach, K. (2010). *The roles of patient-centered medical homes and accountable care organizations in coordinating patient care.* Retrieved from https://pcmh.ahrq.gov/sites/default/files/attachments/Roles%20of%20PCMHs%20And%20ACOs%20in%20Coordinating%20Patient%20Care.pdf

Moini, J. (2009) *Medical assisting review: Passing CMA, RMA, and other exams* (3rd ed.). New York, NY: McGraw-Hill.

Murphy, M. (2015). *Which of these 4 communication styles are you?* Retrieved from http://www.forbes.com/sites/markmurphy/2015/08/06/which-of-these-4-communication-styles-are-you/#53d9d4be1ecb

National Institute on Aging. (2014). *Advance care planning.* Retrieved from https://www.nia.nih.gov/health/publication/advance-care-planning

National Institute on Aging. (2014). *Organ donation and transplantation for older donors and recipients—Resources from the U.S. government.* Retrieved from https://www.nia.nih.gov/health/publication/organ-donation-and-transplantation

National Institutes of Health. (2016). *Probiotics: In depth.* Retrieved from https://nccih.nih.gov/health/probiotics/introduction.htm#hed1

Naylor, M. D., Bowles, K. H., Maislin, G., McCauley, K., Pauly, M. V., & Schwartz, J. S. (2012). *Transitional Care Model (TCM).* Retrieved from http://qio.ipro.org/wp-content/uploads/2012/12/transitional_model_model.pdf

Nelson, J. (2015). *Thallium stress test.* Retrieved from http://www.healthline.com/health/thallium-stress-test#Procedure2

Network for Regional Healthcare Improvement. (2016). *What is MACRA.* Retrieved from http://www.nrhi.org/work/what-is-macra/what-is-macra/

Newtek. (2013). *7 steps for dealing with angry customers.* Retrieved from http://www.forbes.com/sites/thesba/2013/08/02/7-steps-for-dealing-with-angry-customers/#548015e28ad6

Oats, H., & Massey, V. (n.d.). *Employee engagement.* Retrieved from http://www.alchemyformanagers. co.uk/topics/xaXcs3NtqEheNrcM.html

Occupational Safety and Health Administration. (n.d.). *Hazard communication Safety Data Sheets.* Retrieved from https://www.osha.gov/Publications/HazComm_QuickCard_SafetyData.html

Occupational Safety and Health Administration. (n.d.). *Occupational safety and health administration.* Retrieved from https://www.osha.gov/SLTC/personalprotectiveequipment/index.html

Office for Civil Rights. (2008). *Your rights under HIPAA.* Retrieved from http://www.hhs.gov/hipaa/ for-individuals/guidance-materials-for-consumers/index.html

Patient-centered medical homes. (2010). *Health affairs.* Retrieved from http://www.healthaffairs.org/ healthpolicybriefs/brief.php?brief_id=25

Physicians Insurance. (2014). *Improving telephone communication with patients.* Retrieved from https://www.phyins.com/risk-management/taking-care/981/general/ improving-telephone-communication-with-patients/

Plonka, M., Targosz, A., & Brzozowski, T. (2014). Can drinking water serve as a potential reservoir of helicobacter pylori? Evidence for water contamination by helicobacter pylori. In Dr. Bruna Roesler (Ed.), *Trends in Helicobacter Pylori Infection.* doi: 10.5772/57568

Potter, P. A., Perry, A. G., Stockert, P. A., & Hall, A. M. (2017). *Fundamentals of nursing* (9th ed.). Atlanta, GA: Elsevier.

Proctor, D. B., & Adams, A. P. (2014). *Kinn's the medical assistant: An applied learning approach* (12th ed.). St. Louis, MO: Elsevier.

Proctor, D., Niedzwiecki, B., Pepper, J., Madero, P. B., Garrels, M., & Mills, H. (2016). *Kinn's the medical assistant: An applied learning approach* (13th ed.). St. Louis, MO: Elsevier.

Rice, J. (2011) *Principles of pharmacology for medical assisting* (5th ed.). Clifton Park, NY: Delmar.

Richards, E. P., & Rathbun, K. C. (1993). *Intentional torts. Law and the physician: A practical guide.* Retrieved from http://biotech.law.lsu.edu/Books/lbb/x134.htm

Rickert, J. (2012). Patient-centered care: What it means and how to get there. *Heath Affairs Blog.* Retrieved from http://healthaffairs.org/blog/2012/01/24/ patient-centered-care-what-it-means-and-how-to-get-there/

Saint Francis Care. (2013). *Risk management and patient safety.* Retrieved from https://www. stfranciscare.org/uploadedFiles/Saint_Francis_Care_New/Careers/New_Employee_Portal/17%20 RISK%20MANAGEMENT%20AND%20PATIENT%20SAFETY%20May%202011.pdf

Schyve, P. M. (2007). Language differences as a barrier to quality and safety in health care: The Joint Commission perspective. *US National Library of Medicine, 22*(Suppl 2). Retrieved from https://www.ncbi. nlm.nih.gov/pmc/articles/PMC2078554/

Seaward, B. L. (2015). *Managing stress: Principles and strategies for health and well-being* (8th ed.). Burlington, MA: Jones and Bartlett Learning.

Seid, S. (2012). *8 telephone etiquette tips.* Retrieved from http://www.advancedetiquette. com/2012/01/8-telephone-etiquette-tips/

Singer, P. (2015). *Ethics*. Retrieved from https://www.britannica.com/topic/ethics-philosophy

Skidmore-Roth, L. (2016). *Mosby's 2016 nursing drug reference* (29th ed.). St. Louis, MO: Elsevier.

Society for Human Resource Management. (2015). *Communicating with diverse audiences*. Retrieved from https://www.shrm.org/resourcesandtools/hr-topics/behavioral-competencies/communication/pages/communicating-with-diverse-audiences.aspx

Society of Gastroenterology Nurses and Associates (2012). *Standards of infection control in reprocessing of flexible gastrointestinal endoscopes*. Retrieved from http://www.ascquality.org/endoscopereprocessingtoolkit.cfm

Stanfield, P., Hui, Y. H., & Cross, N. (2008). *Essential medical terminology* (3rd ed.). Sudbury, MA: Jones and Bartlett.

The Joint Commission. (2013, November 20). Aseptic versus clean technique. In *Preventing Central Line–Associated Bloodstream Infections: Useful Tools, An International Perspective* (Chapter 3). Retrieved from https://www.jointcommission.org/assets/1/6/CLABSI_Toolkit_Tool_3-8_Aseptic_versus_Clean_Technique.pdf

The Joint Commission. (2015). *Benefits of Joint Commission accreditation*. Retrieved from https://www.jointcommission.org/benefits_of_joint_commission_accreditation/

Thomas, V. (2012). *What works in care coordination? Activities to reduce spending in Medicare fee-for-service*. Retrieved from http://www.academyhealth.org/files/publications/files/RICareCoordination.pdf

Tidy, C. (2014). *Denver development screening test*. Retrieved from http://patient.info/doctor/denver-developmental-screening-test

Townsend, M. C. (2014). *Essentials of psychiatric mental health nursing* (6th ed.). Philadelphia, PA: F. A. Davis Company.

Turley, S. M. (2014). *Medical language: Immerse yourself* (3rd ed.). Upper Saddle River, NJ: Pearson.

United States Department of Agriculture. (2016, January 7). *MyPlate*. Retrieved from http://www.choosemyplate.gov/MyPlate

United States Department of Labor. (2005). *OSHA frequently asked questions*. Retrieved from https://www.osha.gov/needlesticks/needlefaq.html

United States Department of Labor. (2016). *OSHA*. Retrieved from https://www.osha.gov/workers/index.html

United States Drug Enforcement Administration. (2012). *Title 21 United States Code (USC) Controlled Substances Act*. Retrieved from https://www.dea.gov/index.shtml

VanMeter, K. C., & Hubert, R. J. (2014). *Gould's pathophysiology for the health professions* (5th ed.). St. Louis, MO: Elsevier.

Wilkinson, J. M., Treas, L. S., Barnett, K. L., & Smith, M. H. (2015). *Fundamentals of nursing* (3rd ed.). Philadelphia, PA: F. A. Davis.

World Health Organization. (2010). *WHO guidelines on drawing blood: Best practices in phlebotomy*. Retrieved from http://www.who.int/injection_safety/phleb_final_screen_ready.pdf

APPENDIX
Glossary

A

abduct. Move away from the midline of the body

accountable care organization (ACO). An association of providers and third-party payers that assumes a defined range of responsibilities for a specific population and is held accountable, financially as well as through specific quality indicators, for its members' health

account balance. The amount owed on an account

accounts payable. Debts incurred, not yet paid

accounts receivable. Money owed to the provider

ACE inhibitor. Angiotensin-converting enzyme inhibitor, a type of antihypertensive (blood pressure lowering) medication

acquired immunodeficiency syndrome (AIDS). The most advanced stage of infection with the human immunodeficiency virus and resulting in low resistance to disease

active listening. Using techniques that allow the receiver to fully understand the message being communicated

adenoidectomy. The removal of small masses of lymphatic tissue near the opening into the pharynx

administrative law. The body of law in the form of decisions, rules, regulations, and orders created by administrative agencies under the direction of the executive branch of the government, used to carry out the duties of such agencies

advance directives. A document that communicates a patient's specific wishes for end-of-life care should the patient become unable to do so

agent. Someone that acts or exerts power

airborne. Referring to the transmission of diseases from an infected person propelling pathogens through the air on particles smaller than 5 microns in size to a susceptible person's eyes, nose, or mouth. Airborne particles are transmitted as aerosols and can be suspended in the air for long periods of time.

allergic reaction. A hypersensitivity response to a medication, food, or other substance, ranging in intensity from mild itching to severe rash to anaphylaxis

allergy. Adverse reaction caused by an antigen-antibody response

allopathic. Homeopathic medicine; categorized by an effort to counteract the symptoms of a disease by administration of treatments that produce effects opposite to the symptoms

alternating current (AC) interference. 60-cycle interference; an artifact in the EKG tracing caused by electrical interference

ambulatory. Able to walk

ambulatory monitoring. Often referred to as Holter monitoring; an EKG conducted over a period of time while the patient resumes normal activities

amplitude. Also known as gain is the degree of change; in an EKG tracing, it is represented by the vertical axis

ampule. A small, sealed, single-use glass or plastic container containing sterile parenteral medications or solutions

amputation. Surgical removal of all or part of a limb or extremity

anaphylaxis. Life-threatening allergic reaction that leads to circulatory collapse, shock, and death if left untreated

anatomical position. Standing erect, arms at the sides of the body with eyes and palms facing forward, legs parallel with toes pointing forward

antecubital space. The inner bend of the elbow; primary site for phlebotomy procedures

anthropometric measurements. Screening tests that include height and weight (as well as head circumference in infants)

antibiotic. A medication that kills bacteria and thus treats bacterial infections

anticoagulant. A chemical substance that prevents clotting

antiplatelet. A medication that helps delay blood clotting. This medication differs from an anticoagulant because it affects arterial as well as venous blood.

aphasia. Inability to speak

appointment book. A book used to schedule, cancel, and reschedule appointments; can be color-coded or arranged so a week is shown at a glance

arrhythmia. Also known as dysrhythmia; a change from a normal EKG rhythm

artifact. Unwanted external event occurring in an EKG tracing not associated with the heart function

assault. The crime of trying or threatening to hurt someone physically

assets. The entire saleable property of a person, association, corporation, or estate applicable or subject to the payment of debts

atrioventricular (AV) node. The secondary pacemaker located at the junction of the atria and ventricles

audiometry. Test to determine level of hearing

augmented. A unipolar recording that requires assisting in magnifying the tracing by drawing from other poles

auscultation. Listening, usually with a stethoscope

autoclave. An instrument that sterilizes equipment and supplies by subjecting them to high pressure saturated steam

autoimmune. A condition of or related to the immune response of an organism against substances naturally present in the body

automated call routing. A software system that answers phones automatically and routes calls to staff after the caller responds to prompts; also used to call patients to remind them of upcoming appointments

automatic external defibrillator (AED). An external device attached to the chest with which to shock the heart if in asystole or arrhythmia in hopes of restarting or re-establishing a normal heart rhythm

autonomy. The right to make one's own personal decisions, even when those decisions might not be in that person's own best interest

B

basal metabolism. The amount of energy necessary for maintaining life-sustaining activities for a specific period of time

basilic vein. Vein located in the medial antecubital space; superficial to the brachial artery

battery. Intentional touching or using force in a harmful manner, without the person's consent

beta blocker. A medication that, by interfering with specific receptor sites in the heart, can help lower heart rate and blood pressure and treat many other cardiovascular disorders

bile. A yellow-green fluid the liver creates and the gall bladder stores that helps digest fats

biohazard. A biological or chemical substance that is dangerous to human beings and the environment

biopsy. The removal and examination of tissue to diagnose a disease, such as cancer

bipolar. Recording of electrical current involving both a positive and negative pole

bloodborne. Referring to direct contact through nonintact skin or mucous membranes with blood, body fluids, or tissue from an infected person

body language. A method of communication that uses body movements, expressions, or positional changes to express a person's feelings

Braille. A system of writing for blind people that uses raised dots to represent letters of the alphabet

brand/trade name. Assigned by the medication's manufacturer, identifies the medication as the property of the company, begins with a capital letter

breach. Infraction or violation of a law, obligation, tie, or standard

bronchospasm. Narrowing or constriction of the airways that interferes with breathing

bundle of His. A collection of fibers that conduct the electrical impulses from the AV node to the ventricular septum

C

calcium channel blocker. A medication that prevents the entry of calcium ions into the cells of the body, which can lower blood pressure and treat cardiac pain and dysfunction

calorie. A unit that provides a measurement for energy; the amount of heat it takes to raise the temperature of 1 kg of water 1 degree Celsius; also called a kilocalorie

care coordination. The deliberate organization of patient care activities between two or more participants involved in a patient's care to facilitate the appropriate delivery of health care services

Centers for Disease Control and Prevention (CDC). Provides safety guidelines for medical offices and facilities

cephalic vein. Located in the lateral antecubital space; one of two preferred veins for phlebotomy procedures

chain of custody. A series of processes and procedures used to ensure security and accuracy

chemotherapy. Course of treatment with drugs that destroy or inhibit the growth and division of malignant (cancerous) cells; any chemical agents that treat disease, but in common usage generally means cancer treatment

chief complaint. Reason for the office visit

cholesterol. An essential substance in the body that can increase adversely with ongoing fat intake and block blood flow through blood vessels, causing impairment in heart, blood vessel, and brain function

chronic obstructive pulmonary disease. A persistent disorder that impairs breathing

cicatrix. A scar of a healed wound

civil law. Laws that deal with the rights of people rather than with crimes

clarification. Summarizing the information relayed by the sender to clear up any confusion

clean-catch midstream. A urine specimen that is collected in the middle of the urinary stream in a sterile container after perineal cleaning

Clinical Laboratory Improvement Amendments (CLIA). Federal standards that regulate laboratory testing, handling, and processing

closed-ended questions. Questions that have a limited number of possible responses

coagulation. The process by which a clot forms in the blood

colostomy. A surgical procedure in which an opening (stoma) is formed in the large intestine or colon through an incision in the anterior abdominal wall, which will allow stool to pass out of the body

Commission on Office Laboratory Accreditation (COLA). An independent firm that provides accreditation for laboratories and has a goal of meeting CLIA standards

common law. The laws that developed from English court decisions and customs and that form the basis of laws in the U.S.

communication. The process of exchanging information via verbal or nonverbal methods

compliance. Meeting the standards and regulations of the medical practice's established policies and procedures

compound. Combination of atoms of an element; pharmacologically, it refers to a mixture of medications or a medication with a specific base

computerized physician order entry (CPOE). A process of electronic data entry of provider instructions for treatment

conjunctiva. The delicate membrane that lines the eyelids and covers the external surface of the sclerae (the whites of the eyes)

constipation. Condition of having hardened stool that is difficult to eliminate and causes discomfort and excessive straining

contact. Referring to the transmission of diseases by the physical transfer of pathogens from a contaminated object to a susceptible host's body surface

continuity of care. Continuation of care smoothly from one provider to another, so that the patient receives the most benefit and no interruption to care

contract. A legal agreement between two or more parties (e.g., people, companies)

controls. Specific tools used in the laboratory with a known result, used to compare with results of a patient sample to confirm validity of the test and specimen

coronary artery bypass graft. Surgery that eliminates a blockage in an artery going to the heart by replacing it with a section of a blood vessel from another area

coronary artery disease. A disorder that involves partial or complete blockage of the blood vessels that supply oxygen and nutrients to the heart

credit. The monetary balance in an individual's favor

criminal law. Laws that deal with crimes and their punishments

critical value. A laboratory result that is outside of the established reference range and presents potential health risks to a patient

curettage. The removal of tissue or growths from a body cavity, such as the uterus, by scraping with a curette

Current Procedural Terminology (CPT) codes. Five-digit numeric codes used to describe an evaluation/management service rendered by providers

customer service. Providing quality attention and assistance to a consumer of a product or a service

D

debit. An amount owed

deep vein thrombosis (DVT). Formation of a blood clot within a deep vein (most commonly the veins in the legs)

defecation. Excretion (elimination) of solid waste from the body

defendant. A person who is being sued or accused of a crime in a court of law

dementia. A progressive mental disorder characterized by decline of mental functioning and impairment of memory, judgement, and impulse control

Denver Developmental Screening Test. A series of activities used to determine the developmental stage of children

dependence. Caused by repeated use of a medication and will result in withdrawal symptoms when the medication is discontinued

depolarization. Systole; contraction

deposition. A formal statement that someone who has promised to tell the truth makes so that the statement can be used in court

diaphoresis. Profuse sweating

diarrhea. Frequent passage of loose, watery bowel movements

diastolic pressure. The last sound heard during the blood pressure reading

digestion. The process by which the gastrointestinal system breaks down foods to increasingly smaller components to prepare nutrients for absorption

dilation and curettage. Surgery involving the use of an instrument to open the cervix (entrance to the uterus) and then cutting away tissue inside the uterus for therapeutic purposes

disinfect. To clean something (e.g., work area, equipment) using chemicals that kill pathogens but not their spores

diverticula. One of multiple pouches that can form in the walls of the large intestine

diverticulosis. Disorder that involves multiple small pouches forming in the walls of the large intestine

double-booking. Scheduling two patients at the same time with the same provider, often to fit in a patient who has an acute illness

droplet. Referring to the transmission of diseases from an infected person propelling pathogens through the air on particles larger than 5 microns in size to a susceptible person's eyes, nose, or mouth. Droplet transmission is usually limited to a distance of 1 meter or 3 feet.

durable power of attorney for health care. A document in which patients designate someone to make health care decisions for them if they are unable to do so themselves

dysphasia. Difficulty speaking

dyspnea. Difficulty breathing

E

edema. An excessive buildup of fluid in body tissue

ego. A part of the mind that senses and adapts to reality

electrocardiogram. A record of the heart's electrical impulses

electrocardiograph. The machine that records an electrocardiogram

electrocardiography. The process of recording an electrocardiogram

electrodessication. The drying of tissue by a high-frequency electric current applied with a needle-shaped electrode (also called fulguration)

electroencephalogram. A record of the brain's electrical activity

electrolyte. A chemical substance that develops an electrical charge and can conduct an electrical current when placed in water, such as sodium and potassium

electronic health record (EHR). An electronic record of patients' health-related information that conforms to nationally recognized interoperability standards, and can be created, managed, and accessed by authorized individuals from multiple health care organizations

electronic medical record (EMR). An electronic record of health-related information about an individual that can be created, managed, and accessed by authorized individuals within a single health care organization

elixir. A fragrant, sweet, often alcoholic liquid that has a medication in it

empathy. Conveyance of an objective awareness and understanding of the feelings, emotions, and behavior of patients, including trying to envision what it must be like to be in their situation

emulsion. A mixture of water and oil that improves the taste of something distasteful, such as fish oil

endoscope. A medical device consisting of a tube and optical system for observing the inside of a hollow organ, cavity, or tissue plane

enteral. Within or by way of the gastrointestinal tract

enteric-coated. Containing an outer shell that prevents an oral tablet from dissolving until it reaches the intestines, often to prevent stomach irritation

enzyme. A chemical substance in animals and plants that causes or facilitates natural processes such as digestion

etiology. The cause, set of causes, or manner of causation of a disease or condition

expert witness. A witness in a court of law who is an expert on a particular subject

explanation of benefits (EOB). A statement from an insurance carrier describing what services were paid, denied, or reduced in payment

external communication. Sharing information between a business or organization and an outside entity

extract. A concentrated combination of vegetable products and alcohol

F

fasting. Abstinence of food and liquids, except water, for a set number of hours prior to testing

fecal occult blood. Evaluation of a stool specimen for hidden blood

feedback. Information given in response to an action to reinforce or improve the behavior

felony. A crime declared by statute to be more serious than a misdemeanor and deserving of a more severe penalty. Conviction usually requires imprisonment in a penitentiary for longer than 1 year

fistula. An abnormal connection between two body parts; an arteriovenous fistula may be present at birth or surgically created in patients with renal insufficiency to aid with dialysis

fixation. The process of making bone immobile so it can heal

fomite. Any nonliving object or substance capable of carrying infectious organisms

forced expiratory volume. The amount of air that can be forcibly exhaled

fraudulent. Relating to actions that purposely intend to deceive

G

gallstones. The formation of stones in the gall bladder, which is the pear-shaped organ behind the liver that stores and concentrates bile (a substance that helps digest fats)

ganglion. A collection of nerve cell bodies in a place other than the central nervous system

gastroesophageal reflux disease. A disorder that involves chronic or recurrent return of stomach contents into the esophagus, causing a burning sensation under the breastbone, as well as sometimes nausea and coughing

gastrointestinal tract. The organs and structures of the digestive tract, from the mouth to the anus

generativity. The concern for establishing and guiding the next generation that stems from a sense of optimism about humanity

generic name. A noncommercial name for a medication, usually less complex than the medication's chemical name and often more complex than a brand or trade name

genetic. Involving genes, the parts of a cell that control or influence the appearance, growth, and other characteristics of a living thing

genitourinary. Referring to the urinary and reproductive organs

glucocorticoid. One of several hormones that have many functions, both naturally in the body and as a medication, including suppression of inflammation

guilt. A remorseful awareness of having done something wrong

gynecology. The type of medical practice that deals with the female reproductive system

H

healthcare-associated infections (HAI). Infections acquired in a health care setting

Healthcare Common Procedural Coding System (HCPCS). Codes created by the Centers for Medicare and Medicaid Services to report supplies, materials, and other procedures and services not defined in the CPT manual

Health Insurance Portability and Accountability Act (HIPAA). A law implemented in 1996 to improve the portability and continuity of health insurance coverage; contain costs, fraud, and abuse in the health care industry; set a higher standard for electronic health information communications; and promote the privacy of health information

hematocrit. The percentage of a blood sample that is red blood cells

hematological system. The structures and functions relating to the blood

hemoconcentration. Increase in the concentration of red blood cells in the circulating blood, which is commonly caused by exceeding tourniquet time of 60 seconds

hemoglobin. The red, oxygen-carrying pigment of red blood cells

hemolysis. The rupture of red blood cells, which is commonly caused by performing phlebotomy with too small needle gauge or shaking the blood tubes too hard; blood appears a serum cherry color and sample cannot be tested

hemorrhoid. A mass of dilated veins in swollen tissue at the anus or within the rectum

hemostasis. The stoppage of the flow of blood

hepatitis B virus (HBV). Liver infection caused by the hepatitis B virus that is transmitted by blood, semen, or another body fluid from an infected person

hepatitis. Inflammation or infection of the liver

herniation. The protrusion of a loop or portion of an organ or tissue through an abnormal opening

holistic health care. Comprehensive or total patient care that considers the physical, emotional, social, economic and spiritual needs of the person

homeostasis. A balanced, stable state within the body

hospice. A service that provides care in a variety of settings for patients who have terminal illnesses that are not expected to live longer than 6 months

human immunodeficiency virus (HIV). A retrovirus that invades and inactivates helper T-cells of the immune system and is a cause of AIDS and AIDS-related complex

hyperopia. Difficulty seeing things up close; farsightedness

hypertension. A common cardiovascular disorder, often with no symptoms, with which the blood exerts an abnormal amount of force on the inside walls of the arteries persistently so blood pressure readings increase

hyponatremia. A low level of sodium in the blood

hypoxia. Lacking oxygen in the body

I

idiopathic. Of unknown origin

immune system. The organs and structures that regulate the body's immunity, or resistance to disease

implied consent. Voluntary agreement with an action proposed by another

incidence. The rate of new (or newly diagnosed) cases of a disease or injury

incision. A surgical wound that results from cutting into tissue

industry. Competence in performing tasks

infection. The invasion and proliferation of pathogens in body tissues

inferiority. A personal feeling or sense of being inadequate

informed consent. A clear and voluntary indication of preference or choice, usually oral or written, and freely given in circumstances where the available options and their consequences have been made clear

initiative. The ability and tendency to start an action

inorganic. Made from or containing material that does not come from living things

insomnia. Difficulty falling asleep or staying asleep

integrity. The state of being whole, honest, or fair

intentional torts. An intentional wrongful act by a person or entity who means to cause harm, or who knows, or is reasonably certain, that harm will result from the act

internal communication. Sharing information within a business or organization

interrupted baseline. A break in the tracing usually caused by a disconnected or broken lead

ion. An atom or group of atoms that has a positive or negative electric charge

irritable bowel syndrome. A recurrent bowel dysfunction that causes abdominal pain, diarrhea, bloating, and flatulence (expulsion of gas from the rectum)

Ishihara test. A set of templates with patterns or numbers embedded within them to test for color blindness

J

jaundice. Yellowing of the skin, whites of the eyes, mucous membranes, and excretions as a result of liver disease

K

Korotkoff sounds. The five phases of articular relaxation that are audible while obtaining a manual blood pressure

L

laceration. A cut; a torn wound

leading questions. Questions that tend to lead the respondent into the desired answer

leukotriene inhibitor. A specific type of medication that treats asthma by relaxing tight or constricted airways and inflammation in the airways

liabilities. Amounts owed; debts

libel. A false accusation that is made with malicious intent to hurt the reputation of a person who is living or the memory of a person who is dead, resulting in public embarrassment, contempt, ridicule, or hatred

liniment. A liquid or semiliquid preparation containing oil, alcohol, or water for application to the skin, often as a counterirritant

lithotripsy. Destruction of kidney stones using shock waves

litigation. A lawsuit or legal action that determines the legal rights and remedies of the person or party

M

malfeasance. Performance of an unlawful, wrongful act

managed care. An umbrella term for plans that provide health care in return for preset scheduled payments and coordinated care through a defined network of providers and hospitals

mastectomy. Surgical removal of one or both breasts, typically associated with a diagnosis of cancer

matrix. A table used for scheduling

median cubital vein. Located in the center of the antecubital space, most common vein used for phlebotomy procedures

medical asepsis. Clean technique; the practice designed to reduce the number and transfer of pathogens; also helps in breaking the chain of infection

metabolic. Referring to metabolism, the set of processes by which the body uses nutrients it absorbs for energy and to form and maintain the body's structures and functions

metastasis. The spread of disease, usually cancer, to body sites other than where the tumor originated

metered-dose inhaler. A medication-delivery device that disperses the medication as an aerosol spray, mist, or powder into the airways via inhalation

midline. Divides the body into equal halves from head to feet

Mini-Mental State Examination. A tool used to determine the level of awareness of current events and recall of past events to screen for orientation or dementia

misdemeanor. An offense that is considered less serious than a felony and carries a lesser penalty, usually a fine or imprisonment for less than 1 year

misfeasance. The performance of a lawful action in an illegal or improper manner

modified wave scheduling. Allocating two patients to arrive at a specified time and the third to arrive approximately 30 minutes later, repeated throughout the day

Mohs surgery. A method of excising skin cancers and microscopically examining each layer until the entire tumor is removed

mucous membrane. The moist inner lining of various tubular structures, including the mouth, esophagus, stomach, and intestines

myocardial infarction. An interruption of blood flow to the heart, causing heart muscle damage; a heart attack

myopia. Difficulty seeing things far away; nearsightedness

N

nasogastric feedings. Delivery of formula through a tube that goes from the nose to the stomach

nasogastric. From the nose to the stomach

nebulizer. A device for creating and delivering an aerosol spray for inhalation

negative deflection. A downward curvature of waves in an EKG tracing

negligence. The failure to do something that a reasonably prudent individual would do under similar circumstances

nonfeasance. Failure to perform a task, duty, or undertaking that one has agreed to perform or has a legal duty to perform

nonverbal communication. Gestures and actions that leave interpretation up to the receiver

no-show. Appointment that an individual fails to keep without giving notice

Notice of Privacy Practices. A notification by providers required by the HIPAA Privacy Rule that provides an understandable explanation of patients' rights with respect to their personal health information and the privacy practices of their providers

NSAID. Non-steroidal anti-inflammatory medication

O

obese. Having a body mass index of 30 or greater

objective information. Information collected that is observed by someone other than the patient

objective. Referring to data or information the observer can see, measure, or otherwise detect

obstetrics. The type of medical practice that deals with women giving birth

Occupational Safety and Health Administration (OSHA). Agency of the government that oversees and regulates worker safety

off the market. No longer available for purchase or use

open-ended questions. Questions that lead to further explanation (vs. a yes or no response)

organ. Body tissues that work together to perform a specific function

organic. Obtained from living things; not made with artificial chemicals

orthopnea. Difficulty breathing in any position other than standing or sitting

osteopathic. A type of medicine based on the concept that disturbances in the musculoskeletal system affect other bodily parts, causing many disorders that can be improved by various manipulative methods in combination with conventional medical, surgical, pharmacologic, and other therapeutic procedures

over-the-counter. Available for purchase without a prescription

P

palpation. The act of touching

panel. A group of tests that are connected to one particular body system; profile

paralysis. A loss of muscle movement due to nerve damage

parasite. An organism that lives in, on, or at the expense of another organism without contributing to the host's survival

parenteral nutrition. Nutrients delivered intravenously (into a vein)

pathogen. Disease-causing micro-organism.

pathophysiology. The study of physical manifestations of illnesses and disease

patient-centered medical home (PCMH). A model philosophy intended to improve the effectiveness of primary care

pelvic inflammatory disease. A bacterial infection of the female reproductive organs

peripheral edema. Accumulation of fluid causing swelling in tissues, usually in the lower extremities

personal protective equipment (PPE). Barrier equipment used to prevent exposure to blood and other body fluids (gloves, goggles, masks)

pharyngitis. Inflammation of the pharynx, the back of the throat between the mouth and the nasal cavities

phlebotomy. Withdrawal of blood from a vein

physiological. Referring to the body and its functions

plaintiff. A person who files a lawsuit initiating a legal action

plastic needle holder. Adapter that connects to the needle and where the collection tube is inserted during phlebotomy

pneumonia. Inflammation of the lungs

port. A small medical appliance that is installed beneath the skin, used to administer medication or withdraw blood samples

positive deflection. An upward curvature of waves in an EKG tracing

positive reinforcement. Rewarding of a desirable behavior

potassium. A mineral that controls fluid volume, muscle and cardiac activity, and other bodily functions

precertification. Approval obtained by insurance providers that identifies insurance coverage for diagnostic or therapeutic activities

precordial. Located on the chest in front of the heart

presbyopia. A gradual, age-related loss of the eyes' ability to focus actively on nearby objects

prevalence. The number of active cases of a disease or injury

P-R interval. The length of time from the beginning of atrial depolarization to the beginning of ventricular depolarization

professionalism. The skills, behavior, and appropriate judgment that represent the best qualities of a person in a specific profession

proton-pump inhibitor. A specific type of medication that reduces stomach acid

provider-performed microscopy procedure. A CLIA term for microscopic examinations that require the expertise of a physician or mid-level provider qualified in microscopic examinations; falls under CLIA's moderate-complexity category

psychiatrist. A physician with additional medical training and experience in diagnosis, prevention, and treatment of mental disorders

psychologist. A person who specializes in the study of the structure and function of the brain and related mental processes.

psychology. The study of behavior and of the functions and processes of the mind

psychosocial. Referring to the relationship between and interplay of mental health and interpersonal relations

psychotherapy. The treatment of mental or emotional disorders primarily with verbal, therapeutic communication

Purkinje fibers. The fingerlike projections that spread through the ventricular muscle and initiate ventricular contraction

P wave. The first wave in the cardiac cycle representing atria depolarization

pyrexia. Raised body temperature; fever

Q

QRS wave. Also known as QRS complex; the second wave in the cardiac cycle representing ventricular depolarization

QT interval. The length of time from the beginning of the ventricular depolarization to ventricular repolarization

qualitative. Analysis that identifies quality or characteristics of components such as size, shape, and maturity of cells; typically reported as positive or negative

quality assurance. Policies and procedures to maximize patient safety and ensure reliability related to laboratory testing

quality control. Measures incorporated to maximize reliability and accuracy of results while recognizing and eliminating errors in testing

quantitative. Analysis that identifies quantity or actual number counts

R

radioallergosorbent test (RAST). A blood test used to detect antibodies associated with allergens

rales. Clicking or crackling sounds heard on inspiration that can sound moist or dry

random urine. A urine specimen collected in a clean container for screening purposes; no preparation is required

referral. Directing a patient to a specialist

reflection. When the receiver focuses on the main idea of the message but incorporates feelings the sender might be exhibiting or possibly feeling

repolarization. Asystole; relaxation

requisition. A written or computer generated order for laboratory tests

res ipsa loquitur. A doctrine or rule of evidence in tort law that allows an inference or presumption that a defendant was negligent in an accident injuring the plaintiff on the basis of circumstantial evidence if the accident was of a kind that does not usually happen in without negligence

respondeat superior. A doctrine in tort law that makes an employer liable for the wrong of an employee

restatement. Repeating or paraphrasing information relayed by the sender to confirm accuracy

reverse chronological order. Arranged so that the most recent item is on top and older items are filed further back

rheumatoid arthritis. An autoimmune disease that causes pain, swelling, and deformity especially in the hands and feet, due to inflammation in the joints

rhinorrhea. Runny nose

rhonchi. Common rattling snoring sounds often associated with chronic lung diseases

RICE. The treatment for many musculoskeletal system injuries (Rest, Ice, Compression, Elevation)

rugae. Folds within the lining of the stomach that aid in digestion and moving food into the duodenum

S

Safety Data Sheets (SDS). Documents containing necessary information regarding chemicals in the work environment

sanitization. Reducing the number of micro-organisms by removing debris with soap and water prior to disinfecting

scoliosis. Abnormal lateral curvature of the spine

scope of practice. Delegated clinical and administrative duties consistent with education, training, and experience

screening. Examining and separating into groups

sedation. A calm or sleepy state that results from taking a medication

self-consciousness. A feeling of anxiety or constant awareness of others' perception of oneself

sharps container. A puncture-proof container designed specifically to safely dispose of needles, scalpels, and other sharp disposable medical instruments

sinoatrial (SA) node. The natural pacemaker of the heart located in the upper right atrium

slander. To make a false spoken statement that causes people to have a bad opinion of someone

sleep apnea. A disorder in which muscles near the airways relax during sleep and cause a temporary cessation of breathing

SOAP note. Method of charting commonly used in ambulatory care (subjective, objective, assessment, plan)

somatic tremor. Muscle movement causing irregular spike in an EKG tracing

sphygmomanometer. Instrument used to measure blood pressure that has a graduated scale for determining systolic and diastolic pressure by increasing and gradually releasing the pressure in the cuff

stagnation. The result of stopping progression or forward movement

standardization. The universally acceptable speed of the tracing and gain (height) used for accurate interpretation of the tracing

standard of care. The degree of care or competence expected in a particular circumstance or role

sterilization. A technique for destroying pathogens and their spores on inanimate objects, using heat, water, chemicals, or gases

subjective information. Information that is personal or what someone is feeling

subpoena. A written order that commands someone to appear in court to give evidence

suppository. A small, solid, cylinder-shaped medication for insertion into the rectum or vagina; solid at room temperature, dissolves at body temperature

surgical asepsis. The complete removal of micro-organisms and their spores from the surface of an object

suspension. A liquid preparation consisting of solid particles dispersed throughout a liquid in which they are not soluble

sympathy. Feeling compassion, sorrow, or pity for the hardships that another person encounters

syrup. A concentrated solution of sugar in water with a flavoring, sometimes with a medication in it

system. Multiple organs working together to perform a complex function

systolic pressure. The first sound heard during a blood pressure reading

T

tachycardia. Heart rate greater than 100/min

telecommunication. Using of technology to exchange information

template. An outline used to make new pages with a similar design, pattern, or style

therapeutic communication. The purposeful use of verbal and nonverbal actions and interactions to build and maintain helping relationships with patients and families

therapeutic range. The amount of a medication the body must have available to produce the desirable effects for which the provider prescribed it

thermoregulation. The control or maintenance of body temperature

tincture. A medicinal preparation in an alcohol base, sometimes for oral and sometimes for topical use

tonsillectomy. Surgical removal of the tonsils (small masses of lymphatic tissue)

tort. An action that wrongly causes harm to someone but that is not a crime and that is dealt with in a civil court

tourniquet. Flat length of vinyl, rubber, or fabric with Velcro, which restricts blood flow and causes the venous blood to accumulate, enabling better palpation of a vein prior to phlebotomy

toxicity. An adverse medication reaction resulting from excessive dosing

transient ischemic attack. A temporary interruption of blood flow to the brain

triage. Ranking based on the most critical to the least critical

tuberculosis. A highly contagious infectious disease of the lungs that causes necrosis (death) of lung tissues

tumor. An abnormal mass of tissue that grows as a result of excessive cell division, either cancerous (malignant) or noncancerous (benign)

T wave. The third wave in the cardiac cycle representing ventricular repolarization

tympanometry. The process of recording the movement of the tympanic membrane through pressure variances in the external ear canal

type 2 diabetes mellitus. A disorder involving too little insulin (the hormone that regulates blood sugar) secretion and/or a resistance to the effects of insulin, resulting in the need for therapy that includes diet, exercise, oral medications, and possibly injectable medication

tyramine. A substance in some foods and beverages, such as cheese and wine, that can have a life-threatening interaction with a specific type of antidepressant

U

ultraviolet. A type of radiation the sun produces

unipolar. Recording from one location or one pole

urinalysis. A diagnostic examination of urine; a physical, chemical and/or microscopic examination of urine

V

vasovagal response. Fainting because the body overreacts to certain triggers (the sight of blood, extreme emotional distress)

vector. A living thing that carries pathogens

venipuncture. The puncture of a vein for the purposes of withdrawing blood

verbal communication. The use of spoken words to convey information

villus. One of many folds in the intestines

visual acuity testing. Use of tools such as a Snellen chart to screen for visual impairments

vital signs. Also known as cardinal signs; includes temperature, heart rate, respirations, and blood pressure measurements; used to evaluate homeostasis

W

wandering baseline. Inconsistency in the baseline location on the EKG tracing likely caused by poor lead contact or skin applications

wave scheduling. Scheduling three patients at the same time to be seen in the order in which they arrive

wheezing. A whistling sound heard on expiration that is the body's attempt to expel trapped air

whole blood. Total volume of blood including plasma and formed elements; blood that has not been separated by chemical additives or centrifuging

winged infusion. Butterfly style of needle attached to a length of tubing and affixed to a plastic needle holder; used on small or fragile veins such as those of the hands or pediatric and geriatric patients

work ethic. A set of values based on the moral virtues of hard work and diligence

APPENDIX
Index